Public Health 101
Healthy People–Healthy Populations

SECOND EDITION

Richard Riegelman, MD, MPH, PhD
Professor and Founding Dean
The George Washington University
School of Public Health and Health Services
Washington, DC

Brenda Kirkwood, MPH, DrPH
University at Albany, State University of New York
School of Public Health
Albany, NY

JONES & BARTLETT
LEARNING

World Headquarters
Jones & Bartlett Learning
5 Wall Street
Burlington, MA 01803
978-443-5000
info@jblearning.com
www.jblearning.com

Jones & Bartlett Learning books and products are available through most bookstores and online booksellers. To contact Jones & Bartlett Learning directly, call 800-832-0034, fax 978-443-8000, or visit our website, www.jblearning.com.

Substantial discounts on bulk quantities of Jones & Bartlett Learning publications are available to corporations, professional associations, and other qualified organizations. For details and specific discount information, contact the special sales department at Jones & Bartlett Learning via the above contact information or send an email to specialsales@jblearning.com.

Production Credits
Executive Publisher: William Brottmiller
Publisher: Michael Brown
Associate Editor: Chloe Falivene
Associate Production Editor: Rebekah Linga
Senior Marketing Manager: Sophie Fleck Teague
Manufacturing and Inventory Control Supervisor: Amy Bacus
Composition: Cenveo Publisher Services
Cover Design: Theresa Day

Photo Research and Permissions Coordinator: Lauren Miller
Cover and Title Page Image (left to right, top to bottom):
 U.S. Capitol Building: © Orhan Cam/ShutterStock, Inc.;
 Hand washing: © Elena Elisseeva/ShutterStock, Inc.;
 Seat belt: © justasc/ShutterStock, Inc.;
 Vaccine: © Leah-Anne Thompson/ShutterStock, Inc.
Printing and Binding: Edwards Brothers Malloy
Cover Printing: Edwards Brothers Malloy

To order this product, use ISBN: 978-1-284-04528-4

Library of Congress Cataloging-in-Publication Data
Riegelman, Richard K., author.
 Public health 101 : healthy people—healthy populations / Richard Riegelman and Brenda Kirkwood.—Second edition.
  p. ; cm.
 Public health one hundred one
 Includes bibliographical references and index.
 ISBN 978-1-284-04084-5 (pbk.)
 I. Kirkwood, Brenda, author. II. Title. III. Title: Public health one hundred one.
 [DNLM: 1. Public Health. WA 100]
 RA425
 362.1—dc23
                    2013039072

6048

Printed in the United States of America
18 17 16 15 14   10 9 8 7 6 5 4 3 2

Dedication

U.S. Capitol Building: © Orhan Cam/ShutterStock, Inc.; Hand washing: © Elena Elisseeva/ShutterStock, Inc.; Seat belt: © Justasc/ShutterStock, Inc.; Vaccine: © Leah-Anne Thompson/ShutterStock, Inc.

*To Nancy Alfred Persily, whose enthusiasm for
teaching public health to undergraduates inspired* Public Health 101:
Healthy People–Healthy Populations.

Contents

U.S. Capitol Building: © Orhan Cam/ShutterStock, Inc.; Hand washing: © Elena Elisseeva/ShutterStock, Inc.; Seat belt: © Justasc/ShutterStock, Inc; Vaccine: © Leah-Anne Thompson/ShutterStock, Inc.

Acknowledgments

Public Health 101: Healthy People–Healthy Populations, Second Edition, is the culmination of 15 years of effort aimed at introducing public health to undergraduates. The effort originated with the teaching of an introductory course in public health in 1998 at the then newly created The George Washington University School of Public Health and Health Services. The new course, organized by associate dean Nancy Alfred Persily, inspired efforts to teach and to learn from a new generation. The approach was designed as part of a liberal arts education, stimulating the movement that came to be called the Educated Citizen and Public Health.

Efforts to think through the content of an introductory course in public health have involved a large number of people throughout the United States. Public health, arts and sciences, and clinical educators all participated in the 2006 Consensus Conference on Public Health Education, which put forward the framework for Public Health 101 upon which this book is based. Among those who led and continue to lead this effort is Susan Albertine, whose insights into the relationship between public health and liberal education have formed the basis for much of the Educated Citizen and Public Health movement.

I have taught Public Health 101 since 2002, which has provided me with an opportunity to teach and to learn from over 400 undergraduate students at The George Washington University. Their feedback and input has been central to writing and rewriting this book. Madison Hardee and Katie Harter deserve special recognition for their extensive feedback on many chapters of the first edition. Yifen Liu provided important feedback for the second edition. I would also like to thank Alan Greenberg and Dante Verme, the chair and vice chair of the Department of Epidemiology and Biostatistics at The George Washington University School of Public Health and Health Services, for their support of my efforts to expand the audience for undergraduate public health.

A key change in the second edition is the addition of a second author. I am pleased to welcome and acknowledge the contributions of Brenda Kirkwood, MPH, DrPH. I first had the opportunity to work with Brenda while she was a DrPH student at The George Washington University. Dr. Kirkwood has made extraordinary contributions to the second edition. She has taken the primary responsibilities for writing and rewriting several chapters. Her careful reviews and dedication to getting the details right have been key to the quality of this edition. Brenda is truly exceptional and a pleasure to work with, as will be confirmed by all who work with her.

The draft of the second edition went through extensive review and feedback. I am grateful to all those who read chapters and provided constructive input. Mike Brown, Publisher of the Public Health and Health Administration line of products for Jones & Bartlett Learning, has made special contributions to this book and the series as a whole. His vision has helped craft the series, and his publishing expertise made it happen. The production, marketing, and editorial staff of Jones & Bartlett Learning deserve special recognition. Their commitment to this book and the entire *Essential Public Health* series has gone well beyond the expectations of their jobs.

Last, but by no means least, is my wife, Linda Riegelman, who encouraged this book and the *Essential Public Health* series from the beginning. She saw the need to reach out to students and make real the roles that public health plays in their everyday lives. Linda went the extra mile by reading and rereading both the first and the second edition. She deserves the credit for what works, but the blame for what fails is all mine.

Confronting the challenge of putting together *Public Health 101* has been one of the great joys of my professional life. I hope it will bring both joy and challenge to you as you enter into the important and engaging world of public health.

Richard Riegelman, MD, MPH, PhD

Preface: What Is *Public Health 101: Healthy People–Healthy Populations* All About?

Public health is more than a profession; it is a way of thinking. *Public Health 101: Healthy People–Healthy Populations* introduces you to the profession and also the way of thinking that we will call population health. Population health is an important way of looking at the world, whether you are going into public health as a profession, a clinically oriented health profession, business, law, international affairs, or a range of other professions.

Population health is also a key way of thinking, which prepares you for the challenges of citizenship in a democracy. Many of the issues that come before us as a society stem from or benefit from a population health perspective. Whether we are dealing with AIDS, the impact of aging, climate change, or the costs of health care, the population perspective can help us frame the issues and analyze the options to intervene.

In addition, the population perspective leads us to look broadly at the way issues intertwine and interact with each other. We call this systems thinking. In population health, systems thinking is taking center stage as we increasingly struggle with complex problems that require us to look beyond the traditional boundaries of health and disease.

Until recently, public health was considered a discipline taught only at the graduate level. Today, undergraduate public health is booming at four-year colleges and is beginning to take hold at community colleges as well. Its roots in general and liberal education go back to the 1980s, when David Fraser, the president of Swarthmore and an epidemiologist who led the investigation of Legionnaires' disease, wrote a now classic article called "Epidemiology as a Liberal Art."[1]

In 2003, the Institute of Medicine of the National Academies of Sciences recommended that "all undergraduates should have access to education in public health."[2] That recommendation encouraged the development of the Educated Citizen and Public Health initiative, a collaboration of undergraduate educators and public health educators to define and stimulate public health curricula for all undergraduates. *Public Health 101* was written to implement the recommendations that came out of this initiative and continue to form the basis for undergraduate education in public health.

This second edition of *Public Health 101* has been thoroughly updated and expanded. Each chapter includes new material designed to expand your understanding of public health. Two new chapters have been added, one on food and drugs as public health issues and the other on systems thinking as the future of population health. These chapters are designed to keep *Public Health 101* at the cutting edge of new developments and ways of thinking. In addition, each of the five sections includes new case studies challenging you to apply what you have learned.

Public Health 101: Healthy People–Healthy Populations will not try to overload your mind with facts. It is about providing you with frameworks for thinking, and applying these frameworks to real situations and thought-provoking scenarios. Each chapter begins and ends with vignettes designed to show you the types of situations you will confront in public health. After each section, there are cases studies that relate to one or more chapters in the section. They provide realistic, engaging exercises and open-ended questions to help you think through the application of the key concepts presented in each section.

Public Health 101 is designed as a gateway to the world of public health. It provides an introduction to the *Essential Public Health* series, a comprehensive series designed primarily for undergraduate public health education. You should take advantage of the *Essential Public Health* series' website at www.essentialpublichealth.com. It provides information on all the books in the series.

Hopefully, you will come away from reading *Public Health 101* with an appreciation of how the health of the public is influenced by and can be improved by efforts directed at the population level, as well as at the individual level. Let us begin in Chapter 1 by exploring the ways that public health affects everyone's daily life.

REFERENCES

1. Fraser DW. Epidemiology as a liberal art. *N Engl J Med*. 1987;316:309–314.
2. Gebbie K, Rosenstock L, Hernandez LM. *Who Will Keep the Public Healthy? Educating Public Health Professionals for the 21st Century*. Washington DC: National Academy Press; 2003.

About the Authors

Richard Riegelman, MD, MPH, PhD, is professor of epidemiology–biostatistics, medicine, and health policy, and founding dean of The George Washington University School of Public Health and Health Services. His education includes an MD from the University of Wisconsin, plus an MPH and PhD in epidemiology from The Johns Hopkins University. Dr. Riegelman practiced primary care internal medicine for over 20 years.

Dr. Riegelman has over 70 publications, including 6 books for students and practitioners of medicine and public health. He is editor of the Jones & Bartlett Learning *Essential Public Health* series. The series provides books and ancillary materials for the full spectrum of curricula for undergraduate public health education.

Dr. Riegelman has spearheaded efforts to fulfill the Institute of Medicine's recommendation that "all undergraduates should have access to education in public health." His work with national public health and arts and sciences organizations has developed into the Educated Citizen and Public Health movement. This movement now includes efforts by the Association of Schools and Programs of Public Health (ASPPH) and the Association of American Colleges and Universities (AAC&U) to implement undergraduate public health education. He also co-chairs the Community College and Public Health project, which aims to incorporate public health education into community colleges as part of the continuum of public health education.

Richard Riegelman teaches medical school, undergraduate, and graduate public health courses, which include Public Health 101 and Epidemiology 101.

Brenda Kirkwood, MPH, DrPH, has experience in higher education spanning public and private institutions on the associate, baccalaureate, and graduate levels, including development and teaching of undergraduate and graduate public health courses, development and management of public health academic programs, student mentorship, and contributions to national educational initiatives. She has held faculty and administrative positions at the University at Albany, State University of New York, School of Public Health, The George Washington University School of Public Health and Health Services, American University College of Arts and Sciences, and George Mason University College of Health and Human Services. She currently works in academic administration at the University at Albany, State University of New York, School of Public Health.

Prior to her career in higher education, Dr. Kirkwood held positions with the New York State Cancer Registry and the Bureaus of Sexually Transmitted Disease Control and Injury Prevention within the New York State Department of Health. She received a bachelor of science from Ithaca College, master of public health from the University at Albany, State University of New York, and doctor of public health degree from The George Washington University.

Dr. Kirkwood has been actively involved in national efforts to expand public health education and strengthen the public health workforce. As a researcher and educator, she has collaborated with a number of academic and public health workforce organizations. Her recent research explored the adoption of public health curricula in community colleges, contributing to *Healthy People 2020*, a collaborative initiative of the U.S. Department of Health and Human Services. Her publications and presentations at numerous national professional conferences have focused on undergraduate public health education, contributing to the Educated Citizen and Public Health movement.

SECTION I

Principles of Population Health

Section I of *Public Health 101: Healthy People—Healthy Populations* introduces you to the ways that public health affects your every waking moment, from the food you eat, to the water you drink, to the car you drive. Even sleep matters. In public health, we use bed nets to prevent malaria, we use beds that prevent back pain, and we put infants to sleep on their backs to prevent sudden infant death syndrome (SIDS).

In Section I, we will examine a range of approaches to public health that have been used over the centuries. Then we will focus on a 21st century approach known as population health. Population health includes the full range of options for intervention to address health problems, from community control of communicable disease and environmental health, to healthcare delivery systems, to public policies such as taxation and laws designed to reduce cigarette smoking. We will also look at how populations are changing by examining three important transitions that are affecting population health today and will continue to do so for years to come.

In this section, we will also examine an evidence-based approach to population health that focuses on defining the problem, establishing the etiology, making evidence-based recommendations, implementing these recommendations into practice, and evaluating the impacts of interventions. The population health and evidence-based approaches introduced in Section I provide an underpinning for all that follows.

At the end of Section I, as with each section, there are cases with discussion questions that draw on chapters from the section. Each case is designed as a realistic description of the types of problems we face as we seek to achieve healthy people and healthy populations.

So with no further ado, let us take a look at how public health can and does affect all of our daily lives.

CHAPTER 1

Public Health:
The Population Health Approach

LEARNING OBJECTIVES

By the end of this chapter, the student will be able to:

- identify multiple ways that public health affects daily life.
- define eras of public health from ancient times to the early 2000s.
- define the meaning of "population health."
- illustrate the uses of health care, traditional public health, and social interventions in population health.
- identify a range of determinants of disease.
- identify ways that populations change over time, which affects health.

I woke up this morning, got out of bed, and went to the bathroom, where I used the toilet, washed my hands, brushed and flossed my teeth, drank a glass of water, and took my blood pressure medicine, cholesterol medication, and an aspirin. Then I did my exercises and took a shower.

On the way to the kitchen, I didn't even notice the smoke detector I passed or the old ashtrays in the closet. I took a low-fat yogurt out of the refrigerator and prepared hot cereal in the microwave oven for my breakfast.

Then I walked out my door into the crisp clean air and got in my car. I put on my seat belt, saw the light go on for the airbag, and safely drove to work. I got to my office, where I paid

little attention to the new defibrillator at the entrance, the "no smoking" signs, or the absence of asbestos. I arrived safely in my well-ventilated office and got ready to teach Public Health 101.

It wasn't a very eventful morning, but then it's all in a morning's work when it comes to public health.

© kak2s/ShutterStock, Inc.

This rather mundane morning is made possible by a long list of achievements that reflect the often-ignored history of public health.[1] We take for granted the fact that water chlorination, hand washing, and indoor plumbing largely eliminated the transmission of common bacterial diseases, which so often killed the young and not-so-young for centuries. Do not overlook the impact of prevention on our teeth and gums. Teeth brushing, flossing, and fluoridation of water have made a dramatic impact on the dental health of children and adults.

The more recent advances in the prevention of heart disease have been a major public health achievement. Preventive successes include the reduction of blood pressure and cholesterol, cigarette smoking prevention and cessation efforts, the use of low-dose aspirin, an understanding of the role of exercise, and the widespread availability of defibrillators. These can be credited with at least half the dramatic reductions in heart disease that have reduced the death rate from coronary artery disease by approximately 50% in the United States and most other developed countries in the last half century.

The refrigerator was one of the most important advances in food safety, which illustrates the impact of social change and innovation not necessarily intended to improve health. Food and product safety are public health achievements that require continued attention. It was public pressure for food safety that in large part brought about the creation of the U.S. Food and Drug Administration. The work of this public health agency continues to affect all of our lives from the safety of the foods we eat to the drugs and cosmetics we use.

Radiation safety, like radiation itself, usually goes unnoticed, from the regulation of microwave ovens to the reduction of radon in buildings. We rarely notice when disease does not occur.

Highway safety illustrates the wide scope of activities required to protect the public's health. From seat belts, child restraints, and airbags to safer cars, highways, designated driver programs, and enforcement of drunk driving laws, public health efforts require collaboration with professionals not usually thought of as having a health focus.

The physical environment too has been made safer by the efforts of public health. Improvement in the quality of the air we breathe both outdoors and indoors has been an ongoing accomplishment of what we will call "population health." Our lives are safer today because of interventions ranging from installation of smoke detectors to removal of asbestos from buildings.

However, the challenges continue. Globalization increases the potential for the spread of existing and emerging diseases and raises concerns about the safety of the products we use. Climate change and ongoing environmental deterioration continue to produce new territory for "old" diseases, such as malaria and dengue fever. Overuse of technologies, such as antibiotics, has encouraged the emergence of resistant bacteria.

The 1900s saw an increase in life expectancy of almost 30 years in most developed countries, much of it due to the successes of public health initiatives.[2] We cannot assume that these trends will continue indefinitely. The epidemic of obesity already threatens to slow down or reverse the progress we have been making. The challenges of 21st century public health include the protection of health and continued improvement in quality of life, not just quantity of years individuals are living.

To understand the role of public health in these achievements and ongoing challenges, let us start at the beginning and ask: What do we mean by "public health"?

WHAT DO WE MEAN BY "PUBLIC HEALTH"?

Ask your parents what "public health" means and they might say, "Health care for the poor." Well, they are right that public health has always been about providing services for those with special vulnerabilities, either directly or through the health-care system. But that is only one of the ways that public health serves the most needy and vulnerable in our population. Public health efforts often focus on the most vulnerable populations, from reducing exposure to lead paint in deteriorating buildings to food supplementation to prevent birth defects and goiters. Addressing the needs of vulnerable populations has always been a cornerstone of public health. As we will see, however, the definition of "vulnerable populations" continues to change, as do the challenges of addressing their needs.

Ask your grandparents what "public health" means and they might say, "Washing your hands." Well, they are right too—public health has always been about determining risks to health and providing successful interventions that are applicable to everyone. But hand washing is only the tip of the iceberg. The types of interventions that apply to everyone and benefit everyone span an enormous range: from food and drug safety to controlling air pollution, from measures to prevent the spread of tuberculosis to vaccinating against childhood diseases, from prevention and response to disasters to detection of contaminants in our water.

The concerns of society as a whole are always in the forefront of public health. These concerns keep changing and the methods for addressing them keep expanding. New technologies and global, local, and national interventions are becoming a necessary part of public health. To understand what public health has been and what it is becoming, let us look at some definitions of "public health." The following are two definitions of "public health"—one from the early 1900s and one from more recent years.

> Public health is "the science and art of preventing disease, prolonging life and promoting health through organized community effort."[3]

> The substance of public health is the "organized community efforts aimed at the prevention of disease and the promotion of health."[4]

These definitions show how little the concept of public health changed throughout the 1900s; however, the concept of public health in the 2000s is beginning to undergo important changes in a number of ways, including:

- The goal of prolonging life is being complemented by an emphasis on the quality of life.
- Protection of health when it already exists is becoming a focus along with promoting health when it is at risk.
- Use of new technologies, such as the Internet, are redefining "community," as well as offering us new ways to communicate.
- The enormous expansion in the options for intervention, as well as the increasing awareness of potential harms and costs of intervention programs, require a new science of "evidence-based" public health.
- Public health and clinical care, as well as public and private partnerships, are coming together in new ways to produce collaborative efforts rarely seen in the 1900s.
- Complex public health problems need to be viewed as part of larger health and social systems, which require efforts to simultaneously examine multiple problems and multiple solutions rather than one problem or one solution at a time.

Thus, a new 21st century definition of public health is needed. One such definition might read as follows:

> The totality of all evidence-based public and private efforts that preserve and promote health and prevent disease, disability, and death.

This broad definition recognizes public health as the umbrella for a range of approaches that need to be viewed as a part of a big picture or population perspective. Specifically, this definition enlarges the traditional scope of public health to include:

- An examination of the full range of environmental, social, and economic determinants of health—not just those traditionally addressed by public health and clinical health care.
- An examination of the full range of interventions to address health issues, including the structure and function of healthcare delivery systems, plus the role of public policies that affect health even when health is not their intended effect.

If your children ask you what public health is, you might respond: "It is about the big picture issues that affect our own health and the health of our community every day of our lives. It is about protecting health in the face of disasters, preventing disease from addictions such as cigarettes, controlling infections such as the human immunodeficiency virus (HIV), and developing systems to ensure the safety of the food we eat and the water we drink."

A variety of terms have been used to describe this big picture perspective that takes into account the full range of factors that affect health and considers their interactions.[5] A variation of this approach has been called the social-ecological model, systems thinking, or the population health approach. We will use the latter term. Before exploring what we mean by the **population health approach** (also known as the **ecological approach** or **socioecological approach**), let us examine how the approaches to public health have changed over time.[a]

HOW HAS THE APPROACH OF PUBLIC HEALTH CHANGED OVER TIME?

Organized community efforts to promote health and prevent disease go back to ancient times.[6, 7] The earliest human civilizations integrated concepts of prevention into their culture, their religion, and their laws. Prohibitions against specific foods—including pork, beef, and seafood—plus customs for food preparation, including officially designated methods of killing cattle and methods of cooking, were part of the earliest practices of ancient societies. Prohibitions against alcohol or its limited use for religious ceremony have long been part of societies' efforts to control behavior, as well as prevent disease. Prohibition

---

[a] Turnock[2] has described several meanings of "public health." These include the system and social enterprise, the profession, the methods, the government services, and the health of the public. The population health approach used in this text may be thought of as subsuming all of these different perspectives on public health.

of cannibalism, the most universal of food taboos, has strong grounding in the protection of health.[b]

The earliest civilizations have viewed sexual practices as having health consequences. Male circumcision, premarital abstinence, and marital fidelity have all been shown to have impacts on health.

Quarantine or isolation of individuals with disease or exposed to disease has likewise been practiced for thousands of years. The intuitive notion that isolating individuals with disease could protect individuals and societies led to some of the earliest organized efforts to prevent the spread of disease. At times, they were successful, but without a solid scientific basis. Efforts to separate individuals and communities from epidemics sometimes led to misguided efforts, such as the unsuccessful attempts to control the black plague by barring outsiders from walled towns and not recognizing that it was the rats and fleas that transmitted the disease.

During the 1700s and first half of the 1800s, individuals occasionally produced important insights into the prevention of disease. In the 1740s, British naval commander James Lind demonstrated that lemons and other citrus fruit could prevent and treat scurvy, a then-common disease among sailors, whose daily nourishment was devoid of citrus fruit, the best source of vitamin C.

In the last years of the 1700s, English physician Edward Jenner recognized that cowpox, a common mild ailment of those who milked cows, protected those who developed it against life-threatening smallpox. He developed what came to be called a vaccine—derived from the Latin *vacca*, meaning "cow." He placed fluid from cowpox sores under the skin of recipients, including his son, and exposed them to smallpox. Despite the success of these smallpox prevention efforts, widespread use of vaccinations was slow to develop, partially because at that time, there was not an adequate scientific basis to explain the reason for its success.

All of these approaches to disease prevention were known before organized public health existed. Public health awareness began to emerge in Europe and the United States in the mid-1800s. The U.S. public health movement has its origins in Europe, where concepts of disease as the consequence of social conditions took root in the 1830s and 1840s. This movement, which put forth the idea that disease emerges from social conditions of inequality, produced the concept of **social justice**. Many attribute public health's focus on vulnerable populations to this tradition.

While early organized public health efforts paid special attention to vulnerable members of society, they also focused on the hazards that affected everyone, such as contamination of the environment. This focus on sanitation and public health was often called the hygiene movement, although it began even before the development of the germ theory of disease. Despite the absence of an adequate scientific foundation, the hygiene movement made major strides in controlling communicable diseases, such as tuberculosis, cholera, and waterborne diseases, largely through alteration of the physical environment.

The fundamental concepts of epidemiology also developed during this era. In the 1850s, John Snow, often called the father of epidemiology, helped establish the importance of careful data collection and documentation of rates of disease before and after an intervention in order to evaluate effectiveness. He is known for his efforts to close down the Broad Street pump, which supplied water contaminated by cholera to a district of London. His actions quickly terminated that epidemic of cholera. John Snow's approach has become a symbol of the earliest formal epidemiological thinking.

Ignaz Semmelweis, an Austrian physician, used much the same approach in the mid-1800s to control puerperal fever—or fever of childbirth—then a major cause of maternal mortality. Noting that physicians frequently went from the autopsy room to the delivery room without washing their hands, he instituted a hand-washing procedure and was able to document a dramatic reduction in the frequency of puerperal fever. Unfortunately, he was unable to convince many of his contemporaries to accept this intervention without a clear mechanism of action. Until the acceptance of the germ theory of disease, puerperal fever continued to be the major cause of maternal deaths in Europe and North America.

The mid-1800s in England also saw the development of birth and death records, or vital statistics, which formed the basis of population-wide assessment of health status. From the beginning of this type of data collection, there was controversy over how to define the cause of death. Two key figures in the early history of organized public health took opposing positions that reflect this continuing controversy. Edwin Chadwick argued that specific pathological conditions or diseases should be the basis for the cause of death. William Farr argued that underlying factors, including what we would today call risk factors and social conditions, should be seen as the actual causes of death.

Thus, the methods of public health were already being established before the development of the germ theory of

---

[b] In recent years, this prohibition has been indirectly violated by feeding beef products containing bones and brain matter to other cattle. The development of "mad cow" disease and its transmission to humans has been traced to this practice, which can be viewed as analogous to human cannibalism.

disease by Louis Pasteur and his European colleagues in the mid-1800s. The revolutions in biology that they ignited ushered in a new era in public health. U.S. physicians and public health leaders often went to Europe to study new techniques and approaches and brought them back to the United States to use at home.

After the Civil War, U.S. public health began to produce its own advances and organizations. In 1872, the American Public Health Association (APHA) was formed. According to its own historical account, "the APHA's founders recognized that two of the association's most important functions were advocacy for adoption by the government of the most current scientific advances relevant to public health, and public education on how to improve community health."[8]

The biological revolution of the late 1800s and early 1900s that resulted from the germ theory of disease laid the groundwork for the modern era of public health. An understanding of the contributions of bacteria and other organisms to disease produced novel diagnostic testing capabilities. For example, scientists could now identify tuberculosis cases through skin testing, bacterial culture, and the newly discovered chest X ray. Concepts of vaccination advanced with the development of new vaccines against toxins produced by tetanus- and diphtheria-causing bacteria. Without antibiotics or other effective cures, much of public health in this era relied on prevention, isolation of those with disease, and case-finding methods to prevent further exposure.

In the early years of the 1900s, epidemiology methods continued to contribute to the understanding of disease. The investigations of pellagra by Goldberger and the United States Public Health Service overthrew the assumption of the day that pellagra was an infectious disease and established that it was a nutritional deficiency that could be prevented or easily cured with vitamin B-6 (niacin) or a balanced diet. Understanding the role of nutrition was central to public health's emerging focus on prenatal care and childhood growth and development. Incorporating key scientific advances, these efforts matured in the 1920s and 1930s and introduced a growing alphabet of vitamins and nutrients to the U.S. vocabulary.

A new era of effective medical intervention against active disease began in force after World War II. The discovery of penicillin and its often miraculous early successes convinced scientists, public health practitioners, and the general public that a new era in medicine and public health had arrived.

During this era, public health's focus was on filling the holes in the healthcare system. In this period, the role of public health was often seen as assisting clinicians to effec-

tively deliver clinical services to those without the benefits of private medical care and helping to integrate preventive efforts into the practice of medicine. Thus, the great public health success of organized campaigns for the eradication of polio was mistakenly seen solely as a victory for medicine. Likewise, the successful passage of Medicaid and Medicare, outgrowths of public health's commitment to social justice, was simply viewed as efforts to expand the private practice of medicine.

This period, however, did lay the foundations for the emergence of a new era in public health. Epidemiological methods designed for the study of noncommunicable diseases demonstrated the major role that cigarette smoking plays in lung cancer and a variety of other diseases. The emergence of the randomized controlled trial and the regulation of drugs, vaccines, and other interventions by the Food and Drug Administration developed the foundations for what we now call evidence-based public health and evidence-based medicine.

The 1980s and much of the 1990s were characterized by a focus on individual responsibility for health and interventions at the individual level. Often referred to as health promotion and disease prevention, these interventions targeted individuals to effect behavioral change and combat the risk factors for diseases. As an example, to help prevent coronary artery disease, efforts were made to help individuals address high blood pressure and cholesterol, cigarette smoking, and obesity. Behavioral change strategies were also used to help prevent the spread of the newly emerging HIV/AIDS epidemic. Efforts aimed at individual prevention and early detection as part of medical practice began to bear some fruit with the widespread introduction of mammography for detection of breast cancer and the worldwide use of Pap smears for the detection of cervical cancer. Newborn screening for genetic disease became a widespread and often legally mandated program, combining individual and community components.

Major public health advances during this era resulted from the environmental movement, which brought public awareness of the health dangers of lead in gasoline and paint. The environmental movement also focused on reducing cancer by controlling radiation exposure from a range of sources, including sunlight and radon, both naturally occurring radiation sources. In a triumph of global cooperation, governments worked together to address the newly discovered hole in the ozone layer. In the United States, reductions in air pollution levels and smoking rates during this era had an impact on the frequency of chronic lung disease, asthma, and most likely coronary artery disease.

The heavy reliance on individual interventions that characterized much of the last half of the 1900s changed rapidly in the beginning of the 2000s. A new era in public health that is often called "population health" has begun to transform professional and public thought about health. From the potential for bioterrorism to the high costs of health care to the control of pandemic influenza and AIDS, the need for community-wide or population-wide public health efforts have become increasingly evident. This new era is characterized by a global perspective and the need to address international health issues. It includes a focus on the potential impacts of climate change, emerging and reemerging infectious diseases, and the consequences of trade in potentially contaminated or dangerous products, ranging from food to toys.

Table 1-1 outlines these eras of public health, identifies their key defining elements, and highlights important events that symbolize each era.[9]

TABLE 1-1 Eras of Public Health

Eras of public health	Focus of attention/paradigm	Action framework	Notable events and movements in public health and epidemiology
Health protection (Antiquity–1830s)	Authority-based control of individual and community behaviors	Religious and cultural practices and prohibited behaviors	Quarantine for epidemics; sexual prohibitions to reduce disease transmission; dietary restrictions to reduce food-borne disease
Hygiene movement (1840–1870s)	Sanitary conditions as basis for improved health	Environmental action on a community-wide basis distinct from health care	Snow on cholera; Semmelweis and puerperal fever; collection of vital statistics as empirical foundation for public health and epidemiology
Contagion control (1880–1940s)	Germ theory: demonstration of infectious origins of disease	Communicable disease control through environmental control, vaccination, sanatoriums, and outbreak investigation in general population	Linkage of epidemiology, bacteriology, and immunology to form TB sanatoriums; outbreak investigation, e.g., Goldberger and pellagra
Filling holes in the medical care system (1950s–mid-1980s)	Integration of control of communicable diseases, modification of risk factors, and care of high-risk populations as part of medical care	Public system for control of specific communicable diseases and care for vulnerable populations distinct from general healthcare system, beginning of integrated healthcare systems with integration of preventive services into general healthcare system	Antibiotics; randomized controlled trials; concept of risk factors; surgeon general reports on cigarette smoking; Framingham study on cardiovascular risks; health maintenance organizations and community health centers with integration of preventive services into general healthcare system
Health promotion/ Disease prevention (Mid-1980s–2000)	Focus on individual behavior and disease detection in vulnerable and general populations	Clinical and population-oriented prevention with focus on individual control of decision making and multiple interventions	AIDS epidemic and need for multiple interventions to reduce risk; reductions in coronary heart disease through multiple interventions
Population health (2000s)	Coordination of public health and healthcare delivery based upon shared evidence-based systems thinking	Evidence-based recommendations and information management, focus on harms and costs as well as benefits of interventions, globalization	Evidence-based medicine and public health; information technology; new approaches to avoid medical errors; antibiotic resistance; global collaboration, e.g., SARS; tobacco control; climate change

Data from Awofeso N. What's New About the "New Public Health"? *American Journal of Public Health.* 2004;94(5):705–709.

Thus, today we have entered an era in which a focus on the individual is increasingly coupled with a focus on what needs to be done at the community and population level. This era of public health can be viewed as "the era of population health."

WHAT IS MEANT BY "POPULATION HEALTH"?

The concept of population health has emerged in recent years as a broader concept of public health that includes all the ways that society as a whole or communities within society are affected by health issues and how they respond to these issues. Population health provides an intellectual umbrella for thinking about the wide spectrum of factors that can and do affect the health of individuals and the population as a whole. **Figure 1-1** provides an overview of what falls under the umbrella of population health. Population health also provides strategies for considering the broad range of potential **interventions** to address these issues. By "intervention" we mean the full range of strategies designed to protect health and prevent disease, disability, and death. Interventions include preventive efforts, such as nutrition and vaccination; curative efforts, such as antibiotics and cancer surgery; and efforts to prevent complications and restore function—from chemotherapy to physical therapy. Thus, population health is about healthy people and healthy populations.

The concept of population health can be seen as a comprehensive way of thinking about the modern scope of public health. It utilizes an evidence-based approach to analyze the determinants of health and disease and the options for intervention to preserve and improve health. Population health requires us to define what we mean by "health issues" and what we mean by "population(s)." It also requires us to define what we mean by "society's shared health concerns," as well as "society's vulnerable groups."

To understand population health, we therefore need to define what we mean by each of these four components:

- Health issues
- Population(s)
- Society's shared health concerns
- Society's vulnerable groups

WHAT ARE THE IMPLICATIONS OF EACH OF THE FOUR COMPONENTS OF PUBLIC HEALTH?

All four of the key components of public health have changed in recent years. Let us take a look at the historical, current, and emerging scopes of each component and consider their implications.

For most of the history of public health, the term "health" focused solely on physical health. Mental health has now been recognized as an important part of the definition; conditions such as depression and substance abuse make enormous contributions to disability in populations throughout the world. The boundaries of what we mean by "health" continue to expand, and the limits of health are not clear. Many novel medical interventions—including modification of genes and treatments to increase height, improve cosmetic appearance, and improve sexual performance—confront us with the question: Are these health issues?

The definition of "population," likewise, is undergoing fundamental change. For most of recorded history, a population was defined geographically. Geographic communities, such as cities, states, and countries, defined the structure and functions of public health. The current definition of "population" has expanded to include the idea of a global community, recognizing the increasingly interconnected issues of global health. The definition of "population" is also focusing more on nongeographic communities. Universities now include the distance-learning community, health care is delivered to members of a health plan community, and the Internet is creating new social media communities. All of these new definitions of "population" are affecting the thinking and approaches needed to address public health issues.

What about the meaning of society-wide concerns—have they changed as well? Historically, public health and communicable disease were nearly synonymous, as symbolized by the field of epidemiology, which actually derives its name from the study of communicable disease epidemics. In recent decades, the focus of society-wide concerns has greatly expanded to include toxic exposures from the physical environment, transportation safety, and the costs of health care. However, communicable disease never went away as a focus of public health, and the 2000s are seeing a resurgence in

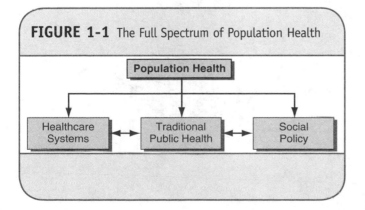

FIGURE 1-1 The Full Spectrum of Population Health

Population Health

Healthcare Systems ↔ Traditional Public Health ↔ Social Policy

TABLE 1-2 Components of Population Health

	Health	Population	Examples of society-wide concerns	Examples of vulnerable groups
Historical	Physical	Geographically limited	Communicable disease	High-risk maternal and child, high-risk occupations
Current	Physical and mental	Local, state, national, global, governmentally defined	Toxic substances, product and transportation safety, communicable diseases, costs of health care	Disabled, frail elderly, uninsured
Emerging	Cosmetic, genetic, social functioning	Defined by local, national, and global communications	Disasters, climate change, technology hazards, emerging infectious diseases	Immunosuppressed, genetic vulnerability

concern over emerging infectious diseases, including HIV/AIDS, pandemic flu, and newly drug-resistant diseases, such as staph infections and tuberculosis. Additional concerns, ranging from the impact of climate change to the harms and benefits of new technologies, are altering the meaning of society-wide concerns.

Finally, the meaning of "vulnerable populations" continues to transform. For most of the 1900s, public health focused on maternal and child health and high-risk occupations as the operational definition of "vulnerable populations." While these groups remain important to public health, additional groups now receive more attention, including the disabled, the frail elderly, and those without health insurance. Attention is also beginning to focus on the immuno-suppressed among those living with HIV/AIDS, who are at higher risk of infection and illness, and those whose genetic code documents their special vulnerability to disease and reactions to medications.

Public health has always been about our shared health concerns as a society and our concerns about vulnerable populations. These concerns have changed over time, and new concerns continue to emerge. **Table 1-2** outlines historical, current, and emerging components of the population health approach to public health. As is illustrated by communicable diseases, past concerns cannot be relegated to history.

SHOULD WE FOCUS ON EVERYONE OR ON VULNERABLE GROUPS?

Public health is often confronted with the potential conflict of focusing on everyone and addressing society-wide concerns versus focusing on the needs of vulnerable populations.[10] This conflict is reflected in the two different approaches to addressing public health problems. We will call them the **high-risk approach** and the **improving-the-average approach**.

The high-risk approach focuses on those with the highest probability of developing disease and aims to bring their risk close to the levels experienced by the rest of the population. **Figure 1-2A** illustrates the high-risk approach.

The success of the high-risk approach, as shown in **Figure 1-2B**, assumes that those with a high probability of

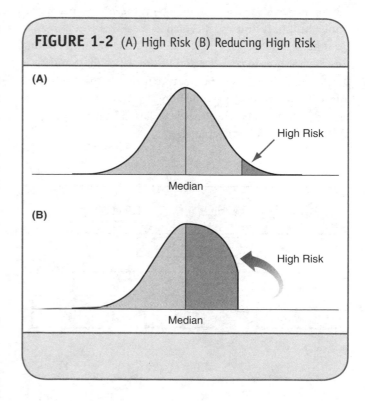

FIGURE 1-2 (A) High Risk (B) Reducing High Risk

(A)

High Risk

Median

(B)

High Risk

Median

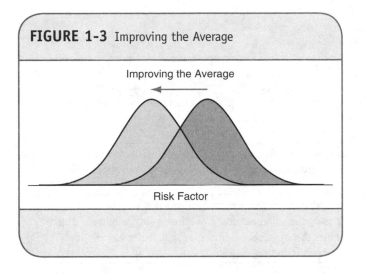

FIGURE 1-3 Improving the Average

Improving the Average

Risk Factor

developing disease are heavily concentrated among those with exposure to what we call **risk factors**. Risk factors include a wide range of exposures, from cigarette smoke and other toxic substances to high-risk sexual behaviors.

The improving-the-average approach focuses on the entire population and aims to reduce the risk for everyone. **Figure 1-3** illustrates this approach.

The improving-the-average approach assumes that everyone is at some degree of risk and the risk increases with the extent of exposure. In this situation, most of the disease occurs among the large number of people who have only modestly increased exposure. The successful reduction in average cholesterol levels through changes in the U.S. diet and the anticipated reduction in diabetes via a focus on weight reduction among children illustrate this approach.

One approach may work better than the other in specific circumstances, but in general, both approaches are needed if we are going to successfully address today's and tomorrow's health issues. These two approaches parallel public health's long-standing focus on both the health of vulnerable populations and society-wide health concerns.[c]

Now that we understand what is meant by "population health," let us take a look at the range of approaches that may be used to promote and protect health.

---

[c] An additional approach includes reducing disparities by narrowing the curve so that the gap is reduced between the lowest of the low-risk and the highest of the high-risk. For instance, this might be accomplished by transferring financial resources and/or health services from the low-risk to the high-risk category through taxation or other methods. Depending on the distribution of the factors affecting health, this approach may or may not reduce the overall frequency of disease more than the other approaches. The distribution of risk in Figures 1-2 and 1-3 assumes a bell-shaped or normal distribution. The actual distribution of factors affecting health may not follow this distribution.

WHAT ARE THE APPROACHES AVAILABLE TO PROTECT AND PROMOTE HEALTH?

The wide range of strategies that have been, are being, and will be used to address health issues can be divided into three general categories: health care, traditional public health, and social interventions.

Health care includes the delivery of services to individuals on a one-on-one basis. It includes services for those who are sick or disabled with illness or diseases, as well as for those who are asymptomatic. Services delivered as part of clinical prevention have been categorized as vaccinations, behavioral counseling, screening for disease, and preventive medications.[11]

Traditional public health efforts have a population-based preventive perspective utilizing interventions targeting communities or populations, as well as defined high-risk or vulnerable groups. Communicable disease control, reduction of environmental hazards, food and drug safety, and nutritional and behavioral risk factors have been key areas of focus of traditional public health approaches.

Both health care and traditional public health approaches share a goal to directly affect the health of those they reach. In contrast, social interventions are primarily aimed at achieving other nonhealth goals, such as increasing convenience, pleasure, economic growth, and social justice. Social interventions range from improving housing, to improving education and services for the poor, to increased global trade. These interventions may have dramatic and sometimes unanticipated positive or negative health consequences. Social interventions, like increased availability of food, may improve health, while the availability of high-fat or high-calorie foods may pose a risk to health.

Table 1-3 describes the characteristics of health care, traditional public health, and social approaches to population health and provides examples of each approach.

None of these approaches is new. However, they have traditionally been separated or put into silos in our thinking process, with the connections between them often ignored. Thinking in systems and connecting the pieces is an important part of the 21st century challenge of defining public health.

Now that we have explained what we mean by "public health" and seen the scope and methods that we call "population health," let us continue our big-picture approach by taking a look at what we mean by the "determinants of health and disease."

WHAT FACTORS DETERMINE THE OCCURRENCE OF DISEASE, DISABILITY, AND DEATH?

To complete our look at the big picture issues in public health, we need to gain an understanding of the forces that determine disease and the outcome of disease, including

TABLE 1-3 Approaches to Population Health

	Characteristics	Examples
Health care	Systems for delivering one-on-one individual health services, including those aimed at prevention, cure, palliation, and rehabilitation	Clinical preventive services, including vaccinations, behavioral counseling, screening for disease, and preventive medications
Traditional public health	Group- and community-based interventions directed at health promotion and disease prevention	Communicable disease control, control of environmental hazards, food and drug safety, reduction in risk factors for disease
Social interventions	Interventions with another non-health-related purpose, which have secondary impacts on health	Interventions that improve the built environment, increase education, alter nutrition, or address socioeconomic disparities through changes in tax laws; globalization and mobility of goods and populations

what in public health has been called morbidity (disability) and mortality (death).[d]

We need to establish what are called contributory causes based on evidence. **Contributory causes** can be thought of as immediate causes of disease. For instance, the HIV virus and cigarette smoking are two well-established contributory causes of disease, disability, and death. They directly produce disease, as well as disability and death. However, knowing these contributory causes of disease is often not enough. We need to ask: What determines whether people will smoke or come in contact with the HIV virus? What determines their course once exposed to cigarettes or HIV? In public health, we use the term **determinants** to identify these underlying factors, or "causes of causes" that ultimately bring about disease.

Determinants look beyond the known contributory causes of disease to factors that are at work often years before a disease develops.[12, 13] These underlying factors may be thought of as "upstream" forces. Like great storms, we know the water will flow downstream, often producing flooding and destruction along the way. We just do not know exactly when and where the destruction will occur.

There is no official list or agreed-upon definition of what is included in determinants of disease.[e] Nonetheless, there is

wide agreement that the following factors are among those that can be described as determinants in that they increase or at times decrease the chances of developing conditions that threaten the quantity and/or quality of life. Some but not all of these factors are related to socioeconomic status and are categorized as social determinants of health.

Behavior
Infection
Genetics

Geography
Environment
Medical care
Socioeconomic-cultural

BIG GEMS provides a convenient device for remembering these determinants of disease. Let us see what we mean by each of the determinants.

Behavior—Behavior implies actions that increase exposure to the factors that produce disease or protect individuals from disease. Actions such as smoking cigarettes, exercising, eating a particular diet, consuming alcohol, having unprotected intercourse, and using seat belts are all examples of the ways that behaviors help determine the development of disease.

Infection—Infections are often the direct cause of disease. In addition, we are increasingly recognizing that early or long-standing exposures to infections may contribute to the development of disease or even protection against disease. Diseases as diverse as gastric and duodenal ulcers, gallstones, and hepatoma or cancer originating in the liver are increasingly suspected to have infection as an important determinant. Early exposure to infections may actually reduce diseases ranging from polio to asthma.

---

[d] We will use the term "disease" as shorthand for the broad range of outcomes that includes injuries and exposures that result in death and disability.

[e] Health Canada[12] has identified 12 determinants of health, which are: 1) income and social status, 2) employment, 3) education, 4) social environments, 5) physical environments, 6) healthy child development, 7) personal health practices and coping skills, 8) health services, 9) social support networks, 10) biology and genetic endowment, 11) gender, and 12) culture. Many of these are subsumed under socioeconomic-cultural determinants in the BIG GEMS framework. The World Health Organization's Commission on Social Determinants of Health has also produced a list of determinants that is consistent with the BIG GEMS framework.[13]

Genetics—The revolution in genetics has focused our attention on roles that genetic factors play in the development and outcome of disease. Even when contributory causes, such as cigarettes, have been clearly established as producing lung cancer, genetic factors also play a role in the development and progression of the disease. While genetic factors play a role in many diseases, they are only occasionally the most important determinant of disease.

Geography—Geographic location influences the frequency and even the presence of disease. Infectious diseases such as malaria, Chagas disease, schistosomiasis, and Lyme disease occur only in defined geographic areas. Geography may also imply local geological conditions, such as those that produce high levels of radon—a naturally occurring radiation that contributes to the development of lung cancer. Geography implies that special locations are required to produce disease, such as frostbite in the arctic or snake bites in the tropics.

Environment—Environmental factors determine disease and the course of disease in a number of ways. The unaltered or "natural" physical world around us may produce disability and death from sudden natural disasters, such as earthquakes and volcanic eruptions, to iodine deficiencies due to low iodine content in the food-producing soil. The altered physical environment produced by human intervention includes exposures to toxic substances in occupational or nonoccupational settings. The physical environment built for use by humans—the **built environment**—produces determinants ranging from indoor air pollution, to "infant-proofed" homes, to hazards on the highway.

Medical care—Access to and the quality of medical care can be a determinant of disease. When a high percentage of individuals is protected by vaccination, nonvaccinated individuals in the population may be protected as well. Cigarette smoking cessation efforts may help smokers to quit, and treatment of infectious disease may reduce the spread to others. Medical care, however, often has its major impact on the course of disease by attempting to prevent or minimize disability and death once disease develops.

Socioeconomic-cultural—In the United States, socioeconomic factors have been defined as education, income, and occupational status. These measures have all been shown to be determinants of diseases as varied as breast cancer, tuberculosis, and occupational injuries. Cultural and religious factors are increasingly being recognized as determinants of diseases because beliefs sometimes influence decisions about treatments, in turn affecting the outcome of the disease. While most diseases are more frequent in lower socioeconomic groups, others, such as breast cancer, may be more common in higher socioeconomic groups.

Determinants of disease come up again and again as we explore the work of population health. Historically, understanding determinants has often allowed us to prevent diseases and their consequences even when we did not fully understand the mechanism by which the determinants produced their impact. For instance:

- Scurvy was controlled by citrus fruits well before vitamin C was identified.
- Malaria was partially controlled by clearing swamps before the relationship to mosquito transmission was appreciated.
- Hepatitis B and HIV infections were partially controlled even before the organisms were identified through the reduction in use of contaminated needles and the establishment of standards for blood transfusions.
- Tuberculosis death rates were greatly reduced through less crowded housing, the use of TB sanitariums, and better nutrition.

Using asthma as an example, **Box 1-1** illustrates the many ways that determinants can affect the development and course of a disease.

BOX 1-1 Asthma and the Determinants of Disease

Jennifer, a teenager living in a rundown urban apartment in a city with high levels of air pollution, develops severe asthma. Her mother also has severe asthma, yet both of them smoke cigarettes. Her clinician prescribed medications to prevent asthma attacks, but she takes them only when she experiences severe symptoms. Jennifer is hospitalized twice with pneumonia due to common bacterial infections. She then develops an antibiotic-resistant infection. During this hospitalization, she requires intensive care on a respirator. After several weeks of intensive care and every known treatment to save her life, she dies suddenly.

Asthma is an inflammatory disease of the lung coupled with an increased reactivity of the airways, which together produce

(continues)

BOX 1-1   Asthma and the Determinants of Disease (*continued*)

a narrowing of the airways of the lungs. When the airways become swollen and inflamed, they become narrower, allowing less air through to the lung tissue and causing symptoms such as wheezing, coughing, chest tightness, breathing difficulty, and predisposition to infection. Once considered a minor ailment, asthma is now the most common chronic disorder of childhood. It affects over 6 million children under the age of 18 in the United States alone.

Jennifer's tragic history illustrates how a wide range of determinants of disease may affect the occurrence, severity, and development of complications of a disease. Let us walk through the BIG GEMS framework and see how each determinant had impacts on Jennifer.

Behavior—Behavioral factors play an important role in the development of asthma attacks and in their complications. Cigarette smoking makes asthma attacks more frequent and more severe. It also predisposes individuals to developing infections such as pneumonia. Treatment for severe asthma requires regular treatments along with more intensive treatment when an attack occurs. It is difficult for many people, especially teenagers, to take medication regularly, yet failure to adhere to treatment greatly complicates the disease.

Infection—Infection is a frequent precipitant of asthma, and asthma increases the frequency and severity of infections. Infectious diseases, especially pneumonia, can be life-threatening in asthmatics, requiring prompt and high-quality medical care. The increasing development of antibiotic-resistant infections poses special risks to those with asthma.

Genetics—Genetic factors predispose people to childhood asthma. However, many children and adults without a family history develop asthma.

Geography—Asthma is more common in geographic areas with high levels of naturally occurring allergens due to

flowering plants. However, today even populations in desert climates in the United States are often affected by asthma, as irrigation results in the planting of allergen-producing trees and other plants.

Environment—The physical environment, including that built for use by humans, has increasingly been recognized as a major factor affecting the development of asthma and asthma attacks. Indoor air pollution is the most common form of air pollution in many developing countries. Along with cigarette smoke, air pollution inflames the lungs acutely and chronically. Cockroaches often found in rundown buildings have been found to be highly allergenic and predisposing to asthma. Other factors in the built environment, including mold and exposure to pet dander, can also trigger wheezing in susceptible individuals.

Medical care—The course of asthma can be greatly affected by medical care. Management of the acute and chronic effects of asthma can be positively affected by efforts to understand an individual's exposures, reducing the chronic inflammation with medications, managing the acute symptoms, and avoiding life-threatening complications.

Socioeconomic-cultural—Disease and disease progression are often influenced by an individual's socioeconomic status. Air pollution is often greater in lower socioeconomic neighborhoods of urban areas. Mold and cockroach infestations may be greater in poor neighborhoods. Access to and the quality of medical care may be affected by social, economic, and cultural factors.

Thus, asthma is a condition that demonstrates the contributions made by the full range of determinants included in the BIG GEMS framework. No one determinant alone explains the bulk of the disease. The large number of determinants and their interactions provide opportunities for a range of health care, traditional public health, and social interventions.

Determinants of health may change over time, and the composition of populations may change in ways that affects health. Let us take a look at some of the ways that populations have changed and are changing that affect population health.

WHAT CHANGES IN POPULATIONS OVER TIME CAN AFFECT HEALTH?

A number of important trends or transitions in the composition of populations that affect the pattern of disease have been described in recent years. These transitions have

implications for what we can expect to happen throughout the 2000s. We will call these the demographic, epidemiological, and nutritional transitions.

The **demographic transition** describes the impact of falling childhood death rates and extended life spans on the size and the age distribution of populations.[14] During the first half of the 1900s, death rates among the young fell dramatically in today's developed countries. Death rates continued their dramatic decline in most parts of the developing world during the second half of the 1900s.

Birth rates tend to remain high for years or decades after the decline in deaths. High birth rates paired with lower death rates lead to rapid growth in population size, as we have seen in much of the developing world. This trend continues today and is expected to go on in many parts of the world well into the 2000s. **Figure 1-4** illustrates how the population of the Nigeria is expected to grow during the first half of the 2000s due to a high birth rate and a lowered death rate.

Despite the delay, a decline in birth rates reliably occurs following the decline in childhood deaths. This decline in births gradually leads to aging of the population. We are now seeing societies in much of Europe and Japan with growing elderly populations. Improved health care and extended life spans for the elderly have magnified this trend. Take a look at **Figure 1-5**, which shows what is expected to occur in the coming years in much of Europe and Japan. Japan is used as an example of the emergence of an inverted population pyramid, with a smaller young population and a larger older population. Populations with a large number of elderly relative to the number of younger individuals have a heavier burden of disease and create the conditions for aging to become a public health issue.

The large number of immigrants to the United States and their generally higher birth rates has slowed this process in the United States, but the basic trend of a growing elderly population continues. The U.S. baby boom, which occurred between 1946 and 1964, is expected to have major impacts on the numbers of elderly in coming years, as illustrated in **Figure 1-6**.

A second transition has been called the **epidemiological transition**,[15] or **public health transition**. The epidemiological or public health transition implies that as social and economic development occurs, different types of diseases become prominent. Deaths in less developed societies are often dominated by epidemic communicable diseases and diseases associated with malnutrition and childhood infections. As a country develops, communicable diseases often come under control, and noncommunicable and chronic diseases, such as heart disease, often predominate.

A related transition known as the **nutritional transition**[16] implies that countries frequently move from poorly balanced diets often deficient in nutrients, proteins, and calories to a diet of highly processed food, including fats, sugars, and salt. The consequences of both under- and overnutrition affect and will continue to affect the public's health well into the 2000s.

As we have seen population health focuses on the big picture issues and the determinants of disease. Increasingly, public health also emphasizes a focus on research evidence as

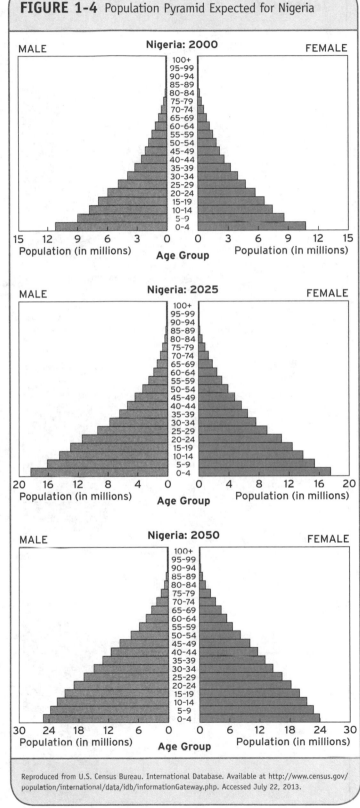

FIGURE 1-4 Population Pyramid Expected for Nigeria

Reproduced from U.S. Census Bureau. International Database. Available at http://www.census.gov/population/international/data/idb/informationGateway.php. Accessed July 22, 2013.

FIGURE 1-5 Population Pyramid Expected for Japan

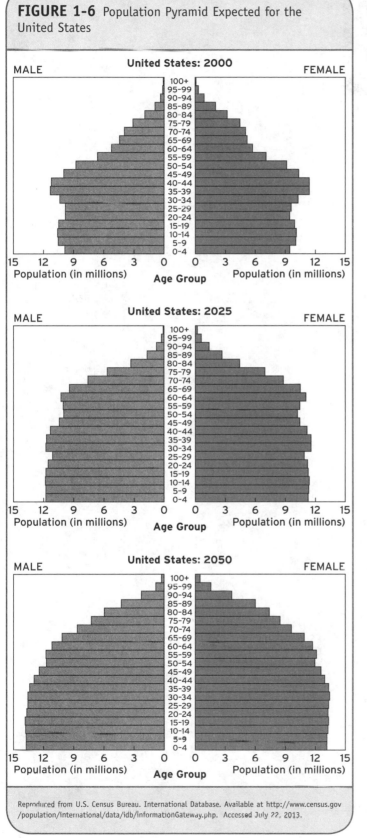

FIGURE 1-6 Population Pyramid Expected for the United States

a basis for understanding the cause or etiology of disease and the interventions that can improve the outcome. Let us now explore what we mean by "evidence-based public health."

KEY WORDS

- **Population health approach**
- **Social justice**
- **Interventions**
- **High-risk approach**
- **Improving-the-average approach**
- **Risk factor**
- **Contributory causes**
- **Determinants**
- **BIG GEMS**
- **Built environment**
- **Demographic transition**
- **Epidemiological transition or public health transition**
- **Nutritional transition**

Discussion Question

1. Think about a typical day in your life and identify ways that public health affects it.

REFERENCES

1. Pfizer Global Pharmaceuticals. *Milestones in Public Health: Accomplishments in Public Health over the Last 100 Years.* New York, NY: Pfizer Global Pharmaceuticals; 2006.

2. Turnock BJ. *Public Health: What It Is and How It Works.* 4th ed. Sudbury, MA: Jones and Bartlett Publishers; 2009.

3. Winslow CEA. The untilled field of public health. *Mod. Med.* 1920;920(2):183–191.

4. Institute of Medicine. *The Future of Public Health.* Washington, DC: National Academy Press; 1988:41.

5. Young TK. *Population Health: Concepts and Methods.* New York, NY: Oxford University Press; 1998.

6. Rosen G. *A History of Public Health.* Baltimore, MD: Johns Hopkins University Press; 1993.

7. Porter D. *Health, Civilization, and the State: A History of Public Health from Ancient to Modern Times.* Oxford: Rutledge; 1999.

8. American Public Health Association. APHA history and timeline. http://www.apha.org/about/news/presskit/aphahistory.htm?NRMODE=Published&NRNODEGUID=%7b8AF0A3FE-8B29-4952-87EF-2757B9B2668F%7d&NRORIGINALURL=%2fabout%2fnews%2fpresskit%2faphahistory.htm&NRCACHEHINT=NoModifyGuest&PF=true. Accessed July 19, 2013.

9. Awofeso N. What's new about the "New Public Health"? *American Journal of Public Health.* 2004;94(5):705–709.

10. Rose G, Khaw KT, Marmot M. *Rose's Strategy of Preventive Medicine.* New York, NY: Oxford University Press; 2008.

11. Agency for Healthcare Research and Quality. Preventive services. http://www.ahrq.gov. Accessed July 22, 2013.

12. Public Health Agency of Canada. Population health approach—what determines health? http://www.phac-aspc.gc.ca/ph-sp. Accessed July 22, 2013.

13. Commission on Social Determinants of Health. Closing the gap in a generation: health equity through action on the social determinants of health. *Final Report of the Commission on Social Determinants of Health.* Geneva: World Health Organization; 2008.

14. U.S. Census Bureau. International database. http://www.census.gov/ipc/www/idb/pyramids.html. Accessed July 22, 2013.

15. Omran AR. The epidemiologic transition: a theory of the epidemiology of population change. *The Milbank Memorial Fund Quarterly.* 1971;49(4): 509–538.

16. Skolnik R. *Global Health 101.* 2nd ed. Burlington, MA: Jones & Bartlett Learning; 2012.

CHAPTER 2

Evidence-Based Public Health

LEARNING OBJECTIVES

By the end of this chapter, the student will be able to:

- explain the steps in the evidence-based public health process.
- describe a public health problem in terms of morbidity and mortality.
- describe the course of a disease in terms of incidence, prevalence, and case-fatality.
- describe how the distribution of disease may be used to generate hypotheses about the cause of a disease.
- describe the approach used in public health to identify a contributory cause of a disease or other condition and establish the efficacy of an intervention.
- describe the process of grading evidence-based recommendations.
- use an approach to identify options for intervention based on "when, who, and how."
- explain the role that evaluation plays in establishing effectiveness as part of evidence-based public health.

Tobacco was introduced to Europe as a new world crop in the early 1600s. Despite the availability of pipe tobacco and, later, cigars, the mass production and consumption of tobacco through cigarette smoking did not begin until the development of the cigarette rolling machine by James Duke in the 1880s. This invention allowed mass production and distribution of cigarettes for the first time. Men were the first mass consumers of cigarettes. During World War I, cigarettes were widely distributed free of charge to U.S. soldiers.

Cigarette smoking first became popular among women in the 1920s—an era noted for changes in the role and attitudes of women—and at this time, advertising of cigarettes began to focus on women. The mass consumption of cigarettes by women, however, trailed that of men by at least two decades. By the 1950s, over 50% of adult males and approximately 25% of adult females were regular cigarette smokers.

The health problems of cigarette smoking were not fully recognized until decades after the habit became widespread. As late as the 1940s, R.J. Reynolds advertised that "more doctors smoke Camels than any other cigarette."

Epidemiologists observed that lung cancer deaths were increasing in frequency in the 1930s and 1940s. The increase in cases did not appear to be due to changes in efforts to recognize the disease, the ability to recognize the disease, or the definition of the disease. Even after the increasing average life span and aging of the population was taken into account, it was evident that the rate of death from lung cancer was increasing—and more rapidly for men than women. In addition, it was noted that residents of states with higher rates of smoking had higher rates of lung cancer. In the 1950s, the number of lung cancer deaths in females also began to increase, and by the 1960s, the disease had become the most common cause of cancer-related deaths in males and was still rising among women.[1, 2]

© RetroClipArt/ShutterStock, Inc.

This type of information was the basis for describing the problems of cigarette smoking and lung cancer and developing ideas or hypotheses about its etiology, or cause. Let us take a look at how the evidence-based public health approach has been used to address the problem of cigarette smoking. There are five basic questions that we need to ask that together make up what we will call the evidence-based public health approach.[3]

1. **P**roblem: What is the health problem?
2. **E**tiology: What is/are the contributory cause(s)?
3. **R**ecommendations: What works to reduce the health impacts?
4. **I**mplementation: How can we get the job done?
5. **E**valuation: How well does/do the intervention(s) work in practice?

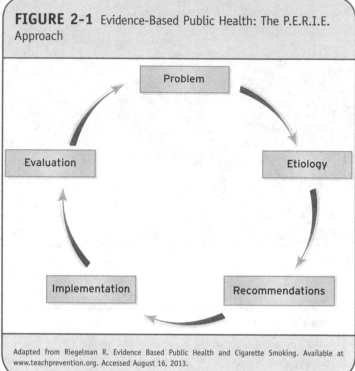

FIGURE 2-1 Evidence-Based Public Health: The P.E.R.I.E. Approach

Adapted from Riegelman R. Evidence Based Public Health and Cigarette Smoking. Available at www.teachprevention.org. Accessed August 16, 2013.

These five questions provide a framework for defining, analyzing, and addressing a wide range of public health issues and can be applied to cigarette smoking for the purposes of this chapter.[4] We will call this framework the **P.E.R.I.E. process**. This process is actually circular, as illustrated in **Figure 2-1**. If the evaluation suggests that more needs to be done, the cycle can and should be repeated. Thus, it is an ongoing process.

Using cigarette smoking as an example, we will illustrate the steps needed to apply the evidence-based public health approach.

HOW CAN WE DESCRIBE A HEALTH PROBLEM?

In describing a health problem, we need to address what we will call the burden of disease, the course of disease, and the distribution of disease. The first step in addressing a health problem is to describe its **burden of disease**, which is the occurrence of disability and death due to a disease. In public heath, disability is often called **morbidity** and death is called **mortality**. We will want to know the current burden of disease and whether there has been a recent change in the burden of the disease.

In addition to describing the burden of disease, it is important to describe what we call the **course of a disease**. The course of the disease asks how often the disease occurs, how likely it is to be present currently, and what happens once it occurs. Describing the course of a disease as well as the burden of disease requires us to use measurements known as rates. **Box 2-1** discusses what we mean by "rates" and how we can use them to describe the burden and course of disease.

In addition to describing the burden and the course of a disease or other health problem, we need to ask: What is the **distribution of disease**? Distribution of disease asks such questions as: Who gets the disease? Where are they located? When does the disease occur? Let us see how understanding

---

BOX 2-1　Rates and the Description of a Health Problem

The term "**rate**" is often used to describe any type of measurement that has a numerator and a denominator where the numerator is a subset of the denominator—that is, the numerator includes only individuals who are also included in the denominator. In a rate, the numerator measures the number of times an event, such as the diagnosis of lung cancer, occurs. The denominator measures the number of times the event could occur. We often use the entire population in the denominator, but at times, we may only use the **at-risk population**. For instance, when measuring the rate of cervical cancer, we would only use the population of women in the denominator, and when measuring rates of prostate cancer, we would only use the population of men in the denominator.[a]

There are two basic types of rates that are key to describing a disease.[5, 6] These are called **incidence rates** and **prevalence**. Incidence rates measure the chances of developing a disease over a period of time—usually one year. That is, incidence rates are the number of new cases of a disease that develop during a year divided by the number of people in the at-risk population at the beginning of the year, as in the following equation:

$$\text{Incidence rate} = \frac{\text{\# of new cases of a disease in a year}}{\text{\# of people in the at-risk population}}$$

We often express incidence rates as the number of events per 100,000 people in the denominator. For instance, the incidence rate of lung cancer might be 100 per 100,000 per year. In evidence-based public health, comparing incidence rates is often a useful starting point when trying to establish the **etiology**, or cause, of a problem.

Mortality rates are a special type of incidence rate that measure the incidence of death due to a disease during a particular year. Mortality rates are often used to measure the burden of disease. When most people who develop a disease die from the disease, as is the situation with lung cancer, the mortality rate and the incidence rates are very similar. Thus, if the incidence rate of lung cancer is 100 per 100,000 per year, the mortality rate might be 95 per 100,000 per year. When mortality rates and incidence rates are similar and mortality rates are more easily or more reliably obtained, epidemiologists may substitute mortality rates for incidence rates.[b]

The relationship between the incidence rate and the mortality rate is important because it estimates the chances of dying from the disease once it is diagnosed. We call this the **case-fatality**. In our example, the chances of dying from lung cancer—the morality rate divided by the incidence rate—is 95%, which indicates that lung cancer results in a very poor prognosis once it is diagnosed.

Prevalence is the number of individuals who have a disease at a particular time divided by the number of individuals who could potentially have the disease. It can be represented by the following equation:

$$\text{Prevalence} = \frac{\text{\# living with a particular disease}}{\text{\# in the at-risk population}}$$

Thus, prevalence tells us the **proportion** or percentage of individuals who have the disease at a point in time.[5, 6]

Despite the fact that lung cancer has become the most common cancer, the prevalence will be low—perhaps one-tenth of 1% or less—because those who develop lung cancer do not generally live for a long period of time. Therefore, you will rarely see people with lung cancer. The prevalence of chronic

---

[a] When talking about the term "rate," many epidemiologists also include a unit of time, such as a day or a year, over which the number of events in the numerator is measured. This may also be called a **true rate**. The term "rate" as used in this text includes true rates, as well as proportions. A proportion is a fraction in which the numerator is a subset of the denominator. A time period is not required for a proportion; however, it often reflects the situation at one point in time.

[b] This is an example of the pragmatic approach that is often taken by epidemiologists when they are limited by the available data. The question facing epidemiologists is frequently: Is the data good enough to address the question? Thus, epidemiology can be thought of as an approximation science.

(continues)

BOX 2-1   Rates and the Description of a Health Problem (Continued)

diseases of prolonged duration, such as asthma or chronic obstructive pulmonary disease (COPD), is often relatively high, hence you will often see people with these diseases.[c]

Prevalence is often useful when trying to assess the total impact or burden of a health problem in a population and can help identify the need for services. For example, knowledge

that there is a high prevalence of lung cancer in a certain region may indicate that there is a need for healthcare services in that area. Prevalence is also very useful in clinical medicine as the starting point for screening and diagnosis.

When using rates to describe a problem, we often use the rates of mortality and morbidity to describe the burden of disease. We use the incidence, prevalence, and case-fatality as the three key rates that together provide a description of the course of disease. Together, these three rates address the key issues that we need to know in describing the course of a health problem: How likely it is to occur, how likely it is to be present currently, and what happens once it occurs. Thus, understanding the burden of disease and the course of disease require us to understand and use rates. As we will see, rates are also key to understanding the distribution of disease.

[c] The relationship between incidence and prevalence rates is approximately the incidence rate x average duration of the disease = the prevalence rate. Both the incidence rate and the average duration affect the prevalence of the disease. Together, the incidence, prevalence, and case-fatality rates provide a population-based summary of the course of a disease. Incidence reflects the chance of developing the disease, prevalence indicates the chances of having the disease, and case-fatality indicates the prognosis or chance of dying from the disease.

---

the distribution of disease may help generate ideas or hypotheses about the disease's etiology (cause).

HOW CAN UNDERSTANDING THE DISTRIBUTION OF DISEASE HELP US GENERATE IDEAS OR HYPOTHESES ABOUT THE CAUSE OF DISEASE?

Public health professionals called **epidemiologists** investigate factors known as "person" and "place" to see if they can find patterns or **associations** in the frequency of a disease. We call these **group associations** or **ecological associations**. Group associations may suggest ideas or hypotheses about the cause, or etiology, of a disease.

"Person" includes demographic characteristics that describe people, such as age, gender, race, and socioeconomic factors. It also includes behaviors or exposures, such as cigarette smoking, exercise, radiation exposure, and use of medications. "Place" implies geographic location, such as a city or state, but it also includes connections between people, such as a university community or a shared Internet site. When these types of factors occur more frequently among groups with the disease than among groups without the disease, we call them **risk indicators** or **risk markers**.[a]

Box 2-2 illustrates how person and place can be used to generate hypotheses about the cause of a disease.

In looking at the distribution of lung cancer and the potential risk factors, epidemiologists found some important relationships. In terms of person, the increases in lung cancer mortality observed in the 1930s through 1950s were far more dramatic among men than among women, though by the 1950s, the mortality rate among women had begun to increase as well. It was noted that cigarette use had increased first in men and later among women. There appeared to be a delay of several decades between the increase in cigarette smoking and the increase in lung cancer mortality among both men and women. This illustrates that "time" along with "person" and "place" is important in generating hypotheses.

In terms of place, it was found that the relationship between cigarette smoking and lung cancer mortality was present throughout the United States, but was strongest in those states where cigarette smoking was most common. Therefore, changes over time and the distribution of disease using person and place led epidemiologists to the conclusion that there was an association between groups of people who smoked more frequently and the same group's mortality rates due to lung cancer. These relationships generated the idea that cigarettes might be a cause of lung cancer.

It is important to realize that these mortality rates are group rates. These data did not include any information about whether those who died from lung cancer were

[a] The term "risk indicator" or "risk marker" needs to be distinguished from the term "risk factor." A risk factor is a candidate for being a contributory cause and implies that at least an association at the individual level has been established.

BOX 2-2   Generating Hypotheses from Distributions of Person and Place

An increased frequency of disease based upon occupation has often provided the initial evidence of a group association based upon a combination of "person" and "place." The first recognized occupational disease was found among chimney sweeps often exposed for long periods of time to large quantities of coal dust and who were found to have a high incidence of testicular cancer.

The Mad Hatter described in *Alice's Adventures in Wonderland* by Lewis Carroll made infamous the 19th century recognition that exposure to mercury fumes was associated with mental changes. Mercury fumes were created when making the felt used for hats, hence the term "mad as a hatter."

The high frequency of asbestosis among those who worked in shipyards suggested a relationship decades before the dangers of asbestos were fully recognized and addressed. A lung disease known as silicosis among those who worked in the mining industry likewise suggested a relationship that led to in-depth investigation and greater control of the risks.

More recently, a rare tumor called angiosarcoma was found to occur among those exposed over long periods to polyvinyl chloride (PVC), a plastic widely used in construction. The initial report of four cases of this unusual cancer among workers in one PVC plant was enough to strongly suggest a cause-and-effect relationship based upon place alone.

An important example of the impact that place can have on generating ideas or hypotheses about causation is the history of fluoride and cavities. In the early years of the 1900s, children in the town of Colorado Springs, Colorado, were found to have a very high incidence of brown discoloration of the teeth. It was soon recognized that this condition was limited to those who obtained their water from a common source. Ironically, those with brown teeth were also protected from cavities. This clear relationship to place was followed by over two decades of research that led to the understanding that fluoride in the water reduces the risk of cavities, while very high levels of the compound also lead to brown teeth. Examination of the levels of fluoride in other water systems eventually led to the establishment of levels of fluoride that could protect against cavities without producing brown teeth.

Such strong and clear-cut relationships are important, but relatively unusual. Often, examinations of the characteristics of person and place in populations suggests hypotheses that can be followed up among individuals to establish cause-and-effect relationships.[5, 6]

---

smokers. It merely indicated that groups who smoked more, such as males, also had higher mortality rates from lung cancer. The most that we can hope to achieve from these data is to generate hypotheses based on associations between groups, or group associations. When we try to establish causation or etiology, we will need to go beyond group association and focus on associations at the individual level.

Finally, epidemiologists take a scientific approach to addressing public health problems. They are often skeptical of initial answers to a question and ask: Could there be another explanation for the differences or changes in the distribution of disease?

HOW DO EPIDEMIOLOGISTS INVESTIGATE WHETHER THERE IS ANOTHER EXPLANATION FOR THE DIFFERENCE OR CHANGES IN THE DISTRIBUTION OF DISEASE?

Epidemiologists ask: Are the differences or changes real or are they **artifactual**? There are three basic reasons that changes in rates may be artifactual rather than real:

- Differences or changes in the interest in identifying the disease

- Differences or changes in the ability to identify the disease
- Differences or changes in the definition of the disease

For some conditions, such as HIV/AIDS, these changes have all occurred. New and effective treatments have increased the interest in detecting the infection. Improved technology has increased the ability to detect HIV infections at an earlier point in time. In addition, there have been a number of modifications of the definition of AIDS based on new opportunistic infections and newly recognized complications. Therefore, with HIV/AIDS, we need to be especially attentive to the possibility that artifactual changes have occurred.

Thus in describing the distribution of a problem, epidemiologists ask: Are the differences or changes used to suggest group associations and generate hypotheses artifactual or real?

Let us see how this applies to our lung cancer example. As we have seen, lung cancer is a disease with a very poor prognosis; therefore, the burden of disease is high as measured by its high mortality rate. This was the situation in the past and to a large extent continues to be the situation.

Mortality rates have been obtained from death certificates for many years. The cause of death on death certificates is classified using a standardized coding system known as the International Classification of Diseases (ICD). No equally complete or accurate system has been available for collecting data on the incidence rates of lung cancer. However, as we learned in our discussion of rates, the incidence rates and mortality rates for lung cancer are very similar. Therefore, we can use mortality data as a substitute for incidence data when evaluating the overall burden of lung cancer in a population.

By the 1930s, epidemiologists had concluded from the study of death certificates that lung cancer deaths were rapidly increasing. This increase continued through the 1950s—with the increase in lung cancer occurring two decades or more after the increase in consumption of cigarettes. Therefore, it was not immediately obvious that the two were related. In order to hypothesize that cigarettes are a cause of lung cancer, one needed to conclude that there was a long delay and/or a need for long-term exposure to cigarettes before lung cancer developed. There was a need for more **evidence** linking cigarettes and lung cancer.

From the 1930s through the 1950s, a large number of studies established that lung cancer deaths were increasing among men, but not among women. That is, there was a change over time and a difference between groups. Epidemiologists, therefore, considered whether the changes or differences in rates were real, or whether they could be artificial or artifactual.

With lung cancer, the diagnosis at the time of death has been of great interest for many years. The ability to diagnose the disease has not changed substantially over the years. In addition, the use of ICD codes on death certificates has helped standardize the definition of the disease. Epidemiologists concluded that it was unlikely that changes in interest, ability, or definition explained the changes in the rates of lung cancer observed in males, thus they concluded that the changes were not artifactual, but real.[b]

Box 2-3 discusses age adjustment, which is one additional step that epidemiologists frequently make when looking at rates.

WHAT IS THE IMPLICATION OF A GROUP ASSOCIATION?

Group associations are established by investigations that use information on groups or a population without having information on the specific individuals within the group.

---

[b] There are actually several types of lung cancer defined by the ICD codes. Most, but not all, types of lung cancer are strongly associated with cigarette smoking.

BOX 2-3   Age Adjustment

Despite the existence of a real change in the rates of lung cancer between 1930 and 1960, it was still possible that the increased mortality rates from lung cancer were due to the increasing life span that was occurring between 1930 and 1960, leading to the aging of the population and an older population on average. Perhaps older people are more likely to develop lung cancer and the aging of the population itself explains the real increase in the rates. To address this issue, epidemiologists use what is called **age adjustment**. To conduct age adjustment, epidemiologists look at the rates of the disease in each age group and also the **age distribution**, or the number of people in each age group in the population. Then they combine the rates for each age group, taking into account or adjusting for the age distribution of a population.[a]

Taking into account the age distribution of the population in 1930 and 1960 did have a modest impact on the changes in the mortality rates from lung cancer, but large differences remained. As a result, epidemiologists concluded that lung cancer mortality rates changed over this period, especially among men; the changes in rates were real; and the changes could not be explained simply by the aging of the population. Thus, epidemiologists had established the existence of a group association between groups that smoked more cigarettes and groups that developed lung cancer.

---

[a] Adjustment for age is often performed by combining the rates in each age group using the age distribution of what is called a **standard population**. The age distribution of the U.S. population in 2000 is currently used as the standard population. Adjustment is not limited to age and may at times be conducted using other characteristics that may differ among the groups, such as gender or race, which may affect the probability of developing a disease.

These studies have been called **population comparisons** or **ecological studies**. Having established the existence of a group association, we still do not know if the individuals who smoke cigarettes are the same ones who develop lung cancer. We can think of a group association as a hypothesis that requires investigation at the individual level. The group association between cigarettes and lung cancer was the beginning of a long road to establish that cigarettes are a cause of lung cancer.

Not all group associations are also individual associations. Imagine the following situation: the mortality rates from drowning are higher in southern states than in northern states. The per capita consumption of ice cream is also higher in southern states than in northern states. Thus, a group association was established between ice cream consumption and drowning. In thinking about this relationship, you will soon realize that there is another difference between southern and northern states. The average temperature is higher in southern states, and higher temperatures are most likely associated with more swimming and also more ice cream consumption. Ice cream consumption is therefore related both to swimming and to drowning. We call this type of factor a **confounding variable**. In this situation, there is no evidence that those who drown actually consumed ice cream. That is, there is no evidence of an association at the individual level. Thus, group associations can be misleading if they suggest relationships that do not exist at the individual level.

Epidemiology research studies that look at associations at the individual level are key to establishing etiology, or cause. Etiology is the second component of the P.E.R.I.E. approach. Let us turn our attention to how to establish etiology.

ETIOLOGY: HOW DO WE ESTABLISH CONTRIBUTORY CAUSE?

Understanding the reasons for disease is fundamental to the prevention of disability and death. We call these reasons etiology or causation. In evidence-based public health, we use a very specific definition of causation—**contributory cause**. The evidence-based public health approach relies on epidemiological research studies to establish a contributory cause. This requires that we go beyond group association and establish three definitive requirements.[7]

1. The "cause" is associated with the "effect" at the individual level. That is, the potential "cause" and the potential "effect" occur more frequently in the same individual than would be expected by chance. Therefore, we need to establish that individuals with lung cancer are more frequently smokers than individuals without lung cancer.
2. The "cause" precedes the "effect" in time. That is, the potential "cause" is present at an earlier time than the potential "effect." Therefore, we need to establish that cigarette smoking comes before the development of lung cancer.
3. Altering the "cause" alters the "effect." That is, when the potential "cause" is reduced or eliminated, the potential "effect" is also reduced or eliminated. Therefore, we need to establish that reducing cigarette smoking reduces lung cancer rates.

Box 2-4 illustrates the logic behind using these three criteria to establish a cause-and-effect relationship, as well as what the implications of a contributory cause are.

These three definitive requirements are ideally established using three different types of studies, all of which relate potential "causes" to potential "effects" at the individual level. That is, they investigate whether individuals who smoke cigarettes are the same individuals who develop lung cancer.[6] The three basic types of investigations are called **case-control** or

BOX 2-4 Lightning, Thunder, and Contributory Cause

The requirements for establishing the type of cause-and-effect relationship known as contributory cause used in evidence-based public health can be illustrated by the cause-and-effect relationship between lightning and thunder that human beings have recognized from the earliest times of civilization.

First, lightning is generally associated with thunder; that is, the two occur together far more often than one would expect if there were no relationship. Second, with careful observation, it can be concluded that the lightning is seen a short time before the thunder is heard. That is, the potential "cause" (the lightning) precedes in time the "effect" (the thunder). Finally, when the lightning stops, so does the thunder—thus, altering the "cause" alters the "effect."

Notice that lightning is not always associated with thunder. Heat lightning may not produce audible thunder, or the lightning may be too far away for the thunder to be heard. Lightning is not sufficient in and of itself to guarantee that our ears will subsequently always hear thunder. Conversely, in recent years, it has been found that the sound of thunder does not always require lightning. Other reasons for the rapid expansion of air, such as an explosion or volcanic eruption, can also create a sound similar or identical to thunder.

The recognition of lightning as a cause of thunder came many centuries before human beings had any understanding of electricity or today's appreciation for the science of light and sounds. Similarly, cause-and-effect relationships established by epidemiological investigations do not always depend on understanding the science behind the relationships.

retrospective studies, **cohort studies** or **prospective studies**, and **randomized controlled trials** or **experimental studies**.

Case-control studies are most useful for establishing requirement number one, that is, the "cause" is associated with the "effect" at the individual level. Case-control studies can demonstrate that cigarettes and lung cancer occur together more frequently than would be expected by chance alone. To accomplish this, cases with the disease (lung cancer) are compared to controls without the disease to determine whether the cases and the controls previously were exposed to the potential "cause" (cigarette smoking).

When a factor such as cigarettes has been demonstrated to be associated on an individual basis with an outcome such as lung cancer, we often refer to that factor as a **risk factor**.[c]

During the 1940s and early 1950s, a number of case-control studies established that individuals who developed lung cancer were far more likely to be regular smokers compared to similar individuals who did not smoke cigarettes. These case-control studies established requirement number one—the "cause" is associated with the "effect" at the individual level. They established that cigarettes are a risk factor for lung cancer.

Cohort studies are most useful for establishing requirement number two—the "cause" precedes the "effect." Those with the potential "cause" or risk factor (cigarette smoking) and those without the potential "cause" are followed over time to determine who develops the "effect" (lung cancer).[d]

Several large scale cohort studies were conducted in the late 1950s and early 1960s. One conducted by the American Cancer Society followed nearly 200,000 individuals over 3 or more years to determine the chances that smokers and nonsmokers would develop lung cancer. Those who smoked regularly at the beginning of the study had a greatly increased chance of developing lung cancer over the course of the study, thus establishing requirement number two, the "cause" precedes the "effect" in time.

Randomized controlled trials are most useful for establishing requirement number three—altering the "cause" alters the "effect." Using a chance process known as **randomization** or **random assignment**, individuals are assigned to be exposed or not exposed to the potential "cause" (cigarette smoking). Individuals with and without the potential "cause" are then followed over time to determine who develops the "effect." Conducting a randomized controlled trial of cigarettes and lung cancer would require investigators to randomize individuals to smoke cigarettes or not smoke cigarettes and follow them over many years. This illustrates the obstacles that can occur in seeking to definitively establish contributory cause. Once there was a strong suspicion that cigarettes might cause lung cancer, randomized controlled trials were not practical or ethical as a method for establishing cigarette smoking as a contributory cause of lung cancer. Therefore, we need to look at additional **supportive** or **ancillary criteria** that we can use to help us establish the existence of contributory cause.[e]

Figure 2-2 illustrates the requirements for definitively establishing contributory cause and the types of studies that may be used to satisfy each of the requirements. Notice that the requirements for establishing contributory cause are the same as the requirements for establishing **efficacy**. Efficacy implies that an intervention works, that is, it increases positive outcomes or benefits in the population being investigated.

WHAT CAN WE DO IF WE CANNOT DEMONSTRATE ALL THREE REQUIREMENTS TO DEFINITIVELY ESTABLISH CONTRIBUTORY CAUSE?

When we cannot definitively establish a contributory cause, we often need to look for additional supportive evidence.[7] In evidence-based public health, we often utilize what have been called supportive or ancillary criteria to make scientific judgments about cause and effect. A large number of these

---

[c] A risk factor, as we just discussed, usually implies that the factor is associated with the disease at the individual level. At times, it may be used to imply that the factor not only is associated with the disease at the individual level, but that it precedes the disease in time. Despite the multiple uses of the term, a risk factor does not in and of itself imply that a cause-and-effect relationship is present, though it may be considered a possible cause.

[d] It may seem obvious that cigarette smoking precedes the development of lung cancer. However, the sequence of events is not always so clear. For instance, those who have recently quit smoking cigarettes have an increased chance of being diagnosed with lung cancer. This may lead to the erroneous conclusion that stopping cigarette smoking is a cause of lung cancer. It is more likely that early symptoms of lung cancer lead individuals to quit smoking. The conclusion that stopping cigarette smoking causes lung cancer is called **reverse causality**. Thus, it was important that cohort studies followed smokers and nonsmokers for several years to establish that the cigarette smoking came first.

[e] At times, a special form of a cohort study called a **natural experiment** can help establish that altering the cause alters the effect. A natural experiment implies that an investigator studies the results of a change in one group, but not in another similar group that was produced by forces outside the investigator's control. For instance, after the surgeon general's 1964 *Report on Smoking and Health* was released, approximately 100,000 physicians stopped smoking. This did not happen among other professionals. Over the next decade, the rates of lung cancer among physicians dropped dramatically, but not among other professionals. Despite the fact that natural experiments can be very useful, they are not considered as reliable as randomized controlled trials. Randomization, especially in large studies, eliminates differences between groups or potential confounding differences, even when these differences in characteristics are not recognized by the investigators.

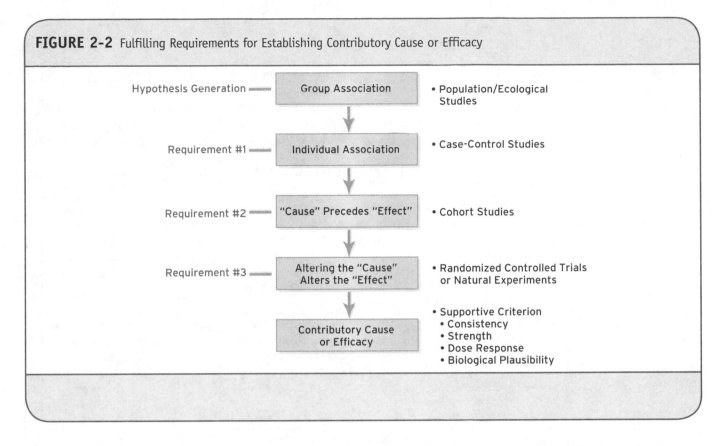

FIGURE 2-2 Fulfilling Requirements for Establishing Contributory Cause or Efficacy

criteria have been used and debated. However, four of them are widely used and pose little controversy. They are:

- Strength of the relationship
- Dose-response relationship
- Consistency of the relationship
- Biological plausibility

Let us examine what we mean by each of these criteria.

The **strength of the relationship** implies that we are interested in knowing how closely related the risk factor (cigarette smoking) is to the disease (lung cancer). In other words, we want to know the probability of lung cancer among those who smoke cigarettes compared to the probability of lung cancer among those who do not smoke cigarettes. To measure the strength of the relationship, we calculate what we call the **relative risk**. The relative risk is the probability of developing the disease if the risk factor is present compared to the probability of developing the disease if the risk factor is not present. Therefore, the relative risk for cigarette smoking is calculated as:

$$Relative\ risk = \frac{probability\ of\ lung\ cancer\ for\ cigarette\ smokers}{probability\ of\ lung\ cancer\ for\ nonsmokers}$$

The relative risk for cigarette smoking and lung cancer is approximately 10. A relative risk of 10 is very large. It tells us that the chances or probability of developing lung cancer are 10 times as great for the average smoker compared to the average nonsmoker.[f]

In addition to looking at the strength of the overall relationship between smoking cigarettes and lung cancer, we can ask whether smoking more cigarettes is associated with a greater chance of developing lung cancer. If it is, then we say there is a **dose-response relationship**. For instance, smoking one pack of cigarettes per day over many years increases the chances of developing lung cancer compared to smoking half a pack per day. Similarly, smoking two packs per day increases the chances of developing the disease compared to smoking one pack per day.

---

[f] A relative risk of 10 does not tell us the **absolute risk**. The absolute risk is the actual chance or probability of developing the disease (lung cancer) in the presence of the risk factor (cigarette smoking), expressed numerically— for example, as 0.03 or 3%. A relative risk of 10 might imply an increase from 1 in 1,000 individuals to 1 in 100 individuals. Alternatively, it might imply an increase from 1 in 100 individuals to 1 in 10 individuals. A relative risk can be calculated whenever we have follow-up data on groups of individuals; therefore, it does not in and of itself imply that a contributory cause is present. We need to be careful not to imply that the risk factor will increase the chances of developing the disease or that reducing or eliminating the risk factor will reduce or eliminate the disease unless we have evidence of contributory cause. For case-control studies, a measure known as the **odds ratio** can be calculated and is often used as an approximation of relative risk.

TABLE 2-1 Supportive or Ancillary Criteria—Cigarettes and Lung Cancer

Criteria	Meaning of the criteria	Evidence for cigarettes and lung cancer	Cautions in using criteria
Strength of the relationship	The risk for those with the risk factor is greatly increased compared to those without the risk factor.	The relative risk is large or substantial. The relative risk is greater than 10 for the average smoker, implying that the average smoker has more than 10 times the probability of developing lung cancer compared to nonsmokers.	Even relatively modest relative risks may make important contributions to disease when the risk factor is frequently present. A relative risk of 2, for instance, implies a doubling of the probability of developing a disease.
Dose-response relationship	Higher levels of exposure and/or longer duration of exposure to the "cause" is associated with increased probability of the "effect."	Studies of cigarettes and lung cancer establish that smoking half a pack a day over an extended period of time increases the risk compared to not smoking. Smoking one pack per day and two packs per day further increase the risk.	No dose-response relationship may be evident between no smoking and smoking one cigarette a day or between smoking three and four packs per day.
Consistency of the relationship	Studies at the individual level produce similar results in multiple locations among populations of varying socioeconomic and cultural backgrounds.	Hundreds of studies in multiple locations and populations consistently establish an individual association between cigarettes and lung cancer.	Consistency requires the availability of numerous studies that may not have been conducted.
Biological plausibility	Known biological mechanisms can convincingly explain a cause-and-effect relationship.	Cigarette smoke directly reaches the areas where lung cancer appears.	Exactly which component(s) of cigarette smoking produce lung cancer are just beginning to be understood.

These examples show that a dose-response relationship is present.[g]

Consistency implies that studies in different geographic areas and among a wide range of groups produce similar results. A very large number of studies of cigarettes and lung cancer in many countries and among those of nearly every race and socioeconomic group have consistently demonstrated a strong individual association between cigarette smoking and lung cancer.

The final supportive criterion is **biological plausibility**. This term implies that we can explain the occurrence of disease based upon known and accepted biological mechanisms. We can explain the occurrence of lung cancer by the

fact that cigarette smoke contains a wide range of potentially toxic chemicals that reach the locations in the body where lung cancer occurs.

Thus, the ancillary criteria add support to the argument that cigarette smoking is a contributory cause of lung cancer. **Table 2-1** summarizes the use of ancillary or supportive criteria in making scientific judgments about contributory cause and illustrates these principles using the cigarette smoking and lung cancer scenario. It also cautions us to use these criteria carefully because a cause-and-effect relationship may be present even when some or all of these criteria are not fulfilled.[7]

We have now summarized the approach used in evidence-based public health to establish a contributory cause. We started with the development of group associations that generate hypotheses and moved on to look at the definitive requirements for establishing contributory cause. We also looked at the ancillary or supportive criteria that are often

---

[g] A dose-response relationship may also imply that greater exposure to a factor is associated with reduced probability of developing the disease, such as with exercise and coronary artery disease. In this case, the factor may be called a **protective factor** rather than a risk factor.

TABLE 2-2 Cigarettes and Lung Cancer—Establishing Cause and Effect

Requirements for contributory cause	Meaning of the requirements	Types of studies that can establish the requirement	Evidence for cigarette smoking and lung cancer
Associated at a population level (group association)	A group relationship between a "cause" and an "effect".	Ecological study or population comparison study: a comparison of population rates between an exposure and a disease.	Men began mass consumption of cigarettes decades before women and their rates of lung cancer increased decades before those of women.
Individual association: "requirement one"	Individuals with a disease ("effect") also have an increased chance of having a potential risk factor ("cause").	Case-control studies: cases with the disease are compared to similar controls without the disease to see who had the exposure.	Lung cancer patients were found to have 10 times or greater chance of smoking cigarettes regularly compared to those without lung cancer.
Prior association: "requirement two"	The potential risk factor precedes—in time—the outcome.	Cohort studies: exposed and similar nonexposed individuals are followed over time to determine who develops the disease.	Large cohort studies found that those who smoke cigarettes regularly have a 10 times or greater chance of subsequently developing lung cancer.
Altering the "cause" alters the "effect": "requirement three"	Active intervention to expose one group to the risk factor results in a greater chance of the outcome.	Randomized controlled trials allocating individuals by chance to be exposed or not exposed are needed to definitively establish contributory cause. Note: these studies are not always ethical or practical.	Alternatives to randomized controlled trials, such as "natural experiments," established that those who quit smoking have greatly reduced chances of developing lung cancer. In addition, the four supportive criteria also suggest contributory cause.

needed to make scientific judgments about contributory cause. **Table 2-2** summarizes this process and applies it to cigarette smoking and lung cancer.

WHAT DOES CONTRIBUTORY CAUSE IMPLY?

Establishing a contributory cause on the basis of evidence is a complicated and often time-consuming job. In practice, our minds often too quickly jump to the conclusion that a cause-and-effect relationship exists. Our language has a large number of words that may subtly imply a cause-and-effect relationship, even in the absence of evidence. **Box 2-5** illustrates how we often rapidly draw conclusions about cause and effect.

It is important to understand what the existence of a contributory cause implies and what it does not imply. Despite the convincing evidence that cigarette smoking is a contributory cause of lung cancer, some individuals never smoke and still develop lung cancer. Therefore, cigarettes are not what we call a **necessary cause** of lung cancer. Others smoke cigarettes all their lives and do not develop lung

cancer. Thus, cigarettes are not what we call a **sufficient cause** of lung cancer.

The fact that not every smoker develops lung cancer implies that there must be factors that protect some individuals from lung cancer. The fact that some nonsmokers develop lung cancer implies that there must be additional contributory causes of lung cancer. Thus, the existence of a contributory cause implies that the "cause" increases the chances that the "effect" will develop. Its presence does not guarantee that the disease will develop. In addition, the absence of cigarette smoking does not guarantee that the disease will not develop.

Despite the fact that cigarettes have been established as a contributory cause of lung cancer, they are not a necessary or a sufficient cause of lung cancer. In fact, the use of the concept of necessary and sufficient cause is not considered useful in the evidence-based public health approach because so few, if any, diseases fulfill the definitions of necessary and sufficient cause. These criteria are too demanding to be used as standards of proof in public health or medicine.

BOX 2-5   Words that Imply Causation

Often when reading the newspaper or other media, you will find that conclusions about cause and effect are made based upon far less rigorous examination of the data than we have indicated are needed to definitively establish cause and effect. In fact, we often draw conclusions about cause and effect without even consciously recognizing we have done so. Our language has a large number of words that imply a cause-and-effect relationship, some of which we use rather casually.

Let us take a look at the many ways that a hypothetical newspaper article might imply the existence of a cause-and-effect relationship or a contributory cause even when the evidence is based only upon a group association or upon speculation about the possible relationships.

> Over several decades, the mortality rates from breast cancer in the United States were observed to increase each year. This trend was due to and can be blamed on a variety of factors, including the increased use of estrogens and exposure to estrogens in food. The recent reduction in breast cancer resulted from and can be attributed to the declining use of estrogens for menopausal and postmenopausal women. The declining mortality rate was also produced by the increased use of screening tests for breast cancer that were responsible for early detection and treatment. These trends demonstrate that reduced use of estrogens and increased use of screening tests have contributed to and explain the reduction in breast cancer.

While these conclusions sound reasonable and may well be cause-and-effect relationships, note that they rely heavily on assertions for which there is no direct evidence provided. For instance, the following words are often used to imply a cause-and-effect relationship when evidence is not or cannot be presented to support the relationship:

- due to
- blamed on
- result from
- attributable to
- produced by
- responsible for
- contributed to
- explained by

It is important to be aware of conscious or unconscious efforts to imply cause-and-effect relationships when the data suggests only group associations and does not meet our more stringent criteria establishing cause and effect.

By 1964, the evidence that cigarette smoking was a contributory cause of lung cancer was persuasive enough for the surgeon general of the United States to produce the first surgeon general's *Report on Smoking and Health*. The report concluded that cigarettes are an important cause of lung cancer. Over the following decades, the surgeon general's reports documented the evidence that cigarette smoking causes not only lung cancer, but also other cancers—including cancer of the throat and larynx. Cigarette smoking is also a contributory cause of chronic obstructive pulmonary disease (COPD) and coronary artery disease. Smoking during pregnancy poses risks to the unborn child, and passive or secondhand smoke creates increased risks to those exposed—especially children.[8] Based on the surgeon general's findings, there is clearly overwhelming evidence that cigarette smoking is a contributory cause of lung cancer and a growing list of other diseases. Thus, let us turn our attention to the third component of the P.E.R.I.E. process: recommendations.

RECOMMENDATIONS: WHAT WORKS TO REDUCE THE HEALTH IMPACT?

The evidence for cigarette smoking as a cause of lung cancer, as well as other diseases, was so strong that it cried out for action. In evidence-based public health, however, action should be grounded in **recommendations** that incorporate evidence. That is, evidence serves not only to establish contributory cause, but is also central to determining whether or not specific interventions work.[9, 10] Evidence-based recommendations are built upon the evidence from studies of interventions. Thus, recommendations are summaries of the evidence about which interventions work to reduce the health impacts, and they indicate whether actions should be taken. Evidence-based recommendations utilize the same types of investigations we discussed for contributory cause. In fact, the requirements of contributory cause are the same as those for establishing that an intervention works or has efficacy on the particular population that was studied. Evidence-based recommendations, however, go beyond efficacy or benefits and take into account harms or safety.

In the decades since the surgeon general's initial report, a long list of interventions has been implemented and evaluated. The term "intervention" is a very broad term in public health. Interventions range from individual counseling and prescription of pharmaceutical drugs that aid smoking cessation; to group efforts, such as peer support groups; to social interventions, such as cigarette taxes and a legal restriction on smoking in restaurants.

Recommendations for action have been part of public health and medicine for many years. Evidence-based recommendations, however, are relatively new. They have been contrasted with the traditional eminence-based recommendation, which uses the opinion of a respected authority as its foundation. Evidence-based recommendations ask about the research evidence supporting the benefits and harms of potential interventions. In evidence-based recommendations, the opinions of experts are most important when research evidence does not or cannot provide answers.

Before looking at the evidence-based recommendations on cigarette smoking made by the Centers for Disease Control and Prevention (CDC), let us look at how they are often made and can be graded. Evidence-based recommendations are based upon two types of criteria: the quality of the evidence and the magnitude of the impact. Each of these criteria is given what is called a **score**.[9, 10] The quality of the evidence is scored based in large part upon the types of investigations and how well the investigation was conducted. Well-conducted randomized controlled trials that fully address the health problem are considered the highest quality evidence. Often, however, cohort and case-control studies are needed and are used as part of an evidence-based recommendation.

Expert opinion, though lowest on the hierarchy of evidence, is often essential to fill in the holes in the research evidence.[9, 10] The quality of the evidence also determines whether the data collected during an intervention are relevant to its use in a particular population or setting. Data from young adults may not be relevant to children or the elderly. Data from severely ill patients may not be relevant to mildly ill patients. Thus, high-quality evidence needs to be based not only on the research, which can establish efficacy in one particular population, but also on the **effectiveness** of the intervention in the specific population in which it will be used.

In evidence-based public health, the quality of the evidence is often scored as good, fair, or poor. Good quality implies that the evidence fulfills all the criteria for quality. Poor quality evidence implies that there are fatal flaws in the

evidence and recommendations cannot be made. Fair quality lies in between having no fatal flaws and fulfilling all the criteria for quality.[h]

In addition to looking at the quality of the evidence, it is also important to look at the magnitude of the impact of the intervention. The magnitude of the impact asks the question: How much of the disability and/or death due to the disease can be potentially removed by the intervention? In measuring the magnitude of the impact, evidence-based recommendations take into account the potential benefits of an intervention, as well as the potential harms. Therefore, we can regard the magnitude of the impact as the benefits minus the harms, or the "net benefits."[i]

The magnitude of the impact, like the quality of the evidence, is scored based upon a limited number of potential categories. In one commonly used system, the magnitude of the impact is scored as substantial, moderate, small, and zero/negative.[9] A substantial impact may imply that the intervention works extremely well for a small number of people, such as a drug treatment for cigarette cessation. These are the types of interventions that are often the focus of individual clinical care. A substantial impact may also imply that the intervention has a modest net benefit for any one individual, but can be applied to large numbers of people, such as in the form of media advertising or taxes on cigarettes. These are the types of interventions that are most often the focus of traditional public health and social policy.

Evidence-based recommendations combine the score for the quality of the evidence with the score for the impact of the intervention.[9] **Table 2-3** summarizes how these aspects can be combined to produce a classification of the strength of the recommendation, graded as A, B, C, D, and I.

It may be useful to think of these grades as indicating the following:

A = Must—A strong recommendation.

---

[h] To fulfill the criteria for good quality data, evidence is also needed to show that the outcome being measured is a clinically important outcome. Short-term outcomes called **surrogate outcomes**, such as changes in laboratory tests, may not reliably indicate longer term or clinically important outcomes.
[i] The magnitude of the impact can be measured using the relative risk calculation. When dealing with interventions, the people who receive the intervention are often placed in the numerator. Thus, an intervention that reduces the bad outcomes by half would have a relative risk of 0.5. The smaller the relative risk is, the greater the measured impact of the intervention. If the relative risk is 0.20, then those with the intervention have only 20% of the risk remaining. Their risk of a bad outcome has been reduced by 80%. The reduction in a bad outcome is called the **attributable risk percentage** or the **percent efficacy**. The intervention can only be expected to accomplish this potential reduction in risk when a contributory cause is present and the impact of the "cause" can be immediately and completely eliminated.

TABLE 2-3 Classification of Recommendations

Quality of the evidence	Magnitude of the impact			
	Net benefit: substantial	Net benefit: moderate	Net benefit: small	Net benefit: zero/negative
Good	A	B	C	D
Fair	B	B	C	D
Poor (insufficient evidence)	I	I	I	I

Data from Agency for Healthcare Research and Quality, U.S. Preventive Services Task Force Guide to Clinical Preventive Services Vol 1, AHRQ Pub. No. 02-500.

B = Should—In general, the intervention should be used unless there are good reasons or contraindications for not doing so.

C = May—The use of judgment is often needed on an individual-by-individual basis. Individual recommendations depend on the specifics of an individual's situation, risk-taking attitudes, and values.

D = Don't—There is enough evidence to recommend against using the intervention.

I = Indeterminant, insufficient, or "I don't know"—The evidence is inadequate to make a recommendation for or against the use of the intervention at the present time.

Notice that evidence-based public health and medicine rely primarily on considerations of benefits and harms. However, recently issues of financial cost have begun to be integrated into evidence-based recommendations. At this point, however, cost considerations are generally only taken into account for "close calls." Close calls are often situations where the net benefits are small to moderate and the costs are large.

The evidence-based public health approach increasingly relies on the use of evidence-based recommendations that are graded based on the quality of the evidence and the expected impact of the intervention. The recommendations are made by a wide array of organizations, as discussed in **Box 2-6**. It is important to appreciate the source of the recommendations, as well as the methods used to develop them.[7]

Let us take a look at some examples of how interventions to prevent smoking, detect lung cancer early, or cure lung cancer have been graded. The CDC publishes "The Guide to Community Prevention Services," commonly referred to as "The Community Guide."[10] This guide indicates that the following interventions are recommended, implying a grade of A or B:

- Clean indoor air legislation, prohibiting tobacco use in indoor public and private workplaces
- Federal, state, and local efforts to increase taxes on tobacco products as an effective public health intervention to promote tobacco use cessation and to reduce the initiation of tobacco use among youths
- The funding and implementation of long-term, high-intensity mass media campaigns using paid broadcast times and media messages developed through formative research
- Proactive telephone cessation support services (quit lines)
- Reduced or eliminated copayments for effective cessation therapies
- Reminder systems for healthcare providers (encouraging them to reinforce the importance of cigarette cessation)
- Efforts to mobilize communities to identify and reduce the commercial availability of tobacco products to youths

Additional recommendations encourage clinicians to specifically counsel patients against smoking, prescribe medications for adults, encourage support groups for smoking cessation, and treat lung cancer with the best available treatments when detected.

Of interest is the grade of D for recommending against screening for early detection of lung cancer using traditional chest X rays. The evidence strongly suggests that screening

BOX 2-6   Who Develops Evidence-Based Recommendations?

Evidence-based recommendations may be developed by a range of groups, including the government, practitioner-oriented organizations, consumer-oriented organizations, organized healthcare systems, and even for-profit organizations. Organizations developing evidence-based recommendations, however, are expected to acknowledge their authorship and identify the individuals who participated in the process, as well as their potential conflicts of interest. In addition, regardless of the organization, the evidence-based recommendations should include a description of the process used to collect the data and make the recommendations.

For-profit organizations may make evidence-based recommendations. However, their obvious conflicts of interest often lead them to fund other groups to make recommendations. Thus, the funding source(s) supporting the development of evidence-based recommendations should also be acknowledged as part of the report.

One well-regarded model for the development of evidence-based recommendations is the task force model used by the United States Preventive Services Task Force of the Agency for Healthcare Research and Quality (AHRQ), as well as by the Task Force on Community Preventive Services of the Centers for Disease Control and Prevention (CDC).[9, 10] The task force model aims to balance potential conflicts of interest and ensures a range of expertise by selecting a variety of experts, as well as community participants, based upon a public nomination process. Once the task force members are appointed, their recommendations are made by a vote of the task force and do not require approval by the government agency.

Thus, as a reader of evidence-based recommendations, it is important that you begin by looking at which group developed the recommendations, whether they have disclosed their membership, including potential conflicts of interest, and the groups' procedures for developing the recommendations.

---

using this method may detect cancer at a slightly earlier stage, but not early enough to alter the course of the disease. Therefore, early detection does not alter the outcome of the disease. Research continues to find better screening methods to detect lung cancer in time to make a difference.

Evidence-based recommendations are not the end of the process. There may be a large number of recommendations among which we may need to choose. In addition, we need to decide the best way(s) to put the recommendations into practice. Thus, implementation is not an automatic process. Issues of ethics, culture, politics, and risk-taking attitudes can and should have major impacts on implementation. A fourth step in the evidence-based public health approach requires us to look at the options for implementation and to develop a strategy for getting the job done.

IMPLEMENTATION: HOW DO WE GET THE JOB DONE?

Strong recommendations based upon the evidence are ideally the basis of implementation. At times, however, it may not be practical or ethical to obtain the evidence needed to establish contributory cause and develop evidence-based recommendations. Naturally occurring implementation itself

may be part of the process of establishing causation, as it was for cigarette smoking in the 1960s when 100,000 physicians stopped smoking and their rates of lung cancer declined rapidly, as compared to other similar professionals who did not stop smoking.

Today, there are often a large number of interventions with adequate data to consider implementation. Many of the interventions have potential harms, as well as potential benefits. The large and growing array of possible interventions means that health decisions require a systematic method for deciding which interventions to use and how to combine them in the most effective and efficient ways. One method for examining the options for implementation uses a structure we will call the "When-Who-How" approach.

"When" asks about the timing in the course of disease in which an intervention occurs. This timing allows us to categorize interventions as **primary**, **secondary**, and **tertiary**. Primary interventions take place before the onset of the disease. They aim to prevent the disease from occurring. Secondary interventions occur after the development of a disease or risk factor, but before symptoms appear. They are aimed at early detection of disease or reducing risk factors while the patient is asymptomatic. Tertiary interventions occur after the initial occurrence of symptoms, but before irreversible disability. They aim to prevent irreversible consequences of the disease. In the cigarette smoking and lung cancer scenario, primary interventions aim to prevent cigarette smoking. Secondary interventions aim to reverse the course of disease by smoking cessation efforts or screening to detect early disease. Tertiary interventions diagnose and treat diseases caused by smoking in order to prevent permanent disability and death.

"Who" asks: At whom should we direct the intervention? Should it be directed at individuals one at a time as part of clinical care? Alternatively, should it be directed at groups of people, such as vulnerable populations, or should it be directed at everyone in a community or population?[j]

Finally, we need to ask: How should we implement interventions? There are three basic types of interventions when addressing the need for behavioral change. These interventions can be classified as information (education), motivation (incentives), and obligation (requirements).[k]

An information or education strategy aims to change behavior through individual encounters, group interactions, or the mass media. Motivation implies use of incentives for changing or maintaining behavior. It implies more than strong or enthusiastic encouragement—it implies tangible reward. Obligation relies on laws and regulations requiring specific behaviors. **Table 2-4** illustrates how options for implementation for cigarette smoking might be organized using the "When-Who-How" approach. To better understand the "who" and "how" of the options for intervention when behavior change is needed, refer to **Table 2-5**, which outlines nine different options.

Deciding when, who, and how to intervene depends in large part upon the available options and the evidence that

they work. It also depends in part on our attitudes toward different types of interventions. In U.S. society, we prefer to rely on informational or educational strategies. These approaches preserve freedom of choice, which we value in public, as well as private, decisions. Use of mass media informational strategies may be quite economical and efficient relative to the large number of individuals they reach though messages, but they often need to be tailored to different audiences. However, information is often ineffective in accomplishing behavioral change—at least on its own.

Strategies based upon motivation, such as taxation and other incentives, may at times be more effective than information alone, though educational strategies are still critical to justify and reinforce motivational interventions. Motivational interventions should be carefully constructed and judiciously used, or they may result in what has been called **victim blaming**. For example, victim blaming in the case of cigarette smoking implies that we regard the consequences of smoking as the smokers' own fault.

The use of obligation or legally required action can be quite effective if clear-cut behavior and relatively simple enforcement, such as restrictions on indoor public smoking, are used. These types of efforts may be regarded by some as a last resort, but others may see them as a key to effective use of other strategies. Obligation inevitably removes freedom of choice and if not effectively implemented with regard for individual rights, the strategy may undermine respect for the law. Enforcement may become invasive and expensive, thus obligation requires careful consideration before use as a strategy.

Understanding the advantages and disadvantages of each type of approach is key to deciphering many of the controversies we face in deciding how to implement programs to address public health problems; however, implementation is not the end of the evidence-based public health process.

EVALUATION: HOW DO WE EVALUATE RESULTS?

Public health problems are rarely completely eliminated with one intervention—there are few magic bullets in this field. Therefore, it is important to evaluate whether an intervention or combination of interventions has been successful in reducing the problem. It is also critical to measure how much of the problem has been eliminated by the intervention(s) and what is the nature of the problem that remains.

Traditionally, evaluation has asked before and after questions. For instance, studies of cigarette smoking between the mid-1960s, when cigarettes were first declared a cause of lung cancer, and the late 1990s demonstrated that there was nearly a 50% reduction in cigarette smoking in the United

---

[j] The CDC defines four levels of intervention: the individual, the relationship (for example, the family), the community, and society or the population as a whole. This framework has the advantage of separating immediate family interventions from community interventions. The group or at-risk group relationship used here may at times refer to the family unit or geographic communities. It may also refer to institutions or at-risk vulnerable groups within the community. The use of group or at-risk group relationship provides greater flexibility, allowing application to a wider range of situations. In addition, the three levels used here correlate with the measurements of relative risk, attributable risk percentage, and population attributable percentage, which are the fundamental epidemiological measurements applied to the magnitude of the impact of an intervention.

[k] An additional option is innovation. Innovation implies a technical or engineering solution. The development of a safer cigarette might be an innovation. A distinct advantage of technical or engineering solutions is that they often require far less behavior change. Changing human behavior is frequently difficult. Nonetheless, it is an essential component of most, if not all, successful public health interventions. Certainly, that is the case with cigarette smoking.

TABLE 2-4 Framework of Options for Implementation

	When	Who	How
Levels	1) Primary—Prior to disease or condition 2) Secondary—Prior to symptoms 3) Tertiary—Prior to irreversible complications	1) Individual 2) At-risk group 3) General population/community	1) Information (education) 2) Motivation (incentives) 3) Obligation (requirement)
Meaning of levels	1) Primary—Remove underlying cause, increase resistance, or reduce exposure 2) Secondary—Postexposure intervention, identify and treat risk factors or screen for asymptomatic disease 3) Tertiary—Reverse the course of disease (cure), prevent complications, restore function	1) Individual often equals patient care 2) At-risk implies groups with common risk factors 3) General population includes defined populations with and without the risk factor	1) Information—Efforts to communicate information and change behavior on basis of information 2) Motivation—Rewards to encourage or discourage without legal requirement 3) Obligation—Required by law or institutional sanction
Cigarette smoking example	1) Primary—Prevention of smoking, reduction in secondhand exposure 2) Secondary—Assistance in quitting, screening for cancer if recommended 3) Tertiary—Health care to minimize disease impact	1) Individual smoker 2) At-risk—Groups at risk of smoking or disease caused by smoking, e.g., adolescents as well as current and ex-smokers 3) Population—Entire population, including those who never have or never will smoke	1) Information—Stop smoking campaigns, advertising, warning on package, clinician advice 2) Motivation—Taxes on cigarettes, increased cost of insurance 3) Obligation—Prohibition on sales to minors, exclusion from athletic eligibility, legal restrictions on indoor public smoking

States and that the rates of lung cancer were beginning to fall—at least among males. However, much of the problem still existed because the rates among adolescent males and females remained high and smoking among adults was preceded by smoking as adolescents nearly 90% of the time. Thus, an evaluation of the success of cigarette smoking interventions led to a new cycle of the process. It focused on how to address the issue of adolescent smoking and nicotine addiction among adults. Many of the interventions being used today grew out of this effort to cycle once again through the evidence-based public health process and look for a new understanding of the problem, its etiology, evidence-based recommendations, and options for implementation as illustrated in **Figure 2-3**.

In recent years, this process of evaluation has been extended to attempt to address how well specific interventions work and are accepted in practice. A new framework, called the **RE-AIM** framework, is increasingly being used to evaluate these factors.[12] RE-AIM is a mnemonic that stands for **r**each, **e**ffectiveness, **a**doption, **i**mplementation, and **m**aintenance. You can think of the "RE" factors as evaluating the potential of the intervention for those it is designed to include or reach as well as those it has the potential to reach in practice. It is important to recognize that interventions are often applied far beyond the groups for whom they have been designed or investigated. The "AIM" factors examine the acceptance of the intervention in clinical or public health practice in the short and long term. **Table 2-6** defines the meaning of each of these components and illustrates how a new intervention for cigarette cessation might be evaluated using the RE-AIM framework.

Deciding the best combination of approaches to address a public health problem remains an important part of the judgment needed for the practice of public health. In general, multiple approaches are often needed to effectively address a complex problem like cigarette smoking. Population and high-risk group approaches, often used by public health professionals, and individual approaches, often used as part of health care, should be seen as complementary. Often using both types of interventions is more effective than either

TABLE 2-5 Examples of "Who" and "How" Related to Cigarette Smoking

	Information	Motivation	Obligation
Individual	Clinician provides patient with information explaining reasons for changing behavior	Clinician encourages patient to change behavior in order to qualify for a service or gain a benefit, e.g., status or financial	Clinician denies patient a service unless patient changes behavior
	Example: Clinician distributes educational packet to a smoker and discusses his or her own smoking habit	Example: Clinician suggests that the financial savings from not buying cigarettes be used to buy a luxury item	Example: Clinician implements recommendation to refuse birth control pills to women over 35 who smoke cigarettes
High-risk group	Information is made available to all those who engage in a behavior	Those who engage in a behavior are required to pay a higher price	Those who engage in a behavior are barred from an activity or job
	Example: Warning labels on cigarette packages	Examples: Taxes on cigarettes	Example: Smokers banned from jobs that will expose them to fumes that may damage their lungs
Population	Information is made available to the entire population, including those who do not engage in the behavior	Incentives are provided for those not at risk to discourage the behavior in those at risk	An activity is required or prohibited for those at risk and also for those not at risk of the condition
	Example: Media information on the dangers of smoking	Example: Lower health care costs for everyone results from reduced percentage of smokers	Example: Cigarette sales banned for those under 18

FIGURE 2-3 Evidence-Based Public Health: The Complete P.E.R.I.E. Approach

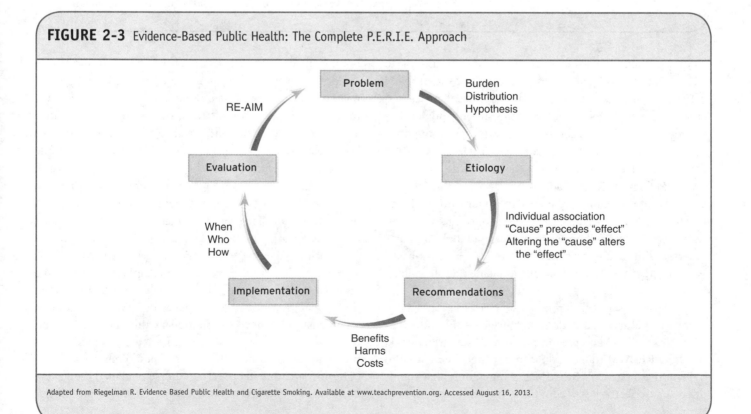

Adapted from Riegelman R. Evidence Based Public Health and Cigarette Smoking. Available at www.teachprevention.org. Accessed August 16, 2013.

TABLE 2-6 Evaluation: RE-AIM Framework

RE-AIM component	Meaning	Example
How well does the intervention work in practice?		
Reach	Asks: Who is the intervention being applied to in practice? May be groups or populations that are different than those on which it was investigated or intended for, i.e., the target population.	New prescription smoking cessation drug along with behavioral intervention approved by FDA and given evidence-based rating of A for long-standing adult smokers. Adverse events include rare depression and liver disease that is reversible with cessation of medication. In practice, being used for short-term smokers and teenagers who experience increased incidence of suicidal ideas.
Effectiveness	Asks: What is the impact in practice on the intended or target population, including beneficial outcomes as well as harm?	When used for long-term adult smokers, follow-up studies demonstrate substantial long-term quit rates similar to those observed in randomized controlled trials with no serious adverse events not identified in preapproval studies. Benefits far exceed harms when used on intended target population.
How well is the intervention accepted in practice?		
Adoption	Asks: How well is the intervention accepted by individuals and providers of services?	The drug is being widely used for long-term adult smokers. The drug is also being widely used for teenagers.
Implementation	Asks: How should the intervention be modified to reach target population and providers of services, but not those for whom the benefits do not exceed the harms?	A "black box" warning is placed on the prescribing information, warning clinicians of the potential suicide risk when used for teenagers.
Maintenance	Asks: How can we ensure long-term continuation of use and success of intervention among individuals and providers of services?	Long-term use of smoking cessation drug is needed and is encouraged by coverage by health insurance plans.

Data from Virginia Tech. RE-AIM. Available at http://www.re-aim.org. Accessed July 23, 2013.

approach alone. Social interventions, such as cigarette taxes and restrictions on public smoking, are also important interventions to consider.

Today, an enormous body of evidence exists on the relationship between tobacco and health. Understanding the nature of the problems, the etiology or cause-and-effect relationships, the evidence-based recommendations, and the approaches for implementing and evaluating the options for interventions remains key to the public health approach to smoking and health.[4] **Figure 2-3** diagrams the full P.E.R.I.E. approach. **Table 2-7** summarizes the questions to ask in the evidence-based public health approach.

The P.E.R.I.E. process summarizes the steps in evidence-based public health. It emphasizes the need to understand the nature of the problem and its underlying causes. It also helps structure the use of evidence to make recommendations and

decide on which options to put into practice. Finally, the circular nature of the P.E.R.I.E. process reminds us that the job of improving health goes on, often requiring multiple efforts to understand and address the problem.[11]

Now that we have an understanding of the basic approach of evidence-based public health, let us turn our attention to the fundamental tools at our disposal for addressing public health problems.

KEY WORDS

- **P.E.R.I.E. process**
- **Burden of disease**
- **Morbidity**
- **Mortality**
- **Course of a disease**
- **Rate**

TABLE 2-7 Questions to Ask—Evidence-Based Public Health Approach

1. Problem—What is the health problem?   • What is the burden of a disease or other health problem?   • What is the course of a disease or other health problem?   • Does the distribution of the health problem help generate hypotheses?
2. Etiology—What are the contributory causes?   • Has an association been established at the individual level?   • Does the "cause" precede the "effect"?   • Has altering the "cause" been shown to alter the "effect"? (If not, use ancillary criteria.)
3. Recommendations—What works to reduce the health impacts?   • What is the quality of the evidence for the intervention?   • What is the impact of the intervention in terms of benefits and harms?   • What grade should be given to indicate the strength of the recommendation?
4. Implementations—How can we get the job done?   • When should the implementation occur?   • At whom should the implementation be directed?   • How should the intervention(s) be implemented?
5. Evaluation—How well does the intervention work in practice?   • How well does the intervention work in practice on the intended or target population?   • How well does the intervention work in practice as actually used?   • How well is the intervention accepted in practice?

Adapted from Riegelman R. Evidence Based Public Health and Cigarette Smoking. Available at www.teachprevention.org. Accessed August 16, 2013.

- **At-risk population**
- **Incidence rate**
- **Prevalence rate**
- **True rate**
- **Etiology**
- **Case-fatality**
- **Proportion**
- **Distribution of disease**
- **Epidemiologists**
- **Associations**
- **Group associations or ecological associations**
- **Risk indicators (or risk markers)**
- **Artifactual**
- **Evidence**
- **Age adjustment**
- **Age distribution**
- **Standard population**
- **Population comparisons**
- **Ecological studies**

- **Confounding variable**
- **Contributory cause**
- **Case-control or retrospective studies**
- **Cohort or prospective studies**
- **Randomized controlled trials or experimental studies**
- **Risk factor**
- **Reverse causality**
- **Randomization or random assignment**
- **Ancillary or supportive criteria**
- **Natural experiment**
- **Efficacy**
- **Strength of the relationship**
- **Relative risk**
- **Absolute risk**
- **Dose-response relationship**
- **Odds ratio**
- **Consistency**
- **Protective factor**

- Biological plausibility
- Necessary cause
- Sufficient cause
- Recommendations
- Score
- Effectiveness

- Surrogate outcomes
- Attributable risk percentage (or the percent efficacy)
- Primary, secondary, and tertiary interventions
- Victim blaming
- RE-AIM

Discussion Questions

1. Use the P.E.R.I.E. framework and the list of questions to outline how each step in the P.E.R.I.E. process was accomplished for cigarette smoking.

2. How would you use the P.E.R.I.E. process to address the remaining problem of cigarette smoking in the United States?

REFERENCES

1. Cable News Network. A brief history of tobacco. http://www.cnn.com/US/9705/tobacco/history/#cigars.htm. Accessed July 16, 2013.

2. Johnson G. A long trail of evidence links cigarette smoking to lung cancer. ON SCIENCE column. http://www.txtwriter.com/Onscience/Articles/smokingcancer2.html. Accessed July 16, 2013.

3. Centers for Disease Control and Prevention. The public health approach to violence prevention. http://www.cdc.gov/violenceprevention/overview/publichealthapproach.html. Accessed July 16, 2013.

4. Riegelman RK. Evidence-based public health and cigarette smoking. http://www.teachprevention.org/browse.php?cid=23-52#. Accessed September 19, 2013.

5. Gordis L. *Epidemiology*. 4th ed. Philadelphia, PA: Elsevier Saunders; 2009.

6. Friis RH, Sellers TA. *Epidemiology for Public Health Practice*. 4th ed. Sudbury, MA: Jones and Bartlett Publishers; 2009.

7. Riegelman RK. *Studying a Study and Testing a Test: Reading Evidence-based Health Research*. 6th ed. Philadelphia, PA: Lippincott, Williams & Wilkins; 2013.

8. United States Department of Health and Human Services. Surgeon general's reports on smoking and tobacco use. http://www.cdc.gov/tobacco/data_statistics/sgr/index.htm. Accessed July 16, 2013.

9. Agency for Healthcare Research and Quality, U.S. Preventive Services Task Force Guide to Clinical Preventive Services. 2002;1 and 2. AHRQ Pub. No. 02-500.

10. Centers for Disease Control and Prevention. The guide to community preventive services. The community guide. http://www.thecommunityguide.org. Accessed July 16, 2013.

11. Centers for Disease Control and Prevention. The social-ecological model: a framework for prevention. http://www.cdc.gov/violenceprevention/overview/social-ecologicalmodel.html. Accessed July 16, 2013.

12. Virginia Tech. RE-AIM. http://www.re-aim.org. Accessed July 23, 2013.

© Elena Elisseeva/ShutterStock, Inc.

SECTION I

Cases and Discussion Questions

HIV/AIDS DETERMINANTS AND CONTROL OF THE EPIDEMIC

A report appeared in the CDC's "Morbidity and Mortality Weekly Report" (MMWR) on June 5, 1981, describing a previously unknown deadly disease in five young homosexual males, all in Los Angeles. The disease was characterized by dramatically reduced immunity, allowing otherwise innocuous organisms to become "opportunistic infections," rapidly producing fatal infections or cancer. Thus, acquired immune deficiency syndrome (AIDS) first became known to the public health and medical communities. It was soon traced to rectal intercourse, blood transfusions, and reuse of injection needles as methods of transmission. Reuse of needles was a common practice in poor nations. It was also widespread among intravenous drug abusers. Within several years, the disease was traced to a previously unknown retrovirus, which came to be called the human immunodeficiency virus (HIV).

A test was developed to detect the disease and was first used in testing blood for transfusion. Within a short period of time, the blood supply was protected by testing all donated blood, and transmission of HIV by blood transfusion became a rare event. Diagnostic tests for HIV/AIDS soon became available for testing individuals. For many years, these were used by clinicians only for high-risk individuals. In recent years, HIV testing has become more widely used, as the testing no longer requires blood drawing and the results are rapidly available. The CDC has put increasing emphasis on testing as part of routine health care.

In subsequent years, much has been learned about HIV/AIDS. Today, it is primarily a heterosexually transmitted disease with greater risk of transmission from male to females than females to males. In the United States, African Americans are at the greatest risk. Condoms have been demonstrated to reduce the risk of transmission. Abstinence and monogamous sexual relationships likewise eliminate or greatly reduce the risk. Even serial monogamy reduces the risk compared to multiple simultaneous partners. Male circumcision has been shown to reduce the potential to acquire HIV infection by approximately 50%.

In major U.S. cities, the frequency of HIV is often greater than 1% of the population, fulfilling the CDC definition of "high risk." In these geographic areas, the risk of unprotected intercourse is substantially greater than in most suburban or rural areas. Nearly everyone is susceptible to HIV infection, despite the fact that a small number of people have well documented protection on a genetic basis.

Maternal-to-child transmission is quite frequent and has been shown to be largely preventable by treatments during pregnancy and at the time of delivery. CDC recommendations for universal testing of pregnant women and intervention for all HIV-positive patients have been widely implemented by clinicians and hospitals and have resulted in greatly reduced frequency of maternal-to-child transmissions in the developed countries and in developing countries in recent years.

Medication is now available that greatly reduces the load of HIV present in the blood. These medications delay the progression of HIV and also reduce the ease of spread of the disease. These treatments were rapidly applied to HIV/AIDS patients in developed countries, but it required about a decade before they were widely used in most developing countries. Inadequate funding from developed countries and controversies over patent protection for HIV/AIDS drugs delayed widespread use of these treatments in developing countries.

New and emerging approaches to HIV prevention include use of antiviral medications during breastfeeding, postcoital treatments, and rapid diagnosis and follow-up to detect and treat those recently exposed.

Discussion Questions

1. Use the BIG GEMS framework to examine the factors in addition to infection that have affected the spread of HIV and the control or failure to control the HIV/AIDS epidemic.

2. What roles has health care played in controlling or failing to control the HIV/AIDS epidemic?

3. What roles has traditional public health played in controlling or failing to control the HIV/AIDS epidemic?

4. What roles have social factors (beyond the sphere of health care or public health) played in controlling or failing to control the HIV/AIDS epidemic?

SMOKING AND ADOLESCENTS—THE CONTINUING PROBLEM

The rate of smoking in the United States has been reduced by approximately one-half since the 1960s. However, the rate of smoking among teenagers increased in the 1980s and 1990s, especially among teenage females. This raised concerns that young women would continue smoking during pregnancy. In addition, it was found that nearly 90% of those who smoked started before the age of 18, and in many cases at a considerably younger age.

In the 1980s and most of the 1990s, cigarette smoking was advertised to teenagers and even preteens, or "tweens," through campaigns by companies such as Joe Camel. In recent years, a series of interventions directed at teenagers and tweens was put into effect. These included elimination of cigarette vending machines, penalties for those who sell cigarettes to those under 18, and elimination of most cigarette advertising aimed at those under 18. In addition, the Truth® campaign aimed to convince adolescents, who often see smoking as a sign of independence from their parents, that not smoking is actually a sign of independence from the tobacco companies who seek to control their behavior. Evaluation studies concluded that these interventions have worked to reduce adolescent smoking by about one-third.

Despite the successes of the early years of the 2000s in lowering the rates of cigarette smoking among adolescents, the rates have now stabilized at over 20%. Evidence indicates that adolescents who smoke generally do not participate in athletics, more often live in rural areas, and are more often white and less often African American. Males and females smoke about the same amount overall, but white females smoke more and Asian females smoke less than their male counterparts.

New drugs have recently been shown to increase the rates of success in smoking cessation among adults with few side effects. Evidence that the benefits are greater than the harms in adolescents is insufficient to recommend them for widespread use because of increased potential for adverse effects, including suicide. A series of interventions has been suggested for addressing the continuing problem of adolescent smoking. These include:

- Expulsion from school for cigarette smoking
- Focus on adolescents in tobacco warning labels
- Selective use of prescriptions for cigarette cessation drugs
- No smoking rules for sporting events, music concerts, and other adolescent-oriented events
- Fines for adolescents who falsify their age and purchase cigarettes
- Higher taxes on tobacco products
- Rewards to students in schools with the lowest smoking rates in a geographic area
- Higher auto insurance premiums for adolescents who smoke
- Application of technology to reduce the quantity of nicotine allowed in tobacco products to reduce the potential for addiction
- Testing of athletes for nicotine and exclusion from competition if they test positive

- Encouragement of the use of e-cigarettes, which utilize smokable nicotine but not cancer-causing components of cigarettes
- Provision of tobacco counseling as part of medical care covered through insurance

Discussion Questions

1. How does this case illustrate the P.E.R.I.E. process?

2. Which of these interventions do you think would be most successful? Explain.

3. How would you classify each of these potential interventions as education (information), motivation (incentives), obligation (required), or innovation (technological change)?

4. What other interventions can you suggest to reduce adolescent smoking?

REYE'S SYNDROME: A PUBLIC HEALTH SUCCESS STORY

Reye's Syndrome is a potentially fatal disease of childhood that typically occurs in the winter months at the end of an episode of influenza, chicken pox, or other acute viral infection. It is characterized by progressive stages of nausea and vomiting, liver dysfunction, and mental impairment that progress over hours to days and result in a range of symptoms, from irritability to confusion to deepening stages of loss of consciousness. Reye's Syndrome is diagnosed by putting together a pattern of signs and symptoms. There is no definitive diagnostic test for the disease.

Reye's Syndrome was first defined as a distinct condition in the early 1960s. By the 1980s, over 500 cases per year were being diagnosed in the United States. When Reye's Syndrome was first diagnosed, there was over a 30% case-fatality rate. Early diagnosis and aggressive efforts to prevent brain damage were shown to reduce the deaths and limit the mental complications, but there is no cure for Reye's Syndrome.

In the late 1970s and early 1980s, a series of case-control studies compared Reye's Syndrome children with similar children who also had an acute viral infection, but did not develop the syndrome. These studies suggested that use of aspirin, then called "baby aspirin," was strongly associated with Reye's Syndrome, with over 90% of those children afflicted with the syndrome having recently used aspirin.

Cohort studies were not practical because they would require observing very large numbers of children who might be given or not given aspirin by their caretakers. Randomized controlled trials were neither feasible nor ethical. Fortunately, it was considered safe and acceptable to reduce or eliminate aspirin use in children because there was a widely used alternative—acetaminophen (often used as the brand name Tylenol)—that was not implicated in the studies of Reye's Syndrome.

As early as 1980, the CDC cautioned physicians and parents about the potential dangers of aspirin. In 1982, the U.S. surgeon general issued an advisory on the danger of aspirin for use in children. By 1986, the U.S. Food and Drug Administration required a Reye's Syndrome warning be placed on all aspirin-containing medications. These efforts were coupled with public service announcements, informational brochures, and patient education by pediatricians and other health professionals who cared for children. The use of the term "baby aspirin" was strongly discouraged.

In the early 1980s, there were over 500 cases of Reye's Syndrome per year in the United States. In recent years, there have often been fewer than 5 per year. The success of the efforts to reduce or eliminate the use of "baby aspirin" and the subsequent dramatic reduction in the frequency of Reye's Syndrome provided convincing evidence that aspirin was a contributory cause of the condition and its removal from use was an effective intervention.

Discussion Questions

1. How does the Reye's Syndrome history illustrate the use of each of the steps in the P.E.R.I.E. process?

2. What unique aspects of Reye's Syndrome made it necessary and feasible to rely on case-control studies to provide the evidence to help reduce the frequency of the syndrome?

3. What types of methods for implementation were utilized as part of the implementation process? Can you classify them in terms of when, who, and how?

4. How does the Reye's Syndrome history illustrate the use of evaluation to demonstrate whether the implementation process was successful?

SUDDEN INFANT DEATH SYNDROME (SIDS)

Sudden infant death syndrome, or SIDS, was first recognized as a distinct public health problem in the late 1960s when over 7,000 infants each year were found to die suddenly and unexpectedly. "Crib deaths" have been recognized for centuries, but until they were formally recorded and investigated, little was known about their cause, leading some to conclude that intentional or unintentional suffocation by parents or caregivers played an important role.

Data from the investigations of SIDS indicated that the syndrome was very rare before babies' first month of life, increased during the second month, and peaked during the third month, before rapidly declining in frequency to again become rare after the fourth month of life. The timing of SIDS suggested that the condition occurs after infants begin to sleep for extended periods but prior to the time in which children can raise themselves up and roll over on their own. Additional evidence suggested a seasonal trend, with more cases of SIDS occurring during cold weather months than during warm weather months.

In the 1980s, several case-control studies of SIDS cases and similar infants without SIDS established that infants who slept on their stomachs were at substantially increased risk of dying from SIDS. The studies indicated that the chances increased four to seven times, suggesting that if a cause-and-effect relationship exists, a clear majority of SIDS cases could be prevented if infants slept on their back. Many parents and clinicians remained skeptical because the traditional teaching emphasized sleeping prone, or on the stomach, to reduce the possibility of choking on regurgitation and vomit. Despite the lack of evidence for this hazard, generations had been raised on this practice and belief.

Additional evidence of the effectiveness of a "back-to-sleep" intervention was provided by the experience of New Zealand, which was the first country to begin a program to encourage caretakers to put infants to sleep on their backs. The rates of SIDS in New Zealand declined rapidly in parallel with the increased rate at which infants were put to sleep on their back. Similar declines in SIDS did not occur in other countries that had not yet instituted similar back-to-sleep programs.

In 1992, the American Academy of Pediatrics made a recommendation that infants be placed on their back to sleep. The initial recommendations also endorsed side sleeping. In 1994, with the support of the American Academy of Pediatrics, the National Institutes of Health (NIH), and the U.S. Public Health Service, the Back-to-Sleep campaign was launched. The educational campaign included public service announcements, brochures and other publications, including information accompanying new cribs, plus efforts for pediatricians and others who care for infants to educate parents and caretakers about the importance of having infants sleep on their backs.

The frequency of infants sleeping prone in the United States was found by survey data to be reduced from approximately 70% to less than 15% during the years immediately following the initiation of the Back-to-Sleep campaign. During these years, the rates of SIDS fell by approximately 50%, an impressive change but less than expected by the initial data. The rate of prone sleeping among African

Americans was found to be over twice as high as the rate among whites, and African American infants continued to have higher rates of SIDS than whites.

Continuing studies suggested that the side position was being commonly used. It was found that many infants moved from the side to the prone position, and movement from the side to the prone position carried a high risk of SIDS. Additional case-control studies suggested that soft objects and loose bedding as well as overheating were associated with SIDS. These relationships are consistent with the initial finding of an increase of SIDS in colder weather months.

Studies of the infants who slept on their back indicated an increasing in flattening of the head, or plagiocephaly. These changes were shown to be reduced by increasing the amount of "tummy time," or play periods in which infants are placed prone under supervision. Guidelines for tummy time are now part of the evidence-based recommendations.

SIDS continues to be an important cause of infant mortality, and new contributory causes continue to be investigated. SIDS reflects the use of evidence-based public health and the importance of continuing to study and develop new approaches to public health problems.

Discussion Questions

1. Discuss how the problem description component of the evidence-based public health approach suggested hypotheses for the etiology of SIDS.

2. Discuss the types of evidence used to support the relationship between sleeping prone and SIDS as well as the limitations of the evidence.

3. Discuss how the evidence-based recommendations incorporated potential benefits and harms.

4. Discuss how implementation and evaluation worked to establish sleeping on the back as a standard intervention to prevent SIDS.

5. Discuss how the continuing presence of the problem of SIDS has produced a new round of use of the evidence-based public health approach.

OXYGEN USE IN PREMATURE INFANTS AND BLINDNESS

Oxygen seemed like just what premature infants needed to address the underdevelopment of their lungs, which often led to pneumonia and death. Thus in the 1940s, after effective means were developed to administer oxygen to pilots in World War II, physicians began to routinely administer high-dose oxygen to nearly all premature infants. The unexpected association between high-dose oxygen and blindness only became established after over 10,000 premature infants, including its most famous victim, Stevie Wonder, developed blindness.

The first hint of a problem came in 1942, when a report of five cases of blindness of premature infants in which no other cause could be determined appeared in the research literature. Once the condition became known, many more cases were identified that met this definition. The process that produced blindness could be seen upon examining the back of the eye during a clinical examination. Proliferation of blood vessels followed by scarring or fibrosis called retrolental fibrosis (RLF), with subsequent detachment of the retina, could be seen in severe cases that had produced blindness.

Using case-control studies, researchers quickly recognized an association between state-of-the-art medical care provided at the most up-to-date medical centers and blindness due to severe RLF. They examined a range of factors associated with state-of-the-art medical care. Reports of constriction of the retinal arteries in fighter pilots given high-dose oxygen led researchers to look for and find similar findings in infants. They found that longer durations of oxygen administration were associated with longer term and more severe retinal artery constriction.

Reinforcing the accumulating clinical evidence were studies of high-dose oxygen use in a variety of animal species. High-dose oxygen used in premature kittens produced retinal damage similar to RLF. The pattern of constriction of the retinal arteries of kittens while on high-dose oxygen was followed by proliferation of new blood vessels similar to that seen leading to scarring or fibrosis in human infants with RLF.

A cohort study was soon conducted in three hospitals in Melbourne, Australia. One had incubators that could give premature infants air with 2 or 3 times the 20% concentration of oxygen in atmospheric air. The second used a less efficient way of delivering oxygen. The third required patients to pay for supplementary oxygen, so oxygen was rarely used. The medical records for 1948 through 1950 revealed that at the hospitals where oxygen was given most intensively, 19% of premature babies developed evidence of RLF. At the other two, where it was used less aggressively, the rate was only 7%.

A large randomized controlled trial was needed to convince clinicians to restrict the use of oxygen for premature infants, especially because clinicians were concerned that restrictions in oxygen use would result in brain damage and a higher mortality rate. A large randomized controlled trial sponsored by NIH was soon conducted at 18 institutions by randomizing infants at 2 days of age to routine supplemental oxygen or to a curtailed-oxygen group that received lower concentration oxygen only as needed.

The study showed that RLF severe enough to produce blindness, if continued, occurred in 17% of the babies receiving routine high oxygen, but in only 5% of the curtailed-oxygen group. The death rate in the two groups was similar. The investigation was continued with all infants assigned to curtailed oxygen. The follow-up study found that the duration of oxygen use was key to the risk of developing RLF and that supplemental oxygen at even low levels increased the risk of developing RLF.

Recommendations of the American Academy of Pediatrics and other authorities, published soon after the release of the study, were key to changing the attitudes and practices of clinicians. By the mid-1950s, follow-up studies showed that the use of routine oxygen for premature infants was on the decline, and so was the rate of RLF. By the late 1950s, RLF had declined to rates seen only before the widespread use of high-dose oxygen.

The evaluation of the impact of oxygen use for premature infants was not over. Soon after the rapid reduction in oxygen use began, the death rates among premature infants began to increase. Investigators in the United States and Britain found an increased mortality rate and rate of brain damage and paralysis among premature infants with underdeveloped lung function. Investigators noted that the randomized controlled trial included only infants who had survived for 2 days, the period of the highest number of deaths from respiratory related causes. Thus, by the early 1960s, it was clear that a trade-off existed between the use of oxygen to reduce early mortality and morbidity and limiting oxygen use to reduce the incidence of RLF.

Evidence-based recommendations encouraged the use of oxygen to limit the impact of too little oxygen while minimizing the level and duration of oxygen. When oxygen was used, clinicians were expected to conduct frequent examinations of the retina to identify early evidence of RLF.

In recent years, there has been an increase in RLF even as clinicians have limited and monitored the use of supplemental oxygen. The increase has been largely attributed to the increased number of premature infants and the ability to keep very premature infants alive. The greater the degree of prematurity, the greater the risk of RLF. In fact, this process may occur in premature infants even without the use of oxygen. Therefore, in recent years, the name of the condition has been changed to retinopathy of prematurity, or ROP.

Clinicians now monitor the retina of premature infants, looking for early signs of ROP. Interventions to treat early ROP, including laser treatments and surgical interventions, are now part of the effort to detect and treat ROP at an early stage to prevent blindness. Evidence-based recommendations of the American Academy of Pediatrics outline this approach and provide specific recommendations for its implementation.

Prevention, detection, and treatment of ROP is now seen as part of an overall approach to the care of premature infants. The success of the current approach requires ongoing evaluation and continued efforts to look for ways to improve the care of newborns.

Discussion Questions

1. What roles did the distribution of disease and biological plausibility play in suggesting the hypothesis that supplemental oxygen causes infant blindness?

2. Discuss the roles played by case-control and cohort studies as well as randomized controlled trials in establishing oxygen supplementation as a contributory cause of blindness in premature infants.

3. Discuss how the evidence-based recommendations sought to balance the benefits and the harms of oxygen use.

4. Discuss how this case illustrates the need for ongoing evaluation and efforts to modify evidence-based recommendations based on new evidence.

SECTION II

Tools of Population Health

In order to protect and promote health and prevent disease, disability, and death, public health uses an array of tools. In this section, we will examine three of the basic tools of public health: public health data and communications; social and behavioral sciences; and health law, policy, and ethics. **Figure S02-1** provides a framework for thinking about the tools used in the population health approach and indicates where they are addressed in this text.

In Chapter 3, we will explore how health information is collected, compiled, and presented, as well as how it is perceived, combined, and used to make decisions in the arena of health communications. Chapter 4 will examine the contributions of the social and behavioral sciences in helping us to understand the sources of health and disease and the strategies available to reduce disease, disability, and death. To do this, we will explore how social and economic factors, or social determinants, affect health. We will also examine how individual and group behavior can be changed to improve health. Finally, in Chapter 5, we will learn how health policies and laws can be used to improve health, as well as how ethical and philosophical issues limit their use.

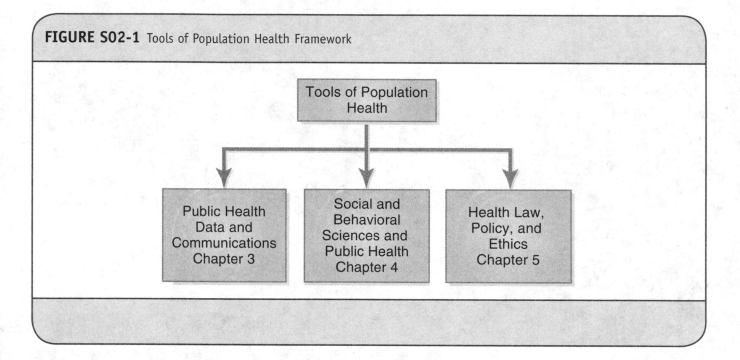

FIGURE S02-1 Tools of Population Health Framework

CHAPTER **3**

Public Health Data and Communications

LEARNING OBJECTIVES

By the end of this chapter, the student will be able to:

- identify six basic types of public health data.
- explain the meaning, use, and limitations of the infant mortality rate and life expectancy measurements.
- explain the meanings and uses of HALEs and DALYs.
- identify criteria for evaluating the quality of information presented on a website.
- explain ways that perceptions affect how people interpret information.
- explain the roles of probabilities, utilities, and the timing of events in combining public health data.
- explain the basic principles for the construction of decision trees and their uses.
- explain how attitudes, such as risk-taking attitudes, may affect decision making.
- identify three different approaches to clinical decision making and their advantages and disadvantages.

You read that the rate of use of cocaine among teenagers has fallen by 50% in the last decade. You wonder where that information might come from.

You hear that life expectancy in the United States is now approximately 80 years. You wonder what that implies about how long

you will live and what that means for your grandmother, who is 82 and in good health.

You hear on the news the gruesome description of a shark attack on a young boy from another state and decide to keep your son away from the beach. While playing at a friend's house, your son nearly drowns after falling into the backyard pool. You ask why so many people think that drowning in a backyard pool is unusual when it is far more common than shark attacks.

"Balancing the harms and benefits is essential to making decisions," your clinician says. The treatment you are considering has an 80% chance of working, but there is also a 20% chance of side effects. "What do I need to consider when balancing the harms and the benefits?" you ask.

You are faced with a decision to have a medical procedure. One physician tells you there's no other choice and you must undergo the procedure, another tells you about the harms and benefits and advises you to go ahead, and the third lays out the options and tells you it's your decision. Why are there such different approaches to making decisions these days?

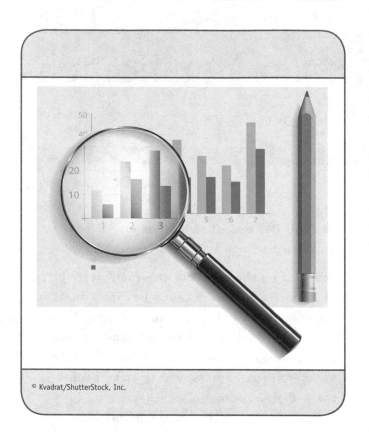

© Kvadrat/ShutterStock, Inc.

These are the types of issues and questions that we will address as we look at health data and communications.

WHAT IS THE SCOPE OF HEALTH COMMUNICATIONS?

The term **health communications** deals with the methods for collecting, compiling, and presenting health information. It also addresses how we perceive information, combine information, and use information to make decisions. Thus, health communication is about information, from its collection to its use. **Figure 3-1** displays how these parts of the process fit into a continuous flow of information.

The field of health communications has been growing at the speed of the Internet. This field has implications for most, if not all, aspects of public health, as well as health care. Therefore, we will focus on key issues in each of the above-mentioned components of this burgeoning field. We will look at the following aspects of health communications and ask the following questions:

- *Collecting data*: Where does public health data come from?
- *Compiling information*: How is public health information compiled or put together to measure the health of a population?
- *Presenting information*: How can we evaluate the quality of the presentation of public health information?
- *Perceiving information*: What factors affect how we perceive public health information?

FIGURE 3-1 Public Health Data, Health Communication, and the Flow of Information

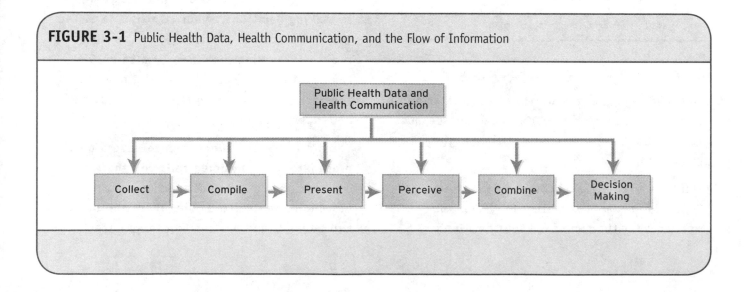

- *Combining information*: What types of information need to be combined to make health decisions?
- *Decision making*: How do we utilize information to make health decisions?

We can only highlight key issues in this complex and evolving field of health communications. To do this, we will use the above questions and provide frameworks and approaches to explore possible answers.

WHERE DOES PUBLIC HEALTH DATA COME FROM?

Public health **data** is collected in a wide variety of ways.[a] These methods are often referred to as **public health surveillance** or **surveillance**. Data from public health surveillance is collected, published, and distributed without identifying specific individuals. Data of this type come from a growing variety of sources. It is helpful, however, to classify these sources according to the way they are collected. **Table 3-1** outlines common types of quantitative public health data, provides examples of each type, and indicates important uses, as well as the advantages and disadvantages of each type of data.

Data from different sources is increasingly being combined to create integrated health data systems or **databases** that can be rapidly and flexibly accessed by computers to address a wide range of questions. These systems have great potential to provide useful information to contribute to evidence-based public health. This information can help describe problems, examine etiology, assist with evidence-based recommendations, and examine the options for implementation, as well as help evaluate the outcomes. Despite their great potential, integrated databases also create the potential for abuse of the most intimate health information. Thus, protecting the privacy of data and ensuring its anonymous collection and distribution is now of great concern as part of the development of integrated databases.

Public health data has traditionally been numerical, or quantitative. In recent years, the importance of nonnumerical, or qualitative, data has received much greater attention in public health. **Box 3-1** discusses some of the important uses of qualitative data.

Data can be used for a wide range of purposes in public health and health care. One particularly important use is the compilation of data to generate summary measurements of the health of a group or population. Let us take a look at how we compile this data.

---

[a] "Data" is usually defined as facts or a representation of facts, while "information" implies that the data is compiled and/or presented in a way designed for a range of uses. Thus, the term "data" is used here only in the context of collection.

HOW IS PUBLIC HEALTH INFORMATION COMPILED TO MEASURE THE HEALTH OF A POPULATION?

Measurements that summarize the health of populations are called **population health status measures**. For over a century, public health professionals have focused on how to summarize the health status of large populations, such as countries and large groups within countries—for example, males and females or large racial groups of a particular nation. In the 1900s, two measurements became standard for summarizing the health status of populations: the **infant mortality rate** and **life expectancy**. These measurements rely on death and birth certificate data, as well as census data. Toward the latter part of the 1900s, these sources of data became widely available and quite accurate in most parts of the world.

The infant mortality rate estimates the rate of death in the first year of life. For many years, it has been used as the primary measurement of child health. Life expectancy has been used to measure the overall death experience of the population, incorporating the probability of dying at each year of life.[1,2] These measures were the mainstay of 20th century population health measurements. Let us look at each of these measures and see why additional health status measurements are needed for the 2000s.

At the turn of the 20th century, infant mortality rates were high even in today's developed countries, such as the United States. It was not unusual for over 100 of every 1,000 newborns to die in the first year of life. In many parts of the world, infant mortality far exceeded the death rate in any later years of childhood. For this reason, the infant mortality rate was often used as a surrogate or substitute measure for overall rates of childhood death. In the first half of the 1900s, however, great improvements in infant mortality occurred in what are today's developed countries. During the second half of the century, many developing countries also saw greatly reduced infant mortality rates. Today, many countries have achieved infant mortality rates below 10 per 1,000, and a growing number of nations have achieved rates below 5 per 1,000.[b]

The degree of success in reducing mortality among children aged 2 to 5 has not been as great.[3] Malnutrition and old and new infectious diseases continue to kill young

---

[b] The infant mortality rate is measured using the number of deaths among those ages 0–1 in a particular year divided by the total number of live births in the same year. If the number of live births is stable from year to year, then the infant mortality rate is a measure of the rate of deaths. Health status measurements of child health have not sought to incorporate disability on the less-than-completely-accurate assumption that disability is not a major factor among children.

TABLE 3-1 The 6 S's of Quantitative Sources of Public Health Data

Type	Examples	Uses	Advantages/Disadvantages
Single case or small series	Case reports of one or a small number of cases, such as SARS, anthrax, mad cow disease and new diseases (e.g., first report of AIDS)	Alert to new disease or resistant disease; alert to potential spread beyond initial area	Useful for dramatic, unusual, and new conditions; requires alert clinicians and rapid ability to disseminate information
Statistics ("Vital Statistics") and reportable diseases	Vital statistics: birth, death, marriage, divorce; reporting of key communicable and specially selected noncommunicable-diseases (e.g., elevated lead levels, child and spouse abuse, etc.)	Required by law—sometimes penalties imposed for non-compliance; births and deaths key to defining leading causes of disease; reportable disease may be helpful in identifying changes over time	Vital statistics very complete because of social and financial consequences; reportable disease often relies on institutional reporting rather than individual clinicians; frequent delays in reporting data
Surveys— sampling	National Health and Nutrition Examination Survey (NHANES); Behavioral Risk Factor Surveillance System (BRFSS)	Drawing conclusions about overall population and subgroups from representative samples	Well-conducted surveys allow inferences to be drawn about larger populations; frequent delays in reporting data
Self-reporting	Adverse effect monitoring of drugs and vaccines as reported by those affected	May help identify unrecognized or unusual events	Useful when dramatic unusual events closely follow initial use of drug or vaccine; tends to be incomplete; difficult to evaluate meaning because of selective process of reporting
Sentinel monitoring	Influenza monitoring to identify start of outbreak and changes in virus type	Early warnings or warning of previously unrecognized events	Can be used for "real-time" monitoring; requires considerable knowledge of patterns of disease and use of services to develop
Syndromic surveillance	Use of symptom patterns (e.g., headaches, cough/fever, or gastrointestinal symptoms, plus increased sales of over-the-counter drugs) to raise alert of possible new or increased disease	May be able to detect unexpected and subtle changes, such as bioterrorism or new epidemic producing commonly occurring symptoms	May be used for early warning even when no disease is diagnosed; does not provide a diagnosis and may have false positives

children. In addition, improvements in the care of severely ill newborns have extended the lives of many children—only to have them die after the first year of life. Children with HIV/AIDS often die not in the first year of life, but in the second, third, or fourth year. Once a child survives to age 5, he or she has a very high probability of surviving into adulthood in most countries. Thus, a new measurement known as **under-5 mortality** has now become the standard health status measure used by the World Health Organization (WHO) to summarize the health of children.

Let us take a look at the second traditional measure of population health status—life expectancy. Life expectancy is a snapshot of a population incorporating the probability of dying at each age of life in a particular year. Life expectancy tells us how well a country is doing in terms of deaths in a particular year. As an example, life expectancy at birth in a developed country may be 80 years. Perhaps in 1900, life expectancy at birth in that same country was only 50 years. In 2020, life expectancy may be 85 years. Thus, this metric allows us to make comparisons between countries and within a single country over time.

BOX 3-1　Qualitative Data and Its Importance to Public Health

Qualitative data can serve a variety of functions in public health. It can generate ideas or hypotheses for further study, provide key information on the reasons for success or failure of an intervention, and provide explanations for findings that cannot be derived from quantitative research. Thus, qualitative research can contribute to the full range of health communications, from data collection to decision making. Qualitative and quantitative research should be seen as complementary, not competitive, as they can work together to provide greater insight and understanding. Quantitative research often includes a large sample and focuses on numbers, whereas qualitative research often looks in depth at a small sample, producing descriptions and allowing for a thorough exploration of the phenomenon of interest.

Focus groups and interviews are increasingly important forms of qualitative research that are being used to gain insight into how and why people come to conclusions or hold opinions. The opinions examined increasingly go beyond commercial products and politicians to include the use of health services, acceptance of new and existing technology, and speculation about the reasons for diseases and health outcomes. The ideas put forward by these types of investigations may generate new hypotheses to be examined using quantitative studies. They may also help assess barriers to implementation and suggest new approaches. Focus groups and interviews are useful when the behavior, thoughts, and interpretations cannot be observed directly but the participants can provide pertinent information on the topic of interest.

Document review and observations are another important method used in qualitative research. Document review includes collection and analysis of existing documents in order to provide context for the issue being explored. Because the documents were developed for purposes other than research, they tend to be objective, shedding light on the culture of the population being studied and revealing intentions and behaviors of the population. Observation can be particularly useful when it is important to understand the real-time behavior of a population in its own environment.

These and other approaches to qualitative research allow us to understand, describe, and explore public health issues in a flexible way to produce richly descriptive and comprehensive findings.

Despite its name, life expectancy cannot be used to accurately predict the future even at the population level—that would require assuming that nothing will change. That is, it assumes that the death rates at all ages will remain the same in future years. We have seen increases in life expectancy in most countries over the last century, but declines occurred in sub-Saharan Africa and countries of the former Soviet Union in the late 1900s.[c]

Life expectancy tells us only part of what we want to know. It reflects the impact of dying, but not the impact of disabilities. When considering the health status of a population in the 2000s, we need to consider disability, as well as death.

Today, the World Health Organization (WHO) uses a measurement known as the **health-adjusted life expectancy (HALE)** to summarize the health of populations.[4] The HALE measurement starts with life expectancy and then incorporates measurements of the quality of health. The WHO utilizes survey data to obtain a country's overall measurement of quality of health. This measurement incorporates key components, including:[d]

- Mobility—the ability to walk without assistance
- Cognition—mental function, including memory
- Self-care—activities of daily living, including dressing, eating, bathing, and use of the toilet
- Pain—regular pain that limits function
- Mood—alteration in mood that limits function
- Sensory organ function—impairment in vision or hearing that impairs function

From these measurements, an overall quality of health score is obtained. In most countries, these range from

---

[c] Life expectancy is greater than you may expect at older ages. For instance, in a country with a life expectancy of 80 years, a 60-year-old may still have a life expectancy of 25 years, not 20 years, because he or she escaped the risks of death during the early years of life. At age 80, the chances of death are very dependent on an individual's state of health because life expectancy combines the probability of death of those in good health and those in poor health. Healthy 80-year-olds have a very high probability of living to 90 and beyond.

[d] It can be argued that use of these measurements associates disability primarily with the elderly. Note that these qualities of health do not specifically include measures of the ability to work, engage in social interactions, or have satisfying sexual relationships, all of which may be especially important to younger populations.

TABLE 3-2 Life Expectancy and Health-Adjusted Life Expectancy for a Range of Large Countries

Country	Life expectancy	Health-adjusted life expectancy (HALE)
Nigeria	49	42
India	64	56
Russian Federation	66	60
Brazil	73	64
China	74	66
United States	78	70
United Kingdom	80	72
Canada	81	73
Japan	83	76

Data from World Health Organization. Healthy life expectancy (HALE) at birth (years). World health report 2009. http://www.who.int/whosis/whostat/EN_WHS09_Full.pdf. Accessed July 17, 2013.

85 to 90%. We may consider a score of less than 85% as poor and greater than 90% as very good. A quality of health measurement of 90% indicates that the average person in the country loses 10% of his or her full health over his or her lifetime to one or more disabilities.

The quality of health measurement is multiplied by the life expectancy to obtain the HALE. Thus, a country that has achieved a life expectancy at birth of 80 years and an overall quality of health score of 90% can claim a HALE of 80.00 × 0.90 = 72.00. **Table 3-2** displays WHO data on life expectancy and HALEs at birth for a variety of large countries.[e]

Today, the under-5 mortality and HALEs are used by the WHO as the standard measures reflecting child health and the overall health of a population. An additional measure, known as the **disability-adjusted life year (DALY)**, has been developed and used by the WHO to allow for comparisons and changes based on categories of diseases and condi-

tions.[5] **Box 3-2** describes DALYs and some of the data and conclusions that have come from using this measurement. **Table 3-3** displays DALYs according to these categories of diseases and conditions for the same large countries for which HALEs are displayed in Table 3-2.

The Global Burden of Disease (GBD) project has produced a number of important conclusions using DALYs, including:

- Depression is a major contributor to most nations' DALYs and may become the number one contributor in the next few decades in developing, as well as developed, countries.
- Chronic disabling diseases, including hookworm, malaria, and HIV, affect the young and working-age population and are the greatest contributors to the burden of disease in many developing countries.
- Cancers, such as breast cancer, hepatomas (primary liver cancer), and colon cancer—which affect the working-age population and are common in many developing countries—have an important impact on the burden of disease as expressed in DALYs.
- Motor vehicle, occupational, and other forms of unintentional injuries have a disproportionate impact on the burden of disease compared to merely measuring deaths because these injuries produce long-term disabilities, as well as death at young ages.
- Obesity is rapidly overtaking malnutrition as a burden of disease in developing countries as early onset diabetes, heart disease, and strokes become major causes of death and disability among younger populations.

We have now looked at important sources of public health data and examined one key way that data is compiled to generate population health status measurements. Now, let us look at a third issue: the presentation of public health information.

HOW CAN WE EVALUATE THE QUALITY OF THE PRESENTATION OF HEALTH INFORMATION?

Having information is not enough. A key role and essential tool of public health is to effectively present the information in ways that serve as a basis for understanding and decision making. Issues of information presentation are increasingly important and increasingly complex. They require the study of a range of disciplines, from mass media, to computer graphics, to statistics.[f] Public health information is often

[e] Not all countries accept the HALE as the method for expressing disabilities. A measurement known as the **health-related quality of life (HRQOL)** has been developed and used in the United States. The HRQOL incorporates a measure of unhealthy days. Unhealthy days are measured by asking a representative sample of individuals the number of days in the last 30 during which the status of either their mental or physical health kept them from their usual activities. It then calculates a measure of the quality of health by adding together the number of unhealthy days due to mental plus physical health. The quality of health is obtained by dividing the number of healthy days by 30. This measurement is relatively easy to collect and calculate, but unlike the HALE, it does not reflect objective measures of disability and cannot be directly combined with life expectancy to produce an overall measure of health. That is, it does not include the impact of mortality.

[f] The use of statistics is one approach to data presentation. It asks questions, such as: What are the strengths of the relationships between risk factors and diseases? This is known as **estimation**. Statistical analysis also draws conclusions from data on small groups (samples) about larger groups or populations—this is called **inference** or statistical significance testing.

BOX 3-2 DALYs

Disability-adjusted life years (DALYs) are designed to examine the impacts that specific diseases and risk factors have on populations, as well as provide an overall measure of population health status. They allow comparisons between countries or within countries over time, based not only on overall summary numbers, such as life expectancy and HALEs, but also on specific diseases and risk factors.

The DALY compares a country's performance to the country with the longest life expectancy, which is currently Japan. Japan has a life expectancy that is approximately 83 years. In a country with zero DALYs, the average person would live approximately 83 years without any disability and would then die suddenly. Of course, this does not occur even in Japan, so all countries have DALYs of greater than zero. The measurement is usually presented as DALYs per 1,000 population in a particular country.[a]

Calculations of DALYs require much more data on specific diseases and disabilities than other measurements, such as life expectancy or HALEs. However, the WHO's Global Burden of Disease (GBD) project has made considerable progress in obtaining worldwide data collected using a consistent approach.[5] Data

a The DALY is a complex and technical measurement. If, in a country with 0 DALYs, 1,000 newborns suddenly died, there would be a loss of as much as 83,000 DALYs from the death of these 1,000 newborns. Thus, the total DALYs a country can lose in a particular year can range from 0 to approximately 83,000 per 1,000 persons. This somewhat overstates the possible loss due to the discounting and weighing that occurs in the calculation of DALYs. Nonetheless, when interpreting a country's total DALYs, it may be useful to compare the number of DALYs to this maximum possible loss.

is often not available on the disability produced by a disease. The WHO then uses expert opinion to estimate the impact.

The GBD project presents data on DALYs divided into the following categories:

- Communicable disease; maternal, neonatal, and nutritional conditions
- Noncommunicable diseases
- Injuries

Data is also available on specific diseases and risk factors, such as the impact of cigarette smoking, alcohol use, or depression.

It is also important to recognize that DALYs require a number of policy decisions that are hidden in the numbers. For instance, it was decided to emphasize the importance of death and disability among those of working age by giving them greater weight or importance in the calculation of this measurement. Working age was defined as age 16–60, which reflects a concept of working age more often used in developing countries. Death and disability at ages greater than the approximately 83 years of life expectancy of Japan do not add to the DALYs. In calculating DALYs, separate maximum life expectancies are used for males (~80 years) and females (~85 years), implying that loss of life among females is given slightly greater importance. These issues illustrate that in order to understand quantitative measures such as DALYs, you need to recognize that policy decisions are often subtly integrated into quantitative measurements. We need to appreciate the policy and sometimes the ethical decisions that are part of what appears to be objective measurements.

TABLE 3-3 DALYs Lost by Disease Categories and Total of All Categories Per 1,000 Population

Country	DALYs lost due to communicable diseases; maternal, neonatal, and nutritional conditions	DALYs lost due to noncommunicable diseases	DALYs lost due to injuries (unintentional + intentional)	Total DALYs lost
Nigeria	41,251	10,279	4,815	56,345
India	12,958	11,824	3,793	28,575
Russian Federation	2,189	18,752	6,411	27,352
Brazil	4,361	13,113	3,247	20,721
China	2,847	10,217	2,314	15,378
United States	941	11,939	1,387	14,267
United Kingdom	855	11,192	744	12,791
Canada	585	10,256	967	11,808
Japan	588	8,791	1,051	10,430

Data from World Health Organization. *Global Burden of Disease Project 2004.* Geneva: World Health Organization; 2004.

presented as graphics. Graphics create a picture in our mind of what is going on, and a picture is truly worth a thousand words. Graphical presentations can accurately inform, but they can also mislead us in a wide variety of ways. The accurate presentation of visual information has become an art as well as a science that deserves attention from all those who use information.[6]

Issues of quality are key to the presentation of information. The Internet is increasingly the primary source of public health information for the user. Thus, when we address issues of quality, we need to have a set of criteria for judging the quality of information presented on the Internet. Before relying on a website for health information, you should ask yourself key questions.[7] These questions are summarized in **Table 3-4**. Try these out the next time that you view a health information website.

The presentation of health information also requires taking into account the audience who will be using the material. Understanding the degree of **health literacy** of the intended audience is so important that a national movement has developed to address these issues. Health literacy is more than the ability to read. It refers to the degree to which individuals have the capacity to obtain, process, and understand basic health information and services needed to make appropriate health decisions.[8]

Even the most accurate data presentation does not tell us how the user will perceive the data. Let us take a look at the rapidly growing component of health communications that deals with how we perceive information.

WHAT FACTORS AFFECT HOW WE PERCEIVE PUBLIC HEALTH INFORMATION?

Regardless of how accurately information is presented, communication also needs to consider how the recipient perceives the information. Therefore, we also need to look at factors known to affect the perception of information or the subjective interpretation of what the information means for an individual.

At least three types of effects can greatly influence our perceptions of potential harms and benefits.[9] We will call them the **dread effect**, the **unfamiliarity effect**, and the **uncontrollability effect**.

TABLE 3-4 Quality Standards for Health Information on the Internet

Criteria	Questions to ask
Overall site quality	• Is the purpose of the site clear?
	• Is the site easy to navigate?
	• Are the site's sponsors clearly identified?
	• Are advertising and sales separated from health information?
Authors	• Are the authors of the information clearly identified?
	• Do the authors have health credentials?
	• Is contact information provided?
Information	• Does the site get its information from reliable sources?
	• Is the information useful and easy to understand?
	• Is it easy to tell the difference between fact and opinion?
Relevance	• Are there answers to your specific questions?
Timeliness	• Can you tell when the information was written?
	• Is it current?
Links	• Do the internal links work?
	• Are there links to related sites for more information?
Privacy	• Is your privacy protected?
	• Can you search for information without providing information about yourself?

Data from American Public Health Association. Criteria for Assessing the Quality of Health Information on the Internet. Available at http://www.apha.org/NR /exeres/412DDD11-42A0-46CB-8705-F9D47A073AF1.htm Accessed July 17, 2013.

The dread effect is present with hazards that easily produce very visual and feared consequences. It explains why we often fear shark attacks more than drowning in a swimming pool. The dread effect may also be elicited by the potential for catastrophic events, ranging from nuclear meltdowns to a poisoning of the water supply.

Our degree of familiarity with a potential harm or a potential benefit can greatly influence how we perceive data and translate it for our own situation. Knowing a friend or relative who died of lung cancer may influence how we perceive the information on the hazards of smoking or the presence of radon. It also may explain why we often see the danger of sun exposure as low and food irradiation as high, despite the fact that the data indicate that the degree of harm is the other way around.

Finally, the uncontrollability effect may have a major impact on our perceptions and actions. We often consider hazards that we perceive as in our control as less threatening than ones that we perceive as out of our control. Automobile collisions, for instance, are often seen as less hazardous than commercial airplane crashes, despite the fact that statistics show that commercial air travel is far safer than travel by automobile.

Perception of bad outcomes (or harms) and good outcomes (or benefits) needs to be considered along with the numbers if we are going to understand the ways information is used to make decisions. Not everyone perceives harms and benefits the same way. The selection of accurate and effective methods for conveying data is key to health communications.[g]

Understanding how we perceive information can help us design effective health messages. **Box 3-3** discusses the SUCCESs approach to developing messages that stick.

One approach to addressing differing perceptions of information is the use of a method known as **decision analysis**. Decision analysis relies on the vast information-processing ability of computers to formally combine information on benefits and harms to reach quantitative decisions. It provides us with insight into the types of information that need to be combined. Let us look at how we combine information—the next question in our flow of health information.

WHAT TYPE OF INFORMATION NEEDS TO BE COMBINED TO MAKE HEALTH DECISIONS?

Decision analysis focuses on three key types of information that need to be combined as the basis for making decisions. We can better understand these types of information by asking the following questions:

- *How likely?*—What is the probability or chance that the particular outcome will occur?
- *How important?*—What is the value or importance we place on a good or a bad outcome?

When expressing the chances that an outcome will occur, we often express the results as a percentage from 0 to 100. Probabilities, on the other hand, range from 0 to 1. Percentages and probabilities are often used interchangeably—the probability of 0.10 can be converted to 10% and vice versa. When faced with a percentage or probability, we need to ask: What period of time is being considered? For instance, if you hear that the chances of developing a blood clot while taking high-dose estrogen birth control pills is 5%, what does that mean? Does it mean 5% per cycle, 5% per year, or 5% over the time period that the average user is on the pill?

Outcomes vary from death to disabilities. Some outcomes greatly affect our function and limit our future, while we can learn to live with other outcomes despite the limitations they impose. When dealing with a quantitative approach, we are forced to place numbers on the value or importance of specific outcomes. A scale known as a **utility scale** is one method to measure and compare the value or importance that different people place on different outcomes. This scale is intended to parallel the scale of probabilities; that is, it extends from 1 to 0 or from 100% to 0%. It defines 1 or 100% as the state of health in which there are no health-related limitations. Zero is defined as immediate death. On the utility scale, there is nothing worse than immediate death. **Figure 3-2** displays the utility scale.[h] **Box 3-4** illustrates how we can use the utility scale to assign numbers to specific outcomes.

Utilities are important, especially when we need to combine potential harms with potential benefits. Probabilities

---

[g] For instance, we generally have difficulty distinguishing between small and very small numbers. The difference between 1 in 10,000 and 1 in 100,000 is difficult for most of us to grasp and incorporate into our decisions. When comparing these types of probabilities, it is tempting to compare the outcomes to ones that are better known, such as those with similar emotional impacts. We may compare the chances of dying from a motorcycle crash with the chances of dying from a truck or automobile crash. Comparison of different types of outcomes, such as between being struck by lightning compared to dying from a chronic exposure to chemicals or radiation, is far less informative.

[h] Many people consider prolonged incapacity or vegetative states as worse than death. The utility scale does not generally take this into account. This is a specific example of the more general limitation of quantitative decision making—that it focuses on the outcome and not on the process of getting there.

BOX 3-3 SUCCESs in Public Health Communications

Effective health communications starts with understanding how information is perceived. In their book *Made to Stick: Why Some Ideas Survive and Others Die*,[10] Chip and Dan Heath have come up with a memory technique they call SUCCESs, which focuses on the perception of ideas and identifies six principles of highly successful communications. SUCCESs stands for:

Simplicity: This first principle requires a short, memorable statement that captures the core of the message. The golden rule, the authors write, "is the ultimate model of simplicity: a one-sentence statement so profound that an individual could spend a lifetime learning to follow it."[11] While public health messages cannot be expected to rival the golden rule, some public health messages say it all. The Back-to-Sleep campaign, for instance, was able to convey the core of its message in just three words.

Unexpectedness: Getting and holding people's attention is often achieved by presenting unexpected facts that are counterintuitive, at least to your audience. Challenging common myths or conventional wisdom may be a good place to start when engaging an audience.

Concreteness: Proverbs often provide specific examples that can be remembered and generalized. For instance, "an apple a day keeps the doctor away" has become a memorable way of conveying the importance of diet in health. Providing concrete, visualizable examples is key. Bad breath and brown teeth may be more convincing reasons for stopping cigarette smoking than the long-term consequences, which are not immediately obvious.

Credibility: Credibility relies not so much on numbers but rather on the source of the information. For instance, news of an epidemic may start with, "Today, the CDC announced..." Credibility is enhanced if people can test out the ideas from their own experience. "Think about the last time you texted while driving. Could it have waited until you stopped?"

Emotions: Connecting with people's emotions is key not only in getting their attention but also for ensuring they will retain the ideas. Emotions connect people with ideas. For instance, the Heaths write, "It's difficult to get teenagers to quit smoking by instilling in them a fear of the consequences, but it's easier to get them to quit by tapping into their resentment of the duplicity of Big Tobacco."[12]

Stories: We remember and relate to stories about real or realistic people. Sharing "war stories" is a classic example of how people relate to the events in each other's lives. Short vignettes and stories help to make the issues real. Hopefully, the vignettes at the beginning of each chapter of *Public Health 101* accomplish this for you.

Putting the SUCCESs principles together as a coherent message is a real but important challenge. As the ideal example, the Heaths cite John F. Kennedy's famous challenge to "put a man on the moon and return him safely by the end of the decade."[13] They conclude that the message is simple, unexpected, amazingly concrete, credible because it is from the president of the United States, full of emotion, and a story in miniature.

It is not so easy to put together such memorable messages, but focusing on how information is perceived and using the SUCCESs principles is a good way to start.

Data from Heath C and Heath D. *Made to Stick: Why Some Ideas Survive and Others Die*. New York, NY: Random House; 2007.

FIGURE 3-2 Scale Used to Measure Utilities

100%   0%

Full Health   Immediate Death

alone often do not give us the answers we need when addressing issues of hazards ranging from environmental toxins to unhealthy behaviors. Utilities are also critical when looking at particular interventions, such as prevention or treatment options that include positive benefits, but also involve side effects or harms. Thus, whenever we need to combine or balance benefits and harms, we need to consider the utility of the outcomes along with the chances or probabilities of the outcomes.

Probabilities and utilities (both on a scale of 0 to 1) are often combined by multiplying the probability by the utility to obtain a probability that takes into account the utility or

BOX 3-4 Obtaining a Utility Score

Let us see how we can use the utility scale to put numbers on a specific outcome: complete and permanent blindness. Using the scale in Figure 3-2, place a number on the importance or value that you give to complete and permanent blindness.

In large groups of individuals, the average utility placed on blindness is quite predictable—about 50%. However, the range of values among a group is generally quite wide ranging, from 20 to 80% and sometimes even wider. Predicting an individual's utility is quite difficult because gender, socioeconomic group, and other predictors have little impact.[a]

Individuals who place a high utility on complete and permanent blindness usually indicate that they can learn to live with blindness and it will not greatly affect their enjoyment of life. Those who place a low utility on blindness generally say just the opposite. Thus, we need to understand that a utility of 50% is an average, including some with a much higher and some with a much lower utility. Therefore, the best way to know the value or utility that an individual places on a particular outcome such as blindness is to ask him or her.

[a] There are at least two predictors that are of some value. Those who have experienced an outcome usually find that they can adapt to it to a certain extent and usually rate its utility as somewhat higher than those who have not experienced the outcome. Second, age does have an impact on the scoring of utility. Younger people generally rate the utility

of an outcome as somewhat worse or lower than older people, perhaps due to the longer-term impact the disability has on their future options. The average utility placed on blindness by college students, for instance, is often closer to 40%. Neither of these impacts is large on average, nor can they be used to successfully predict the utility of any one individual.

what is called **expected utility.** Expected utilities are often displayed using graphical methods called **decision trees**.[14] **Box 3-5** discusses the use of decision trees based on expected utilities.

WHAT OTHER DATA NEEDS TO BE INCLUDED IN DECISION MAKING?

We also need to ask:

How soon?—When, on average, will the particular outcome happen if it is going to happen?

The expected timing of the occurrence of good and bad outcomes can also affect how we view the outcome. Most people view the occurrence of a bad outcome as worse if it occurs in the immediate future compared to years from now. Conversely, we usually view a good outcome as more valuable if it occurs in the immediate future. Thus, whenever we consider harms and benefits and try to combine them, we need to ask: When are the outcomes expected to occur? When both the good and the bad outcomes occur in the immediate future, the timing is not an issue. In public health and medicine, however, this is rarely the case. When dealing with many treatments, the benefits come first while the harms may occur at a later time. When dealing with vaccines and surgery, the pain and side effects often precede the potential gain. The timing of the benefits is rarely the same as the timing of the harms. Thus, we need to take this into account. This process is known as **discounting.** Discounting is a quantitative process in which we give greater emphasis or weight to events that are expected to occur in the immediate

future compared to events that are expected to occur in the distant future.[i]

We have seen that probabilities, utilities, and timing are key components of health communications that need to be combined when making public health and healthcare decisions.[j] However, there are other factors that are characteristic

[i] The exact amount of discounting that should occur is controversial, but there is agreement that we should place less importance on outcomes that occur in the distant future than those that occur in the immediate future. There is also agreement that the rate of discounting for harms and for benefits should be the same. The concept of discounting comes from economics and can be most easily understood with a financial example. Let us imagine that we want to discount at 5% per year. A discount rate of 5% implies that I am willing to give you $95 today if you are willing to give me $100 one year from now. Discounting is above and beyond inflation, so the actual return may be $100 plus the rate of inflation. Note that economists try to set the rate based on the average real return on money invested over a large number of years. In the past, this has been about 3% in most developed countries. When making decisions on a subjective basis, we often discount the future at a much higher rate. This is especially true of those who are very sick and are often focused heavily on the immediate future.

[j] Decision analysis is not the usual method used to combine information. Because the task of combining information is so complex and the ability of our minds to handle large quantities of information is so limited, we often use rules of thumb known as **heuristics.** Heuristics allow us to make decisions more rapidly and often with less information. For instance, we often prefer to structure decisions to allow only one of two choices, rather than choosing from a large number of options presented to us at the same time. Thus, we often narrow the field of candidates in primary elections to allow side-by-side comparisons in the general elections. The one-on-one comparisons allow manipulation of the results by getting rid of candidates in the primaries who might have fared better in the general election.

BOX 3-5 Using Decision Trees to Compare Interventions

Decision trees are a visual method for displaying the benefits and harms of two or more options for intervention. They allow us to directly compare the outcomes, incorporating the probability and the utility of each outcome in a process known as decision analysis. Decision trees are made up of two types of nodes, which reflect points in which decisions are made or events occur by chance. Therefore, we speak of **choice nodes** and **chance nodes**. As indicated in **Figure 3-3**, choice nodes are presented using a square box, while chance nodes are represented using a circle.

Let us see how choice nodes and chance nodes can be put together to develop a decision tree. **Figure 3-4** represents a simple decision tree. For each of the outcomes, a probability is included.

Note that the probability of each of the potential outcomes adds to 1 or 100%. For intervention #1, the potential outcomes are cure and die. For intervention #2, there is a third potential outcome: blindness. To compare intervention #1 and intervention #2, we need to know more than the probabilities of each outcome—we need to know the utility of blindness.

Thus, to compare intervention #1 and intervention #2, we will need to assume that die has a utility of 0 and cure has a utility of 1. Blindness is a more subjective utility. As we have seen, on average, it has been found that people regard blindness as having a utility of about 0.5. However, many people will have a utility that is as high as 0.8 or as low as 0.2. Let us start by using a utility of 0.5. In **Figure 3-5**, the probabilities and utilities of each intervention have been filled in, and the

probability has been multiplied by the utility to produce what is called an expected utility, or a probability that takes into account the utility of the outcomes. We can add together the expected utilities of each potential outcome to produce an overall expected utility. The overall expected utilities allow us to compare one intervention to another.

Notice that when we use a utility of 0.5, the overall expected utilities for the two interventions are the same. At least by decision analysis, these two potential interventions are considered a toss-up.

Now let us see what happens when we change the utility of blindness first to 0.8 and then to 0.2. **Figure 3-6** displays the decision tree and expected utilities when blindness's utility is set at 0.8. **Figure 3-7** displays the decision tree and expected utilities when blindness's utility is set at 0.2.

Notice that when the utility is set at 0.8 in Figure 3-6, the overall expected utility for intervention #2 is greatest. That is, the decision analysis recommends intervention #2 over intervention #1. However, in Figure 3-7, when the utility of blindness is set at 0.2, the overall utility for intervention #1 is

FIGURE 3-4 Decision Tree

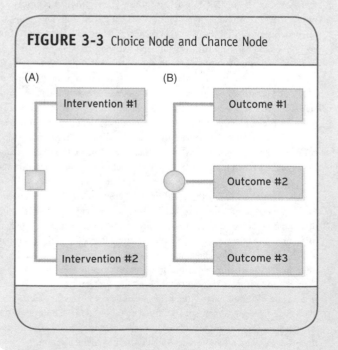

FIGURE 3-3 Choice Node and Chance Node

BOX 3-5 Using Decision Trees to Compare Interventions (*continued*)

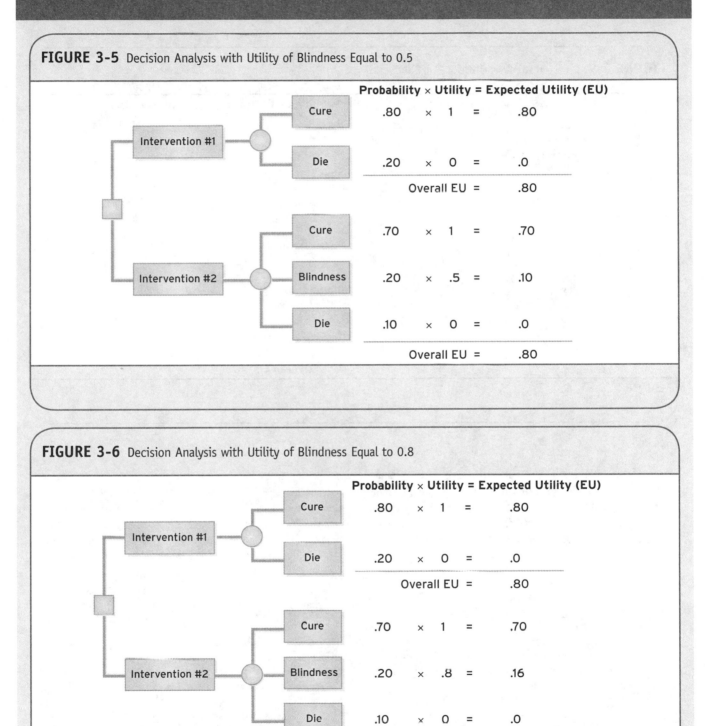

FIGURE 3-5 Decision Analysis with Utility of Blindness Equal to 0.5

Probability × Utility = Expected Utility (EU)

Intervention #1
- Cure: .80 × 1 = .80
- Die: .20 × 0 = .0

Overall EU = .80

Intervention #2
- Cure: .70 × 1 = .70
- Blindness: .20 × .5 = .10
- Die: .10 × 0 = .0

Overall EU = .80

FIGURE 3-6 Decision Analysis with Utility of Blindness Equal to 0.8

Probability × Utility = Expected Utility (EU)

Intervention #1
- Cure: .80 × 1 = .80
- Die: .20 × 0 = .0

Overall EU = .80

Intervention #2
- Cure: .70 × 1 = .70
- Blindness: .20 × .8 = .16
- Die: .10 × 0 = .0

Overall EU = .86

(continues)

BOX 3-5 Using Decision Trees to Compare Interventions (*continued*)

FIGURE 3-7 Decision Analysis of Utility of Blindness Equal to 0.2

greater than intervention #2. That is, the decision analysis rec-ommends intervention #1 over intervention #2. When a factor, such as the utility we place on blindness, produces a change in the recommended choice of intervention, we say that the decision analysis is **sensitive** to the factor, such as blindness.[a]

Decision trees and decision analysis are increasingly being used to display the options for intervention and to compare them based on probabilities and utilities. Decision trees are increasingly used as part of public health decision making for populations and for health policy decisions that affect large groups. Decision trees are often far more complex in an effort to reflect the realities of decision making. Decision analysis can help us compare interventions and help us recognize why individuals or organizations may come to different conclusions about their preferred intervention.[b]

---

[a] Decision trees assume that an outcome is measured by its probability multiplied by its utility. Thus, expected utility focuses on outcomes, not on the process of getting there. Therefore, this approach considers an outcome such as death or blindness to be the same whether it occurs suddenly or after a complicated hospitalization with multiple unsuccessful interventions. Also note that the example used does not take into account the timing of the outcome. It is possible in decision analysis to take into account the timing of outcomes through the process of discounting. Decision analysis assumes that when two chance nodes appear one after another, the probability of the second outcome is not affected by the outcome of the first node; that is, the chances of a good or bad outcome after the first and second chance nodes are independent of each other. The decision trees used in this box are also simplified in that only one choice node is presented. It is possible to introduce choice nodes even after a

chance node. Decision trees may become very complex and may need to become so in order to realistically reflect the choice and chance situations faced in practice. However, the more complex the decision tree, the more data is needed to utilize it to make recommendations.
[b] Decision analysis, which compares interventions for two or more conditions, frequently utilizes a measure of outcome known as **quality adjusted life-years**, or QALYs. QALYs incorporate the increase or decrease in life-expectancy as well as the probabilities and utilities of each outcome. QALYs may be used in decision analysis, but they are expected for cost-effectiveness analysis.

not of the data itself, but of the **decision maker**. A decision maker may be an individual; a health professional; or an organization, such as a nonprofit, a corporation, or a government agency. Let us turn our attention to decision makers and ask how we can go about making decisions. To do this, we need to address issues beyond probability, utility, and timing.

HOW DO WE UTILIZE INFORMATION TO MAKE HEALTH DECISIONS?

There are two key questions that we can ask to gain an understanding of how we use information to make health decisions:

- How do our risk-taking attitudes affect the way we make decisions?
- How do we incorporate information into our decisions?

There are a large number of attitudes that can affect the way we make decisions. One of the most important is known as our **risk-taking attitudes**.[k]

Let us examine what we mean by this term and see what type of risk-taking attitude you use in making decisions. Attitudes toward risk greatly influence the choices that we all make in the prevention and treatment of disease.[9] **Box 3-6** illustrates how you can understand your own attitudes toward risk taking by making some choices. We will assume that you understand what we mean by "utilities" and that you have thought through what a wide range of utilities means to you personally.

Understanding attitudes toward risk is important for analyzing how individuals make decisions about their own lives. It is also key when trying to understand how group decisions are made that require society to balance harms and benefits. Perhaps the most common health decisions that you will make are the decisions related to your health care and that of your family. Therefore, let us complete our examination of health communications by looking at three different approaches that can be used to make clinical healthcare decisions.

HOW CAN WE USE HEALTH INFORMATION TO MAKE HEALTHCARE DECISIONS?

There are three basic approaches to using health information to make healthcare decisions. We will call these approaches **inform of decision, informed consent,** and **shared decision**

making. Preferences for these types of approaches have changed over time, yet all three are currently part of clinical practice.

The inform of decision approach implies that the clinician has all the essential information and can make decisions that are in the patient's best interest. The role of the clinician is then merely to inform the patient of what needs to be done and to prescribe the treatment, or write the orders. At one point in time, this type of decision-making approach was standard for practicing clinicians. In the not-too-distant past, clinicians rarely told patients that they had cancer, justifying their silence by arguments that the knowledge might make the patient depressed, which could interfere with their response to the disease and to the treatment. The decision to administer many tests and receive a range of medications is still often done using the inform of decision approach.

A second type of decision-making approach is called informed consent. It rests on the principle that ultimately, patients need to give their permission or consent before major interventions, such as surgery, radiation, or chemotherapy, can be undertaken. Informed consent may be written, spoken, or implied. Clinically, informed consent implies that individuals have the right to know what will be done, why it will be done, and what the known benefits and harms are. Patients have the right to ask questions, including inquiring about the availability of other options. Informed consent does not mean that all possible options are presented to the patient, but it does imply that a clinician has made a recommendation for a specific intervention.

The third type of decision making is called shared decision making. In this approach, the clinician's job is to provide information to the patient with which he or she can make a decision. This might include directly giving information to the patient; providing consultations; or referring patients to sources of information, often on the Internet. Shared decision making places a far greater burden on the patient to seek out, understand, and use information. Using this approach, clinicians are not required to provide recommendations on specific interventions, though patients are free to ask for a clinician's opinion.[15]

All three types of decision-making approaches are currently in use today. **Table 3-5** outlines the process and roles implied by each of these approaches, as well as some of the potential advantages and disadvantages of each approach.

Health communications provides key tools for population health. We have taken a look at important issues related to each of them. We have asked questions about how public health data and information is collected, compiled, presented, perceived, combined, and used in decision making. Data and information are key public health tools for guiding our decision making. We will find ourselves coming back

---

k In addition to a risk-taking attitude, there are other attitudes that affect our decision making. For instance, decision making may depend on whether we regard an error of omission as equal to an error of commission. Decision analysis and most ethicists regard them as equal, but many people see errors of omission as more acceptable than errors of commission. That is, most people consider a bad outcome resulting from inaction as more tolerable than a bad outcome resulting from their own actions.

BOX 3-6 Risk-Taking Attitudes

Review the following situations and write down your decisions.

Situation A

Imagine that you have coronary artery disease and have a reduced quality of life with a utility of 0.80, compared to your previous state of full health with a utility of 1.00. You are offered the following pair of options. You can select only one option. Which of the following options do you prefer?

OPTION #1: A treatment with the following possible outcomes:

50% chance of raising the quality of your health (your utility) from 0.80 to 1.00

50% chance of reducing the quality of your health (your utility) from 0.80 to 0.60

OPTION #2: Refuse the above treatment and accept a quality of your health (your utility) of 0.80

Situation B

Imagine that you have coronary artery disease and have a reduced quality of life that has a utility of 0.20, compared to your previous state of full health that had a utility of 1.00. You are offered the following pair of options. You can select only one option. Which of the following options do you prefer?

OPTION #1: A treatment with the following possible outcomes:

10% chance of raising the quality of your health (your utility) from 0.20 to 1.00

90% chance of reducing the quality of your health (your utility) from 0.20 to 0.11

OPTION #2: Refuse the above treatment and accept a quality of your health (your utility) of 0.20

What was your answer in situation A? Situation B? To understand the meaning of your answers, you need to appreciate that in terms of the probabilities and utilities presented in each situation, these options are a toss-up. That is, taking into account the probabilities and the utilities, there is no difference between these options. To convince yourself of this, draw

a decision tree including the two options in situation A and the two options in situation B. You will find that they produce the same overall expected utilities.[a]

Thus, the information does not determine your choice; it must be your attitude toward taking chances, which is your attitude toward risk taking.

Did you choose option #2 in situation A and option #1 in situation B? Most, but not all, people make these choices. In situation A, we begin with a utility of 0.80. For many people, this is a tolerable situation and they do not want to take any chances of being reduced to a lower, perhaps intolerable utility. Thus, they want to guarantee a tolerable level of health. We can call this the **certainty effect**. In situation B, we begin with a utility of 0.20. For many people, this is an intolerable situation. Thus, people are usually willing to take their chances of getting even worse in the hopes of a major improvement in their health. When the quality of life is bad enough, most, if not all, people are willing to take their chances and go for it. This risk-taking behavior can be called the **long-shot effect**. Thus, risk-taking and risk-avoiding choices are both common, defensible, and reasonably predictable. Most of us are **risk takers** when conditions are intolerable and **risk avoiders** when conditions are tolerable.

A few people will choose option #1 in both situations A and B. These individuals are willing to take their chances in a range of situations in order to improve their outcome. We call them risk takers. Are you one of them? The only way to know is to ask yourself. Similarly, a few people will choose option #2 in both situations. These individuals seek to avoid taking chances in a range of situations in order to preserve their current state of health. We call them risk avoiders. Are you one of them? Only you can answer that question.[b]

---

[a] Notice that the outcomes occur in the immediate future so there is no issue of timing or need to discount the benefits or the harms.

[b] There is a fourth option, which is to choose option #2 in situation A and option #1 in situation B. The small number of individuals who make this choice usually have a very different perception of what utilities mean to them. For instance, they might perceive little difference between a 0.80 and a 0.20 utility.

TABLE 3-5 Types of Individual Decision Making

Type of decision making	Process/roles	Advantages	Disadvantages
Inform of decision	Clinician has all the essential information to make a decision that is in the patient's best interest	May be efficient and effective when patients seek clear direction provided by an authoritative and trusted source	Patient may not gain information and understanding of the nature of the problem or the nature of the treatment
	Clinician aims to convey his or her decision as a clear and unambiguous action or order	Patients may favor if they do not seek out or feel they can handle independent decision-making responsibilities	Patient may not be prepared to participate in the implementation of the decision
	Patients accept the clinician's recommendation without necessarily understanding or agreeing with the underlying reasoning		Patient may not accept responsibility for the outcome of the treatment
Informed consent	Clinician has the responsibility to convey a recommendation to the patient. The patient must decide whether to accept or reject the recommendation.	Patient gains information and understanding of the nature of the problem or the nature of the treatment	Time consuming compared to informing of the decision
	Harms and benefits of treatment are weighed by the clinician in making a recommendation	Patient may be prepared to participate in the implementation of the decision	May require elaborate paperwork to implement formal informed consent process
	Clinician has a responsibility to provide information on the aim of the recommendation, the potential benefits, the known harms, and the process that will occur; the patient has the right to ask additional questions about the treatment and the availability of other alternatives	Patient may accept responsibility for the outcome of the treatment	May increase emphasis on legal documents and malpractice law
Shared decision making	Clinicians serve as a source of information for patients, including providing it directly or identifying means of obtaining information	May increase the control of the patients over their own lives	May be time consuming for patients and clinicians
	Patients can expect to be informed of the existence of a range of accepted options and be assisted in their efforts to obtain information	May increase the types of information considered in decision making	May increase the costs of health care
	Patients may seek information on experimental or alternative approaches and can discuss the advantages and disadvantages of these approaches with a clinician	May reduce the adversarial nature of the relationship between clinicians and patients	May increase the stress/anxiety for patients
	Considerations besides benefits and harms are part of the decision-making process, including such considerations as cost, risk-taking attitudes, and the distress/discomforts associated with the treatment	May improve the outcome of care by increasing the patient's understanding and commitment to the chosen course of care	May shift the responsibility for bad outcomes from the clinician to the patient, i.e., takes the clinician off the hook/clinician does not need to do the hard work of thinking through the decision and making a recommendation
	Patients are often directly involved in the implementation of care		

again and again to these principles as we study the population health approach. Now, let us turn our attention to the utilization of the social and behavioral sciences as key tools of public health.

KEY WORDS

- Health communications
- Data
- Public health surveillance or surveillance
- Databases
- Estimation
- Population health status measures
- Infant mortality rate
- Inference
- Life expectancy
- Under-5 mortality
- Health-adjusted life expectancy (HALE)
- Disability-adjusted life year (DALY)
- Health-related quality of life (HRQOL)
- Health literacy
- Dread effect
- Unfamiliarity effect
- Uncontrollability effect
- Decision analysis
- Utility scale
- Expected utility
- Decision trees
- Choice nodes
- Chance nodes
- Sensitive
- Quality adjusted life-years (QALYs)
- Discounting
- Heuristics
- Decision maker
- Risk-taking attitudes
- Certainty effect
- Long-shot effect
- Risk takers
- Risk avoiders
- Inform of decision
- Informed consent
- Shared decision making

Discussion Questions

Take a look at the questions posed in the following scenarios, which were presented at the beginning of this chapter. See whether you can now answer these questions.

1. You read that the rate of use of cocaine among teenagers has fallen by 50% in the last decade. You wonder where that information might come from.

2. You hear that life expectancy in the United States is now approximately 80 years. You wonder what that implies about how long you will live and what that means for your grandmother, who is 82 and in good health.

3. You hear on the news the gruesome description of a shark attack on a young boy from another state and decide to keep your son away from the beach. While playing at a friend's house, your son nearly drowns after falling into the backyard pool. You ask why so many people think that drowning in a backyard pool is unusual when it is far more common than shark attacks.

4. "Balancing the harms and benefits is essential to making decisions," your clinician says. The treatment you are considering has an 80% chance of working, but there is also a 20% chance of side effects. "What do I need to consider when balancing the harms and the benefits?" you ask.

5. You are faced with a decision to have a medical procedure. One physician tells you there's no other choice and you must undergo the procedure, another tells you about the harms and benefits and advises you to go ahead, and the third lays out the options and tells you it's your decision. Why are there such different approaches to making decisions these days?

REFERENCES

1. Gordis L. *Epidemiology*. 4th ed. Philadelphia, PA: Elsevier Saunders; 2009.

2. Friis RH, Sellers TA. *Epidemiology for Public Health Practice*. 4th ed. Sudbury, MA: Jones and Bartlett Publishers; 2009.

3. Skolnik R. *Global Health 101*. Burlington, MA: Jones & Bartlett Learning; 2012.

4. World Health Organization. Healthy life expectancy (HALE) at birth (years). World health report 2009. http://www.who.int/whosis/whostat/EN_WHS09_Full.pdf. Accessed July 17, 2013.

5. World Health Organization. *Global Burden of Disease Project 2004*. Geneva: World Health Organization; 2004.

6. Tufte ER. *The Visual Display of Quantitative Information*. 2nd ed. Cheshire, CT: Graphics Press; 2001.

7. American Public Health Association. Criteria for assessing the quality of health information on the internet. http://www.apha.org/NR/exeres/412DDD11-42A0-46CB-8705-F9D47A073AF1.htm. Accessed July 17, 2013.

8. National Network of Libraries of Medicine. Health literacy. http://nnlm.gov/outreach/consumer/hlthlit.html. Accessed July 17, 2013.

9. Dawes RM, Hastie R. *Rational Choice in an Uncertain World*. Thousand Oaks, CA: Sage Publications; 2001.

10. Heath C, Heath D. *Made to Stick: Why Some Ideas Survive and Others Die*. New York: Random House; 2007.

11. Heath C, Heath D. *Made to Stick: Why Some Ideas Survive and Others Die*. New York: Random House; 2007:16.

12. Heath C, Heath D. *Made to Stick: Why Some Ideas Survive and Others Die*. New York: Random House; 2007:18.

13. Heath C, Heath D. *Made to Stick: Why Some Ideas Survive and Others Die*. New York: Random House; 2007:21.

14. Riegelman RK. *Studying a Study and Testing a Test: Reading Evidence-based Health Research*. Philadelphia, PA: Lippincott, Williams and Wilkins; 2013.

15. Riegelman RK. *Measures of Medicine: Benefits, Harms and Costs*. Cambridge, MA: Blackwell Science; 1995.

CHAPTER 4

Social and Behavioral Sciences and Public Health

You travel to a country in Asia and find that this nation's culture affects most parts of life. From the food the people eat and their method of cooking, to their attitudes toward medical care, to their beliefs about the cause of disease and the ability to alter it through public health and medical interventions, this country is profoundly different from the United States. You ask: How does culture affect health?

You are working in a country with strict Islamic practices and find that religion, like culture, can have major impacts on health. Religious practices differ widely—from beliefs about food and alcohol; to sexual practices, such as male circumcision and female sexual behavior; to acceptance or rejection of interventions aimed at women's health. You ask: How does religion affect health?

You are trying to help your spouse quit smoking cigarettes and prevent your kids from starting. You know that gentle encouragement and support on a one-on-one basis are essential, but often not enough because cigarette smoking is an addiction that produces withdrawal and long-term cravings. You wonder what other factors in the social system influence behavior and how they can be addressed.

Your efforts to convince your friends to avoid smoking (or stop smoking) focus on giving them the facts about how cigarettes cause lung cancer, throat cancer, and serious heart disease. You are frustrated by how little impact you have on your friends. You wonder what tools are available to better explain and predict health behavior.

Your classmate, who is first in her family to attend college, received word that her father lost his job at the local factory and she needs to take a leave from school because her family can no longer afford tuition. You wonder how this will affect her and her family.

Your town board just approved extending public transportation services to a wider geographic area. Although there are several opponents to the plan, you learn that a group of public health professionals supports this extension of services. You wonder what this transportation plan has to do with health.

You are in the checkout line at the grocery store, and a pregnant mother is ahead of you. You glance at the sugary cereals, snacks, and sodas she is purchasing and happen to notice that she is using an EBT card from the Supplemental Nutrition Assistance Program (SNAP), formerly known as the Food Stamp program. You wonder what could be done to encourage the consumption of healthy food options.

One of your friends asked for your assistance in helping his aunt move from her farm in the rural part of the state into the city center. He explained that his aunt was recently diagnosed with cancer and required regular chemotherapy treatments. You wonder why this diagnosis necessitates a move from a rural to an urban area.

Every day on your way to work, you pass the same homeless man on the same corner. He does not look very old—you guess he is about 25 years of age. You notice that over the past few weeks, he has been coughing, and you figure he must have a cold. Today when you walk by his usual place on the corner, he is not there, but someone has left a sign that reads, "Rest in peace, Ramón." You are surprised, especially because he was so young. You wonder whether there was anything that could have been done to prevent his death.

As a new parent, you hear from your pediatrician, nurses in the hospital, and even

the makers of your brand of diapers that babies should sleep on their backs. They call it "Back-to-Sleep." You are surprised to find that it is part of the class on baby-sitting given by the local community center and a required part of the training for those who work in registered day care centers. You find out that it is all part of a social marketing campaign that has halved the number of deaths from sudden infant death syndrome. You ask: Why has the Back-to-Sleep campaign been so successful?

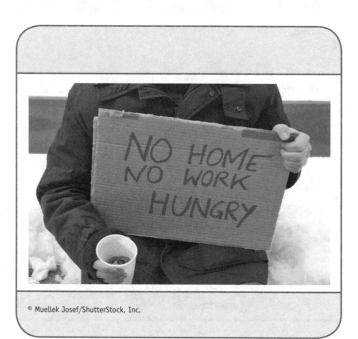

© Muellek Josef/ShutterStock, Inc.

Each of these cases illustrates ways that an understanding of social and behavioral sciences can contribute to an understanding of public health. Let us explore these connections.

HOW IS PUBLIC HEALTH RELATED TO THE SOCIAL AND BEHAVIORAL SCIENCES?

The development of social and behavioral sciences in the 1800s and 1900s is closely connected with the development of public health. These subject areas share a fundamental belief that understanding the organization and motivation behind social forces, along with a better understanding of the behavior of individuals, can be used to improve the lives of individuals, as well as society as a whole.[1]

The 19th century development of social and behavioral sciences, as well as public health, grew out of the Industrial Revolution in Europe, and later in the United States. It was grounded in efforts to address the social and economic inequalities that developed during this period and provided an intellectual and institutional structure for what was and is now called **social justice**. Social justice implies a society that provides fair treatment and a fair share of the rewards of society to individuals and groups of individuals. Early public health reformers advocated for social justice and saw public health as an integral aspect of it.

The intellectual link between social and behavioral sciences and public health is so basic and so deep that it is often taken for granted. For students with opportunities to learn about both social sciences and public health, it is important to understand the key contributions that social sciences make to public health. It is not an exaggeration to view public health as an application of the social sciences, or in other words, as an applied social science. **Table 4-1** summarizes many of the contributions that the social sciences make to public health.

HOW ARE SOCIAL SYSTEMS RELATED TO HEALTH?

Complex Interactions

As humans, we are constantly interacting with our surroundings. Those surroundings include social systems comprised of interactions we have with other people, institutions, communities, and policies. The relationship between individuals and social systems is reciprocal, meaning we influence our social systems and our social systems influence us.

Due to our constant interaction with our surroundings, efforts aimed at improving population health require an understanding of the complex relationship between social systems and health. Medical care is only a piece of the puzzle, considering its focus is to treat disease without addressing the conditions in the social system that contributed to the illness in the first place.

To assist in pulling apart the complex social characteristics that impact health, it is useful to consider different levels of influence within the social system. Socio-ecological models are often employed to gain an understanding of the various social influences on health as well as to assist in

TABLE 4-1 Examples of Contributions of Social and Behavioral Sciences to Public Health

Social science discipline[a]	Examples of disciplinary contributions to public health
Psychology	Theories of the origins of behavior and risk-taking tendencies and methods for altering individual and social behaviors
Sociology	Theories of social development, organizational behavior, and systems thinking; social impacts on individual and group behaviors
Anthropology	Social and cultural influences on individual and population decision making for health with a global perspective
Political science/public policy	Approaches to government and policy making related to public health; structures for policy analysis and the impact of government on public health decision making
Economics	Understanding the micro- and macroeconomic impact on public health and health-care systems
Communications	Theory and practice of mass and personalized communication and the role of media in communicating health information and health risks
Demography	Understanding demographic changes in populations globally due to aging, migration, and differences in birth rates, plus their impact on health and society
Geography	Understanding the impacts of geography on disease and determinants of disease, as well as methods for displaying and tracking the location of disease occurrence

[a] A similar list of contributions of the humanities could be developed including the contributions of literature, the arts, history, philosophy, and ethics. These contributions of the social sciences are in addition to contributions of the sciences, mathematics, and humanities. Biology, chemistry, and statistics underpin much of epidemiology and environmental health. Languages and culture, history, and the arts provide key contributions to health communications and health policy. Thus, a broad arts and sciences education is often considered a key part of preparation for public health.

identifying points at which to intervene. In general, the levels of influence include:

- Individual lifestyle factors: Characteristics of the individual, including knowledge, attitudes, beliefs, and personality traits, as well as age, sex, and hereditary factors.
- Social and community networks: Points at which interaction with other individuals occurs. This sphere of influence can further be divided into the following levels:
  - Interpersonal: Family, friends, and peers who shape social identity, support, and roles.
  - Institutional/organizational: Rules and regulations of institutions, such as schools and places of employment, that may limit or promote healthy behavior.
  - Community: Comprises informal and formal social networks and norms formed among individuals, groups, and organizations, including cultural and religious practices.
- General socioeconomic, cultural, and environmental conditions: Components of the surroundings external to individuals that comprise living and working conditions, such as education, housing, work environment, and healthcare services. These conditions are shaped by public policy and laws at the local, state, and federal levels.

Influencing Behavior

The complex relationship between social systems and individuals affects health through individual behavior. Berkman and Kawachi argue that social systems influence behavior by[2]:

1. Shaping norms: Certain behaviors may become generally accepted among social groups. An attitude of "everyone else is doing it" can have a strong influence on an individual's decision to partake in the activity. For example, in some communities, perhaps it is rare for anyone to wear a helmet while biking. So an individual who has always used a bicycle helmet in the past may decide to forego it because nobody else wears one in his new community.
2. Enforcing patterns of social control: Having rules and regulations in place creates structure for society, which can affect health. For instance, having a curfew for teenagers to be off the streets by 9:00 p.m. unless accompanied by an adult may assist in preventing violence.
3. Providing or not providing opportunities to engage in certain behaviors: The opportunities, or lack thereof, in our surroundings can have a strong influence on our health. For instance, having access to a community pool can encourage individuals to learn to swim, thus preventing drowning, while also serving as a form of physical exercise and social cohesion.
4. Reducing or producing stress for which certain behaviors may be an effective coping strategy, at least in the short term: For example, college students often go through stressful periods throughout their academic career, particularly around exam time. Some students may decide to cope with this stress by "blowing off steam." This can take many forms, from binge drinking to going for a run, each choice having an effect on health.

We have explored the complex relationship between social systems and individuals. Let us now look at three key components of the social system and their relationship to health: socioeconomic status, culture, and religion.

HOW DO SOCIOECONOMIC STATUS, CULTURE, AND RELIGION AFFECT HEALTH?

Socioeconomic Status

Beginning in the 1800s, social scientists developed the concept of **socioeconomic status**. They also developed elaborate systems to operationalize the definition of "socioeconomic status" and classify individuals. In the United States, the definition has generally included measures that are primarily economic, including:[a]

- family income
- educational level or parents' educational level
- professional status or parents' professional status

In developed countries such as the United States, health status, at least as measured by life expectancy, is strongly associated with socioeconomic status.[3, 4] Greater longevity is associated with higher social status, with a gradient of increasing longevity from lowest to highest on the socioeconomic scale. **Box 4-1** provides greater detail on this important relationship.

We understand many, but not all, of the ways that socioeconomic factors affect health. Greater economic wealth usually implies access to healthier living conditions. Improved sanitation, less crowding, greater access to health care, and safer methods for cooking and eating are all strongly associated with higher economic status in developed, as well as developing, countries.

Education is also strongly associated with better health. It may change health outcomes and increase longevity by

---

[a] A more formal social hierarchy has traditionally existed in Europe. European social scientists utilized the concept of social class when categorizing individuals by socioeconomic status. In Europe, economics alone was not thought to be adequate to explain socioeconomic status or categorize individuals.

BOX 4-1 Income and Population Health

Health status as measured by life expectancy has been found to improve with increasing average gross domestic product (GDP), up to a threshold of about $10,000 per person, which is the current level for the many successful middle income developing nations. The United States currently has an average GDP above $40,000.

Once this threshold of adequate income is reached, the health status of countries does not continue to steadily rise as income increases. At these higher levels of GDP, as seen in most developed countries, income disparities are a better predictor of life expectancy than absolute levels of average GDP. Developed countries with lower levels of income disparity, such as Japan, Canada, Sweden, and France, have longer life expectancies than countries such as the United States and the United Kingdom, which have greater income disparities.

Even in countries with modest levels of income disparities, a **socioeconomic gradient** of health status exists such that individuals with a higher socioeconomic status tend to have better health outcomes compared to those with a lower socioeconomic status. This gradient can be viewed as a ladder in that moving down the socioeconomic ladder, more ill health and shorter life expectancy are experienced at each rung. Therefore, socioeconomic determinants of health do not solely affect the very poorest or those in the lowest socioeconomic levels but are rather an issue throughout all income levels.

An argument has been made that poorer health leads to lower income and not the other way around. There is little evidence that this phenomenon explains the socioeconomic factors that affect health. Education level is an even stronger predictor of life expectancy than income, and education levels are usually well established before poor health develops. Education level, income level, and professional status are three key components of socioeconomic status as measured in the United States. Therefore, it may be more accurate to say that disparities in socioeconomic status are associated with poorer population health status.

A measure that has been adapted to calculate economic inequity across populations is the **Gini index**, also known as the Gini coefficient. This is a commonly used measure of income distribution, with an index ranging from 0 to 1, with higher values indicating greater inequality. A Gini index of 0 indicates complete income equality (everyone has the same income), and 1 indicates complete inequality in income (one individual receives all the income). Oftentimes, for ease of reporting and drawing comparisons, the index is multiplied by 100 so that the values range from 0 to 100. The index measures the extent of deviation between an economy's distribution of income among individuals or households and that of perfectly equal distribution.

Among developed countries, income inequality is strongly associated with higher rates of mortality. Countries with a wider gap between the poorest of the poor and richest of the rich (a Gini index closer to 1) experience poorer population health outcomes on measures such as infant mortality and life expectancy, compared to countries with a narrow gap between rich and poor (a Gini index closer to 0).[5, 6]

The U.S. Gini index is approximately 45, compared to 34 in the United Kingdom, 32.7 in France, 32.1 in Canada, 27 in Germany, and 23 in Sweden. The United States has the highest Gini index of major developed countries.[6]

Place matters. Some Americans will die twenty years earlier than others who live just a short distance away because of differences in education, income, race, ethnicity, and where and how they live. One classical study revealed dramatic disparities in life expectancy across U.S. counties overall, and particularly when racial or ethnic differences were also considered. For example, black men in the county with the shortest life expectancy for blacks lived approximately 60 years, while white men in the county with the longest life expectancy for whites could expect to live two decades longer.[7, 8a]

---

[a] The association between socioeconomic status and longevity is most strongly associated with an individual's socioeconomic status as an adult. The socioeconomic status of an individual's parents has a much weaker association. This suggests that genetic factors have little to do with the association between socioeconomic status and life expectancy. Education has a stronger association with health status than income or professional status. Lower socioeconomic status leads to poor health rather than poor health leading to lower socioeconomic status. Socioeconomic factors are associated with an increase in relative risk of death of 1.5 to 2.0 when comparing the lowest and highest socioeconomic groups. This means that those in the lowest group have more than a 50% increase in the death rate compared to the highest group. This relative risk steadily increases as the socioeconomic level decreases. The relationship has a dose-response relationship; that is, there is an increase in longevity with every increase in socioeconomic status. Thus, the impact is not limited to those with the lowest status. The largest contributors to the differences in the death rate are cardiovascular disease, violence, and, increasingly, AIDS; however, the death rate is impacted in general by a wide range of diseases—most being malignancies and infectious diseases.[9]

encouraging behaviors that provide protection against disease and likewise reduce exposure to behaviors that put individuals at risk of disease. Higher education levels, coupled with the increased resources that greater wealth can provide, may increase access to better medical care and provide greater ability to protect against health hazards.

Individuals of lower socioeconomic status are more likely to be exposed to health hazards at work and in the physical environment through toxic exposure in the air they breathe, in the water they drink, and in the food they eat. **Table 4-2** outlines a number of mechanisms by which socioeconomic status can directly and indirectly influence health.

These factors, while important, do not explain the entire observed differences in life expectancy among individuals of different socioeconomic status. For instance, the rates of coronary heart disease are considerably higher among those of lower socioeconomic status—even after taking into account cigarette smoking, high blood pressure, cholesterol levels, and blood sugar counts.[9]

Considerable research is now being directed to better understand these and other effects of socioeconomic status. One theory suggests that social control and social participation may help explain these substantial differences in health. It contends that control over individual and group decision making is much greater among individuals of higher socioeconomic status. The theory holds that the ability to control

one's life may be associated with biological changes that affect health and disease.[9] Additional research is needed to confirm or reject this idea and/or provide an adequate explanation for these important, yet unexplained, differences in health based upon socioeconomic status.

Culture

Culture, in a broad sense, helps people make judgments about the world and decisions about behavior. Culture defines what is good or bad, and what is healthy or unhealthy. This may relate to lifestyle patterns, beliefs about risk, and beliefs about body type—for example, a large body type in some cultures symbolizes health and well-being, not overweight or other negative conditions.

Culture directly affects the daily habits of life. Food choice and methods of food preparation and preservation are all affected by culture, as well as socioeconomic status. The Mediterranean diet, which includes olive oil, seafood, vegetables, nuts, and fruits, has been shown to have benefits for the heart even when used in countries far removed from the Mediterranean.

There are often clear-cut negative and/or positive impacts on disability related to cultural traditions as diverse as feet binding in China and female genital mutilation in some parts of Africa. Some societies reject strenuous physical activity for those who have the status and wealth to be served by others.

TABLE 4-2 Examples of Ways that Socioeconomic Status May Affect Health

Ways	Examples
Living conditions	Increases in sanitation, reductions in crowding, methods of heating and cooking
Overall educational opportunities	Education has the strongest association with health behaviors and health outcomes May be due to better appreciation of factors associated with disease and greater ability to control these factors
Educational opportunities for women	Education for women has an impact on the health of children and families
Occupational exposures	Lower socioeconomic jobs are traditionally associated with increased exposures to health risks
Access to goods and services	Ability to access goods, such as protective devices, and high-quality foods and services, including medical and social services to protect and promote health
Family size	Large family size affects health and is traditionally associated with lower socioeconomic status and lower health status
Exposures to high-risk behaviors	Social alienation related to poverty may be associated with violence, drugs, and other high-risk behaviors
Environmental	Lower socioeconomic status is associated with greater exposure to environmental pollution, "natural" disasters, and dangers of the "built environment"

TABLE 4-3 Examples of Ways that Culture Can Affect Health

Ways that culture may affect health	Examples
Culture is related to behavior—social practices may put individuals and groups at increased or reduced risk	Food preferences—vegetarian, Mediterranean diet Cooking methods History of binding of feet in China Female genital mutilation Role of exercise
Culture is related to response to symptoms, such as the level of urgency to recognize symptoms, seek care, and communicate symptoms	Cultural differences in seeking care and self-medication Social, family, and work structures provide varying degree of social support—low degree of social support may be associated with reduced health-related quality of life
Culture is related to the types of interventions that are acceptable	Variations in degree of acceptance of traditional Western medicine, including reliance on self-help and traditional healers
Culture is related to the response to disease and to interventions	Cultural differences in follow-up, adherence to treatment, and acceptance of adverse outcome

Culture is also related to an individual's response to symptoms and acceptance of interventions. In many cultures, medical care is exclusively for those with symptoms and is not part of prevention. Many traditional cultures have developed sophisticated systems of self-care and self-medication supported by family and traditional healers. These traditions greatly affect how individuals respond to symptoms, how they communicate the symptoms, and the types of medical and public health interventions that they will accept.

Many cultures allow and even encourage the use of traditional approaches alongside Western medical and public health approaches. In some cultures, traditional healers are considered appropriate for health problems whose causes are not thought to be biological, but instead related to spiritual and other phenomena. Recent studies of alternative, or complementary, medicine have provided evidence that specific traditional interventions, such as acupuncture and specific osteopathic and chiropractic manipulation, have measurable benefits. Thus, cultural differences should not be viewed as problems to be addressed, but rather as practices to be understood. **Table 4-3** summarizes a number of the ways that culture can affect health.

Religion

Social factors affecting health include religion along with culture. Religion can have a major impact on health, particularly for specific practices that are encouraged or condemned by a particular religious group. For instance, we now know that male circumcision reduces susceptibility to HIV/AIDS.

Religious attitudes that condone or condemn the use of condoms, alcohol, and tobacco have direct and indirect impacts on health as well.

Some religions prohibit specific healing practices, such as blood transfusions or abortion, or totally reject medical interventions altogether, as is practiced by Christian Scientists. Religious individuals may see medical and public health interventions as complementary to religious practice or may substitute prayer for medical interventions in response to symptoms of disease. **Table 4-4** outlines some of the ways that religion may affect health.

We have examined a number of ways that the broad social influences of socioeconomic status, culture, and religion may affect health and the response to disease. Let us now explore additional social factors that determine health.

WHAT ARE SOCIAL DETERMINANTS OF HEALTH?

A subset of all the determinants of health, **social determinants of health** refer to the conditions in which people are born, grow up, live, learn, work, play, worship, and age, as well as the systems put in place to deal with illnesses that affect health and quality of life. These conditions are shaped by a wider set of forces, including economics, social policies, and politics.[10, 11]

Although there is no universally agreed upon set of social determinants, the following categories highlighted by the World Health Organization encompass many key social determinants that affect health. Each individual has his or her unique combination of influences; however, patterns

TABLE 4-4 Examples of Ways that Religion May Affect Health

Ways that religion affects health	Examples
Religion may affect social practices that put individuals at increased or reduced risk	Sexual: circumcision, use of contraceptives Food: avoidance of seafood, pork, beef Alcohol use: part of religion versus prohibited Tobacco use: actively discouraged by Mormons and Seventh-Day Adventists as part of their religion
Religion may affect the response to symptoms	Christian Scientists reject medical care as a response to symptoms
Religion may affect the types of interventions that are acceptable	Prohibition against blood transfusions Attitudes toward stem cell research Attitudes toward abortion End-of-life treatments
Religion may affect the response to disease and to interventions	Role of prayer as an intervention to alter outcome

have been observed and are summarized in the following sections.[12, 13] Notice that these social determinants should not be viewed in isolation because they often interact with each other.

10 Key Categories of Social Determinants of Health

Social Status

Societies place value on certain characteristics such that a hierarchical social structure is formed. In the United States, value tends to be placed on income, education, and occupation, which collectively form socioeconomic status. Social status interacts and influences many of the other social determinants of health.

Social Support or Alienation

Being part of a social network has benefits to health, including emotional effects associated with feelings of inclusion and tangible benefits, such as having someone to go jogging with or having someone to provide a ride to the doctor's office. Social exclusion can occur due to racism, discrimination, and other forms of marginalization, limiting the opportunities for education, leisure activities, and other community services, either directly through discriminatory practices or as a consequence of cumulative exposure to discrimination resulting in fear, anger, distrust, or stress so that individuals do not seek out such opportunities.

Food

An inadequate or insecure food source remains an issue for disadvantaged populations in the United States and around the world. However, excess calorie intake and the lack of a nutritious diet is a rapidly growing problem. Not only is education important in being aware of what constitutes a good diet, but having access to affordable, healthy food is also a central component of leading a healthy lifestyle. A **food desert** is a term used to describe geographic areas that lack grocery stores and other establishments in which low-income individuals are able to purchase nutritious food due to high prices or inaccessibility. Although these areas may have food available, the options easily accessible via public transportation and price to low-income families often include unhealthy food such as that offered at convenience stores and fast food establishments.

Housing

Having affordable, stable housing influences health in a number of ways. Homelessness can lead to malnutrition, lack of medical care, drug use, and violence. Therefore, those with a home tend to have better overall health compared to those without; however, hazards can also be present in the home, including lack of clean water and sanitation, asthma triggers such as mold and dust, lead paint, cockroaches, inadequate sanitation, and unsafe structural conditions.

Education

Even within the same overall socioeconomic status, those with more education tend to experience better health compared to those with less education. Efforts to address health should, therefore, include making quality education at all levels widely accessible to populations. In the United States, increasing the high school graduation rate is now a leading indicator of *Healthy People 2020,* a collaborative initiative of the United States Department of Health and Human Services which guides the national prevention agenda.

Work

Several aspects of work can affect health. Overall, being employed tends to be better for health compared to being unemployed. This is partially attributed to the connection between socioeconomic status and health. Having an income assists a person's ability to secure resources that may protect and promote health, such as safe housing, food, and education. Being employed can also assist in accessing health services if the employer provides health insurance to its employees. Type of employment can also affect health. Some jobs are more hazardous to health than others. Health effects associated with work are not restricted to physical health because work can also affect mental health. Job satisfaction and stress in the workplace contribute to health. Those who are unemployed also face psychological consequences due to the anxiety and stress that can be associated with lack of job security and inability to adequately provide for their families.

Stress

Stress is a social and psychological response with biological consequences. A variety of circumstances can create anxiety and worry, whether it is an intense work setting or the threat of losing one's home. Sustained periods of stress can negatively affect physical health due to the body's fight or flight response, which increases the heart rate and cortisol levels. Over time, stress can lead to such conditions as cardiovascular disease and depression.

Transportation

A component of environmental health, transportation also affects health in a number of ways. By driving less and walking/cycling more and using mass transit, people increase their physical activity levels. It is becoming even more important to find ways to integrate physical activity into our lives as lifestyles in the United States grow increasingly sedentary and obesity is on the rise. Opting for walking, cycling, and mass transit also increases social contact, which can serve as a protective health factor. Relying less on cars also reduces air and noise pollution, contributing to environmental health as well. Therefore, city planning can have an impact on health.

Place

Where you live affects your health. For example, those living in rural areas have fewer healthcare services available nearby, whereas those living in urban areas are exposed to increased air pollution from factories and vehicles. The built environment also affects health in that it influences whether there are safe places to be physically active, including walking and biking trails and green spaces, as well as easy access to nutritious food.

Access to Health Services

Having access to preventive health services and medical care contributes to overall health. Access to such services is often limited by health insurance. On a broader scale, having an appropriate number and type of healthcare professionals is instrumental to maintaining the health of individuals and populations.

HOW DO SOCIAL DETERMINANTS AFFECT HEALTH?

Social determinants of health contribute to a wide variety of illnesses and diseases rooted in lifestyle, environmental, and social factors. Recent increased attention on social determinants of health has been driven by their connection with **health disparities**. A health disparity is a type of difference in health that is closely linked with social or economic disadvantage. Health disparities negatively affect groups of people who have systematically experienced greater social or economic obstacles to health. These obstacles stem from characteristics historically linked to discrimination or exclusion, such as race or ethnicity, religion, socioeconomic status, gender, disability, mental health, sexual orientation, and geographic location.[b]

Disparities occur in a wide range of health conditions, including communicable and noncommunicable diseases and environmental health and safety. **Table 4-5** provides a few examples of conditions in which disparities occur within the U.S. population.

It is important to note that social determinants affect not only physical health, but mental health as well. **Mental health** is a state of successful performance of mental function, resulting in productive activities, fulfilling relationships with other people, and the ability to adapt to change and to cope with challenges.[14] Mental illness refers to all diagnosable mental disorders, which are health conditions characterized by alterations in thinking, mood, and/or behavior associated with distress and/or impaired functioning. Examples of mental disorders are depression, anxiety, bipolar disorder, schizophrenia, and dementia. Mental disorders are the leading cause of disability in the United States, with approximately 1 in 17 U.S. adults exhibiting a debilitating mental illness in any

---

[b] When discussing differences in health, a variety of terms are used, each with a slightly different focus. In addition to "health disparity," other terms include **healthcare disparity**, **health equity**, **health inequity**, and **health inequality**.

TABLE 4-5 Disparities in Health, United States

Noncommunicable Disease
Coronary heart disease: Black men and women are much more likely to die of heart disease and stroke compared to white men and women.
Colorectal cancer screening: Disparities in colorectal cancer screening rates exist based on education level and income. As education increases, screening for colorectal cancer also increases. The same pattern exists for income level: as income increases, screening rates increase.

Environmental Health and Safety
Air pollution: Local sources of air pollution, often in urban areas, can impact the health of people who live or work near these sources. Everyone in these areas, regardless of socioeconomic status, can experience the negative health effects of air pollution; however, because racial/ethnic minority groups are more likely to live in the most polluted sections of urban areas, they continue to experience a disproportionately larger impact.
Motor vehicle crashes: Men of all races/ethnicities are two to three times more likely to die in motor vehicle crashes than are women, and death rates are twice as high among American Indians/Alaska Natives.

Communicable Disease
HIV: Racial/ethnic minorities, with the exception of Asians/Pacific Islanders, experience disproportionately higher rates of new human immunodeficiency virus diagnoses than whites, as do men who have sex with men (MSM). In addition, rates are increasing among black and American Indian/Alaska Native males, as well as MSM, while rates hold steady or are decreasing in other groups.
Influenza vaccination: Whites aged 65 years and older consistently have higher rates of influenza vaccine coverage compared to all other races/ethnicities in this age group, with non-Hispanic blacks experiencing the lowest rates of flu vaccine coverage.

Data from the Centers for Disease Control and Prevention. CDC Health Disparities and Inequalities Report – United States, 2011. *Morbidity and Mortality Weekly Report.* Supplement / Vol. 60. January 14, 2011.

given year.[14] The suicide rate increased by over 10% among the U.S. population between 1999 and 2008, and it varies by race and ethnicity, with the highest rate observed among the white non-Hispanic population in the United States.[15]

Mental health is not only essential to successful function in and contribution to society but it can also impact physical health. For example, depression may prohibit an individual's desire and motivation to exercise and seek out nutritious food, contributing to chronic conditions such as cardiovascular disease and diabetes. Therefore, understanding the factors, both internal and external to the individual, contributing to emotional, psychological, and social well-being is critical in addressing population health. National objectives, as part of *Healthy People 2020*, have been set to improve mental health status and expand mental health screening and treatment services.

CAN HEALTH BEHAVIOR BE CHANGED?

Much of the preventable disease and disability today in the United States and other developed countries is related to the behavior of individuals. From cigarette smoking to obesity, from intentional to unintentional injuries, from sexual behavior to drug abuse, health issues can be traced to the behavior of individuals.

Consider all the behaviors related to health. Some are intentional health behaviors, while others are not necessarily motivated by health concerns. Getting a mammogram could be an example of an intentional health behavior because it is a behavior most likely undertaken for health benefits—in this case, screening for breast cancer. However, driving the speed limit may be a behavior that has an effect on health but is undertaken not because the individual is concerned about the health benefits of doing so (avoiding injury from a motor vehicle crash) but because he or she wants to avoid getting a ticket. Therefore, in order to have an impact on health, a wide range of behavioral motivations and factors needs to be addressed.

At times, we hear discouraging messages that behavior cannot be changed. However, if we take a relatively long-term view, we find that there are many examples of behavioral change that have occurred for the better. For instance:

- Cigarette smoking in the United States among males has been reduced from approximately 50% in the 1960s to approximately 20% today.

- Infants today generally are placed on their backs for sleeping and napping and not on their stomachs, as was the usual practice in the 1980s and earlier. Back-to-Sleep campaigns are believed to have reduced sudden infant death syndrome (SIDS) by nearly 50% in the United States.
- Seat belt use in the United States has increased from less than 25% in the 1970s to over 80% currently.
- Drunk driving in the United States has been dramatically reduced, with a resulting decline in automobile-related fatalities.
- Mammography use increased by approximately 50% during the 1990s and has been credited with beginning to reduce the previously rising mortality rates from breast cancer.

The potential to change behavior can make health worse as well. The following changes for the worse have also occurred in the United States in recent years:

- Over the last three decades, Americans have increased their caloric intake and reduced their average amount of exercise, resulting in more than doubling the obesity rate to over 33% of all adults.
- Between the 1960s and the 1990s, teenage girls and young adult women increased their cigarette smoking, subjecting their unborn children to additional hazards of low birthweight.

Thus, behavioral change is possible for the better and for the worse. Some behaviors, however, are easier to change than others. Let's take a look at why this is.

WHY ARE SOME INDIVIDUAL HEALTH BEHAVIORS EASIER TO CHANGE THAN OTHERS?

Some behaviors are relatively easy to change, while others are extremely difficult. Being able to recognize the difference is an important place to start when trying to alter behavior. It is relatively easy when one behavior can be substituted for a similar one and results in a potentially large payoff. In these situations, knowledge often goes a long way. For instance, the substitution of acetaminophen (Tylenol) for aspirin to prevent Reye's Syndrome was relatively easy. Similarly, the Back-to-Sleep campaign was quite successful in reducing the rate of death from SIDS. In both of these cases, an acceptable and convenient substitute was available, making the needed behavioral change much easier to accomplish.

Along with knowledge, incentives—such as reduced cost, increased availability, or improvements in ease of use—can encourage rapid acceptance and motivate behavioral

change. For instance, easier-to-install child restraint systems have increased their use. Greater insurance coverage and widespread availability of modern mammography equipment has led to an increase in the number of mammograms performed.

The most difficult behaviors to change are those that have a physiological component, such as obesity, or an addictive element, such as cigarette smoking. Individual interventions aimed at smoking cessation or long-term weight control generally succeed less than 30% of the time—even among motivated individuals. Even intensive interventions with highly motivated individuals cannot be expected to be successful more than 50% of the time, as was illustrated by the Multiple Risk Factor Intervention Trial (MRFIT), which attempted intensive interventions to reduce risk factors for cardiovascular disease.

In addition, physical, social, and economic barriers can stand in the way of behavior change, even if individuals themselves are motivated. If health care is not accessible, or if survival needs require individuals to engage in risks they might not take otherwise, change in behavior may be impeded.

Successful behavioral change requires that we understand as much as we can about how behavior can be changed and what we can do to help.

HOW CAN INDIVIDUAL BEHAVIOR BE CHANGED?

The behavior of individuals is often the final common pathway through which disease, disability, and death can be prevented. The fact that individual behavior has a clearly observable connection with these factors does not necessarily imply that the best or only way to address the behavior of individuals is to focus exclusively on individuals. The forces at work to mold individual behaviors are sometimes referred to as **downstream factors, mainstream factors,** and **upstream factors.** Downstream factors are those that directly involve an individual and can potentially be altered by individual interventions, such as an addiction to nicotine. Mainstream factors are those that result from the relationship of an individual with a larger group or population, such as peer pressure to smoke or the level of taxation on cigarettes. These factors require attention at the group or population level. Finally, upstream factors are often grounded in social structures and policies, such as government-sponsored programs that encourage tobacco production. These require us to look beyond traditional health care and public health interventions to the broader social and economic forces that affect health.

Thus, changes in behavior often require more than individual motivation and determination to change. They require encouragement and support from groups ranging from friends and families to work and peer groups. Behavioral change may also require social policies and expectations that reinforce individual efforts.

HOW CAN HEALTH BEHAVIOR BE EXPLAINED AND PREDICTED?

When addressing issues affecting the health of populations, behaviors contributing to these issues must be explored and understood. But what tools do we have to understand these behaviors? A **theory** is a set of interrelated concepts that presents a systematic view of relationships among variables in order to explain and predict events and situations. Similarly, a **model** is a combination of ideas and concepts taken from multiple theories and applied to specific problems in particular settings. Theories and models are tools commonly used by health researchers and health practitioners to gain insight into why people behave in healthy or unhealthy ways and to guide the development and evaluation of interventions aimed at changing behavior to improve health.

Because theories present a systematic way to understand events or situations, linking various factors and elements together, they provide a useful framework to study health problems, develop appropriate interventions, and evaluate the impact of the interventions. Theory serves as a road map for research and practice, exploring the "why," "what," and "how" of health issues and their solutions. In accordance with evidence-based public health principles, interventions developed based on theory and supported by evidence using these theories are more likely to succeed than those that were not.

Let us take a look at a few examples of theories and their application to health behavior.

WHAT ARE SOME KEY THEORIES AND MODELS USED TO ADDRESS HEALTH BEHAVIOR?

Many theories and models are used in health behavior research and practice. A few key theories and models will be highlighted here. Theories and models are categorized according to three levels of influence:

- Intrapersonal: Focusing on characteristics of the individual, including knowledge, attitudes, beliefs, motivation, self-concept, past experiences, and skills
- Interpersonal: Focusing on relationships between people, acknowledging that other people influence behavior by sharing their thoughts, advice, feelings, emotional support, and other assistance

- Population and community: Focusing on factors within social structures, such as norms, rules, regulations, policies, and laws

Intrapersonal Level

Health promotion and health education efforts set out to raise awareness of health issues among individuals; therefore, a number of intrapersonal theories and models exist, focusing on factors within the individual that influence behavior, such as knowledge, attitudes, beliefs, and skills.

One of the original theories of health behavior that remains among the most widely recognized today is the **Health Belief Model**. The model, developed in the 1950s by a group of U.S. Public Health Service social psychologists, originated out of a desire to understand why so few people were taking advantage of a free mobile x-ray unit to screen for tuberculosis (TB).[16] The social psychologists theorized that people's readiness to act was influenced by their beliefs about whether or not they were susceptible to TB and their perceptions of the benefits of screening for the disease.

The Health Belief Model is an intrapersonal theory, as it focuses on individuals' characteristics, including their perceptions and thought processes prior to taking health-related action. The premise of the model is that personal beliefs influence health behavior. The model proposes that people will be more likely to take action if they believe they are susceptible to the condition; they believe the condition has serious consequences; they believe taking action would benefit them, with the benefits outweighing the harms; and they are exposed to factors that prompt action and believe in their ability to successfully perform the action. **Table 4-6** summarizes the model's constructs and their application to osteoporosis.

Another widely used intrapersonal model is the **Transtheoretical Model**, also referred to as the **Stages of Change Model**. The underlying assumption of this model is that people go through a set of incremental stages when changing behavior rather than making significant changes all at once.[17] c

---

c Designing interventions based upon the Stages of Change model has not been uniformly successful. One potential reason for this may be that individuals are often in different stages of change for different types of interventions. With complex interventions, such as those required to address obesity, an individual may be in one stage of change for exercise, another for adding fruits and vegetables to his/her diet, and a different stage in terms of calorie reduction. A critique of this model is that people do not always go through the set of stages consecutively, but instead may revert back to an earlier stage before moving through the other stages.

TABLE 4-6 Health Belief Model and Osteoporosis

Construct	Description	Example: osteoporosis
Perceived susceptibility	An individual's opinion of getting a condition	"Osteoporosis only happens to old women, not me."
Perceived severity	An individual's opinion of how serious a condition is and its consequences	"Osteoporosis is not a big deal."
Perceived benefits	An individual's belief in the advised action to reduce risk and/or severity of condition	"Screening for osteoporosis will catch it early so I can continue to live an active lifestyle."
Perceived barriers	An individual's belief of the costs (tangible and psychological) of the advised action	"Screening for osteoporosis takes too much time."
Modifying variables	Individual characteristics that influence personal perceptions	"Women in my culture are viewed as strong; therefore, we do not concern ourselves with osteoporosis."
Cues to action	Strategies/events that encourage one's "readiness" to act	"My sister was recently diagnosed with osteoporosis, so I should get screened."
Self-efficacy	Belief in one's ability to take action	"If I am diagnosed with osteoporosis, I know I can manage it."

Data from National Cancer Institute. U.S. Department of Health and Human Services. *Theory at a Glance: A Guide for Health Promotion Practice*. 2nd edition. Available at: http://www.cancer.gov/cancertopics/cancerlibrary/theory.pdf. Accessed August 5, 2013.

The first stage, called precontemplation, implies that an individual has not yet considered changing his or her behavior. At this stage, efforts to encourage change are not likely to be successful. However, efforts to educate and offer help in the future may lay the groundwork for later success.

The second phase, known as contemplation, implies that an individual is actively thinking about the benefits and barriers to change. At this stage, information focused on short- and immediate-term gains, as well as long-term benefits, can be especially useful. In addition, the contemplation stage lends itself to developing a baseline—that is, establishing the current severity or extent of the problem in order to measure future progress.

The third phase is called preparation. During this phase, the individual is developing a plan of action. At this point, the individual may be especially receptive to setting goals, considering a range of strategies, and developing a timetable. Help in recognizing and preparing for unanticipated barriers can be especially useful to the individual during this phase.

The fourth phase is the action phase, when the change in behavior takes place. This is the time to bring together all possible outside support to reinforce and reward the new behavior and help with problems or setbacks that occur.

The fifth—and hopefully final—phase is the maintenance phase, in which the new behavior becomes a permanent part of an individual's lifestyle. The maintenance phase requires education on how to anticipate the long-term nature of behavioral change, especially how to resist the inevitable temptations to resume the old behavior. Using cigarette smoking as illustration again, **Table 4-7** summarizes the stages of behavioral change and the specific actions that can be helpful at each of the stages.

A third widely used intrapersonal theory is the **Theory of Planned Behavior**. This theory is based on the idea that intention is the main predictor of behavior. The theory proposes that behavioral intention is influenced by an individual's attitude toward performing a behavior, his or her beliefs about whether people important to him or her approve or disapprove of the behavior, and his or her beliefs about their control over performing the behavior. According to the theory, intention determines whether someone will engage in a behavior; therefore, interventions based on the Theory of Planned Behavior set out to affect individuals' intention to perform a behavior.[18] **Figure 4-1** illustrates the theory's constructs in relation to getting a flu vaccine.

Interpersonal Level

Interpersonal theories and models take into consideration the influences of other people on an individual's behavior. These other people can include family members, peers, coworkers, healthcare providers, etc., and they can influence

TABLE 4-7 Stages of Change Model and Cigarette Smoking

Stages of change	Actions	Example: cigarette smoking
Precontemplation	*Prognosticate*	
Individual not considering change	Assessing readiness for change— timing is key	Determine individual's readiness to quit. If not ready, indicate receptivity to help in the future. Look for receptive timing, such as during acute respiratory symptoms Social factors, such as workplace and indoor restriction on smoking and taxation, increase likelihood of entering precontemplation phase
Contemplation	*Motivate change*	
Individual thinks actively about the health risk and action required to reduce that risk Issue of change is on the individual's agenda but no action is planned	Provide information focused on short and intermediate gains from behavioral change, as well as long-term benefits Doubtful, dire, and distant impacts are less effective	Reinforce increase in exercise level, reduction in cough, financial savings, serving as example to children, protection of fetus, etc. Continue to inform of longer term effects on health
	Establish baseline to assess severity of the problem; focus attention on the problem and provide basis for comparison	Develop log of timing, frequency, and quantity of smoking, as well as associated events
Preparation	*Plan change*	
Prepare for action, including developing a plan and setting a timetable	Set specific measurable and obtainable goals with deadlines	Quit date or possible tapering if heavy smoker
	Two or more well-chosen simultaneous interventions may maximize effectiveness	Family support, peer support, individual planning, medication, etc., may reinforce and multiply impacts
	Recognize habitual nature of existing behavior and remove associated activities	Remove cigarettes, ashtrays, and other associated smoking equipment Remove personal and environmental impacts of past smoking, such as teeth cleaning and cleaning of drapery Anticipate temptations, such as associations with food, drink, and social occasions
Action	*Reinforce change*	
Observable changes in behavior with potential for relapse	Provide/suggest tangible rewards	Provide rewards, such as alternative use of money, focus on personal hygiene or personal environment
	Positive feedback and encouragement of new behavior Anticipate adverse effects and frustrations	Focus on measurable progress toward new behavior Provide receptive environment, but avoid focus on excuses Take short-term, one-day-at-a-time approach Recognize potential for symptoms to worsen at first before improvement occurs Anticipate potential for weight gain and encourage exercise and other behaviors to reduce potential for weight gain
	Utilize group/peer support	Family and peer reinforcement critical during action phase

TABLE 4-7 Stages of Change Model and Cigarette Smoking (*continued*)

Stages of change	Actions	Example: cigarette smoking
Maintenance	*Maintain change*	
New behavior needs to be consolidated as part of permanent lifestyle change	Practice/reinforce methods for maintaining new behavior	Avoid old associations and prepare/practice response when encountering old circumstances
	Recognize long-term nature of behavioral change and need for supportive peers and social reinforcement	Negative social attitudes toward smoking among peers and society along with social restrictions, such as limiting public indoor smoking, and social actions, such as taxation, help prevent smoking and reinforce maintenance of cessation

Data from Prochaska JO, DiClemente CC. Stages and processes of self-change of smoking: toward an integrative model of change. *J Consult Clin Psychol*. 1983;51:390–395.

FIGURE 4-1 Theory of Planned Behavior and Flu Vaccine

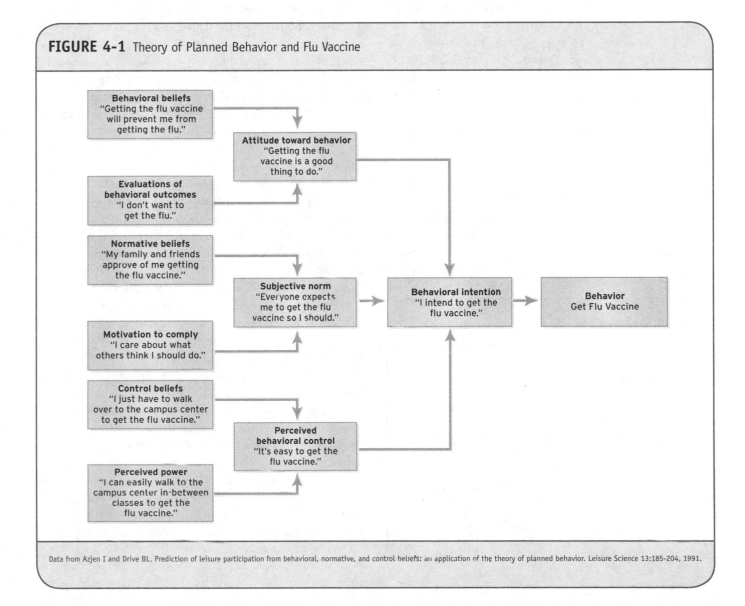

Data from Azjen I and Drive BL. Prediction of leisure participation from behavioral, normative, and control beliefs: an application of the theory of planned behavior. Leisure Science 13:185-204, 1991.

behavior by sharing their advice, feelings, and opinions and through the support and assistance they provide.

One of the most commonly used interpersonal theories is the **Social Cognitive Theory**. The Social Ccognitive Theory, originally known as the Social Learning Theory, focuses on the interaction between individuals and their social systems. According to the theory, changing behavior requires an understanding of:

- Individual characteristics, such as knowledge, skills, and beliefs
- Influences in the social and physical environment, such as peer influence, level of family support, characteristics of the neighborhood, and work and school environments that help or hinder opportunities for health
- Interaction among all these factors

A key concept of the theory is **reciprocal determinism**, the dynamic interplay among personal factors, the environment, and behavior. The theory proposes that changing one of these factors will change them all.[19] **Figure 4-2** illustrates the concept of reciprocal determinism.

Social Cognitive Theory can be applied to a wide variety of public health issues that encompass the complex interactions between individual characteristics, influences in the social system, and individual behavior. Addiction to drugs, alcohol, and tobacco are such public health issues. Illicit drug use, the use and abuse of illegal drugs, has been on the rise in the United States, with 2011 estimates indicating nearly 9% of the U.S. population had used an illicit drug or abused a psychotherapeutic medication in the past month.[20] Over 50% of adults in the United States aged 18 years and older are current regular drinkers, consuming at least 12 drinks in the

past year.[21] Tobacco use in the United States is on the decline, falling from 26% to 22% of the population aged 12 years and older between 2002 and 2011.[20] **Table 4-8** illustrates application of the Social Cognitive Theory to drug addiction.

Population and Community Level

Theories and models on the population, or community, level explore factors within social systems, offering strategies that can be used to alter these factors to address health issues within the population. Theories and models on the community level are typically viewed as change theories guiding strategies that change aspects within the social systems, such as norms, rules, regulations, policies, and laws. This contrasts with theories and models on the intrapersonal and interpersonal levels, which are viewed as explanatory theories because they primarily identify and describe reasons for a problem.

A commonly used community-level theory is the **Diffusion of Innovation**. This theory focuses on how a new idea, product, or social practice (an innovation) is disseminated and adopted in a population. The theoretical constructs include the innovation itself, the time it takes to adopt the innovation, the communication channels used to transmit the innovation, and the social system in which diffusion of the innovation takes place.[22]

The theory proposes that the diffusion and adoption, or rejection, of an innovation is affected by perceived attributes of the innovation, including relative advantage (Is the innovation better than what it will replace?), compatibility (Does the innovation fit with the values and needs of the intended audience?), complexity (Is the innovation easy to understand and use?), trialability (Can the innovation be tried before making a decision to adopt?), and observability (Are the results of the innovation observable and easily measureable?).

The diffusion of innovation theory has contributed the concept of different types of adopters, including early adopters (those who seek to experiment with innovative ideas), early majority adopters (often opinion leaders whose social status frequently influences others to adopt the behavior), and late adopters (or laggards—those who need support and encouragement to make adoption as easy as possible).

A different approach is often needed to engage each of these groups. For instance, marketing efforts may initially target early adopters with an approach encouraging innovation and creativity. This may be followed by an approach to opinion leaders who can help the innovation or behavior change become mainstream. A different approach emphasizing ease of use and widespread acceptance may be most helpful for encouraging late adopters. **Table 4-9** illustrates the innovation-decision process regarding the adoption of the new idea to sneeze into one's elbow as a public health measure.

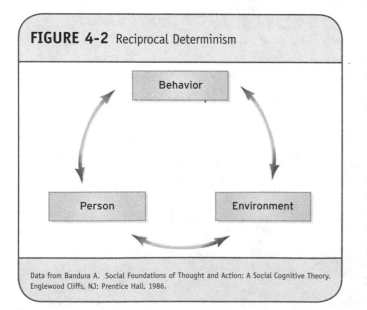

FIGURE 4-2 Reciprocal Determinism

Data from Bandura A. Social Foundations of Thought and Action: A Social Cognitive Theory. Englewood Cliffs, NJ: Prentice Hall, 1986.

TABLE 4-8 Social Cognitive Theory and Drug Addiction

Construct	Description	Example: drug addiction
Self-efficacy	Belief in one's ability to take action	"I am able to stop taking drugs."
Observational learning (modeling)	Learning by watching others	"My best friend has been drug-free for three years."
Expectations	The likely outcome of a particular behavior	"If I quit taking drugs, I will be able to hold a job and earn income."
Expectancies	The value placed on the outcome of the behavior	"Being able to work and have an income is very important to me."
Emotional arousal	Emotional reaction to a situation	"When I take drugs, I feel like I am out of control and that is very frightening."
Behavioral capability	Knowledge and skills needed to engage in a behavior	"I know I need to seek professional assistance to quit my drug addiction and I know where and how to get that assistance."
Reinforcement	Rewards or punishments for performing a behavior	"When I take drugs, people do not want to hang out with me. But when I am not taking drugs, I am surrounded by my friends and family."
Locus of control	One's belief regarding one's personal power over events	"Only I can get myself drug-free."

Data from Bandura A. *Social Foundations of Thought and Action: A Social Cognitive Theory*. Englewood Cliffs, NJ: Prentice Hall, 1986.

TABLE 4-9 Innovation-Decision Process: Diffusion of Innovation of Sneezing into Elbow

Stage	Description	Example
Knowledge	Before people can adopt an innovation, they must know it exists. Communication channels, such as media, friends, family members, and physicians, are influential in this stage.	Knowing sneezing into elbow exists as a public health measure
Persuasion	In the persuasion stage, people develop an opinion about the innovation. That opinion may be positive or negative. The perceived characteristics of the innovation are particularly influential in the persuasion stage.	Considering whether to begin sneezing into elbow Relative advantage: "Sneezing into your elbow is a lot better than sneezing into your hand." Compatibility: "Sneezing into my elbow is consistent with my desire to prevent the spread of disease." Complexity: "Sneezing into your elbow is easy to do." Trialability: "I can give sneezing into my elbow a try." Observability: "I have seen others sneeze into their elbows."
Decision	During the decision stage, people decide to either adopt or reject an innovation.	Deciding to sneeze into elbow
Implementation	During the implementation stage, an innovation is tried.	Sneezing into elbow
Confirmation	During the confirmation stage, support is sought for the decision, so that there is either continued adoption, continued rejection, later adoption, or discontinuance of the innovation.	Continue to sneeze into elbow as a common practice that becomes a habit after continued use

Data from Rogers, E.M. (2003). *Diffusion of Innovations*. New York: Free Press.

HOW CAN THEORIES BE APPLIED IN PRACTICE?

Choosing a Theory/Model

Choosing which theory or model to use requires an understanding of the public health issue and population being addressed, but there is no set formula for which theory or model is most appropriate in every situation. Components from multiple theories and models may be used when addressing particular situations and populations. Even though there are no right and wrong theories and models to use in given situations, some guidance is helpful in selecting the theoretical framework. Hayden offers the following guidance in choosing a theory:[23]

1. Identify the health issue or problem and the population affected.
2. Gather information about the issue, population, or both.
3. Identify possible reasons or causes for the problem.
4. Identify the level of interaction (intrapersonal, interpersonal, or community) under which the reasons or causes most logically fit.
5. Identify the theory or theories that best match the level and the reasons or causes.

Planning Frameworks

Theory is useful in identifying points at which to intervene in an effort to protect and promote the health of populations. These points will vary depending on the issue and the population. For instance, assume that theory-guided research on colon cancer screening suggests that women are unlikely to get screened because they do not think they are susceptible to the disease, while men are unlikely to get screened because they are not encouraged or reminded to do so. Interventions aimed at addressing colon cancer screening would, therefore, vary for women and men. Perhaps an intervention for women would focus on raising awareness of colon cancer among women, whereas an intervention for men may focus on the role of physicians and significant others to encourage them to make an appointment.

A variety of approaches can be undertaken to apply theory to practice. Two useful approaches, social marketing and the PRECEDE-PROCEED framework, will be described.

In recent years, public health has begun to apply marketing approaches to try to better understand and change the health behaviors of groups of people—especially those who are at high risk for the health impacts of their behavior, such as cigarette smokers. **Social marketing**, a use and extension of traditional product marketing, has become a key component of a public health approach to behavioral change.[24] Social marketing campaigns were first successfully used in the developing world for promoting a range of products and behaviors, including family planning and pediatric rehydration therapy. In recent years, social marketing efforts have been widely and successfully used in developed countries, including such efforts as:

- The truth® campaign—Developed by the American Legacy Foundation, it aims to redirect the perception of smoking being seen as a teenage rebellion to the decision to not smoke being a rebellion against the alleged behavior-controlling tobacco industry.
- The National Youth Anti-Drug campaign—It uses social marketing efforts directed at young people, including the "Parents. The Anti-Drug." campaign.
- The VERB™ campaign—It focused on 9- to 13-year-olds, or "tweens," with a goal of making exercise fun and "cool" for everyone, not just competitive athletes.

Social marketing incorporates the "4 Ps," which are widely used to structure traditional marketing efforts. These are:

- **Product**: Identifying the behavior or innovation that is being marketed
- **Price**: Identifying the benefits, the barriers, and the financial costs
- **Place**: Identifying the target audiences and how to reach them
- **Promotion**: Organizing a campaign or program to reach the target audience(s)

Social marketing, like product marketing, often relies on what marketers call **branding**. Branding includes words and symbols that help the target audience identify with the service; however, it goes deeper than just words and symbols. It can be seen as a method of implementing the fourth "P," or promotion. It also builds upon the first three "Ps":

- Branding requires a clear understanding of the product or the behavior to be changed (product).
- Successful branding puts forth strategies for reducing the financial and psychological costs (price).
- Branding identifies the audience and segments of the audience and asks how each segment can be reached (place).

BOX 4-2 VERB™ Campaign

The VERB™ social marketing campaign was funded through the Centers for Disease Control and Prevention (CDC), which worked with advertising agencies to reach tweens and make exercise "cool." After a series of focus groups and other efforts to define and understand the market, it was concluded that the message should not be one of improving health, but rather of having fun with friends, exploring new activities with a sense of adventure, and being free to experiment without being judged on performance.

Marketing efforts also identified barriers, including time constraints and the attraction of other activities, from social occasions to television to computers. In addition, barriers included lack of access to facilities, as well as negative images of competition, embarrassment, and the inability to become an elite athlete.

The VERB™ campaign implied action and used the tagline "It's what you do." Initial messages used animated figures of children covered with verbs being physically active. Later, messages turned these animated verb–covered kids into real kids actively playing. Widely used logos were developed and promoted as part of the branding effort. The VERB™ campaign partnered with television channels that successfully reach tweens, sponsored outreach events, and distributed promotional materials.

During the four years of the VERB™ campaign, tweens developed widespread recognition of the program and rated it highly in terms of "saying something important to me" and "makes me want to get more active," with maximum levels of recognition of 64% and 68%, respectively. Despite the documented success of VERB™, it was discontinued because of cuts in the federal budget.

Data from Wong F, Huhman M, Asbury L, Mueller RB, McCarthy S, Londe P, et al. VERB™—A social marketing campaign to increase physical activity among youth. *Prev Chronic Disease.* 2004;3(1):1–7.

Thus, branding is the public face of social marketing, but it also needs to be integrated into the core of the marketing plan.[d]

Social marketing efforts in developing and developed countries have demonstrated that it is possible to change key health behaviors of well-defined groups of people, including adolescents, who are often regarded as the hardest to reach.

An example of the use of social marketing to reach young people, the VERB™ campaign, is examined in **Box 4-2.**[25]

The **PRECEDE-PROCEED** planning framework provides a structure to design and evaluate health education and health promotion programs through a diagnostic planning process followed by an implementation and evaluation process. There are nine steps of the framework, divided into two phases: PRECEDE and PROCEED.[26e]

Table 4-10 illustrates the nine steps of the PRECEDE-PROCEED framework. Theory is applied in each step of the PRECEDE-PROCEED framework, guiding researchers and practitioners in their decisions.

The diagnostic phase of PRECEDE consists of collecting data and information to understand societal needs (step 1: social assessment), prioritizing community needs (step 2: epidemiological assessment), identifying factors contributing to the health issue (step 3: behavioral and environmental assessment), identifying factors that must be in

---

[d] Social marketing has not only incorporated traditional product marketing approaches; it has extended them to address the special circumstances of not-for-profit and government organizations. The use of social marketing in public health has required modifications and enhancements that have been described using four more "Ps": publics, partnerships, policies, and purse strings. "Publics" refers to the need to reach not only a target audience whose behavior we seek to change, but also those people who influence the target audience—be they parents, employers, or opinion leaders. For example, a campaign to address obesity, cigarettes, or high-risk sexual behavior in schools requires support from parents. "Partnerships" refers to the need for collaborations to achieve most public health goals. The VERB™ campaign, for instance, partnered with television stations appealing to tweens and schools to help get its message out. Successful efforts to reduce adolescent smoking, increase exercise, and reduce drug use also require changing institutional policies, which means reaching adult decision makers. Finally, the "purse string" aspect is money—few public health social marketing campaigns have adequate resources to do the job. Funding issues may require public health marketing teams to incorporate a long-term approach and look for nontraditional sources of funding.

---

[e] PRECEDE is an acronym for **p**redisposing, **r**einforcing, **e**nabling **c**onstructs in **e**ducational/environmental **d**iagnosis, and **e**valuation. PROCEED is an acronym for **p**olicy, **r**egulatory, and **o**rganizational **c**onstructs in **e**ducational and **e**nvironmental **d**evelopment. Combined, these two phases view health behavior as influenced by both individual and environmental factors.

TABLE 4-10 PRECEDE-PROCEED Framework and Application

Step	Description	Example: gun violence
Diagnostic phase: PRECEDE		
1: Social assessment	Assess people's perceptions of their own needs and quality of life through data collection activities such as surveys, interviews, focus groups, and observation.	Gun violence emerged as a major concern among community members through focus groups that were conducted to explore health and safety concerns in the community.
2. Epidemiological assessment	Determine which health problems are most important for which groups in a community, often by analyzing data from vital statistics, state and/or national surveys, etc. This step should assist in identifying subpopulations at high risk and provide data to set measurable objectives for the program.	Data from death certificates and crime reports reveals that the majority of deaths among males aged 24 years and younger in the community are due to gunshot wounds.
3. Behavioral and environmental assessment	Identify factors, internal and external to the individual, that contribute to the health issue of interest. Literature searches and theory application provide guidance during this step.	A literature search provides insight into factors contributing to gun violence among males aged 24 years and younger. Gang-related behavior is found to be frequent in populations with similar socioeconomic status as that of the target population.
4. Educational and organizational assessment	Preceding and reinforcing factors that initiate and sustain behavior change are identified, such as an individual's knowledge, skills and attitudes, social support, peer influence, and availability of services.	Interventions aimed at males 16 years and younger are found to be most successful. Young males with older male role models are more likely to view gangs as negative and more likely to participate in sports and community service.
5. Administrative and policy assessment	Identify policies, resources, and circumstances that may help or hinder implementation of the intervention.	Communication system recently established between school system and law enforcement to report truancy and criminal behavior among student population. May assist in identifying subgroups to target intervention.
Implementation and evaluation phase: PROCEED		
6. Implementation	The intervention is implemented.	After-school program implemented that incorporates educational, service-oriented, and physical activity components, led by males from the community. The program is tailored for males 12–16 years of age.
7. Process evaluation	Process evaluation assesses the extent to which the intervention was implemented as planned.	Evaluate how program activities were delivered.
8. Impact evaluation	Impact evaluation assesses the change in the factors identified in steps 3 and 4.	Evaluate gang associations among participants in the after-school programming.
9. Outcome evaluation	Outcome evaluation assesses the effect of the intervention on the health issue of interest.	Evaluate deaths due to gun violence in the community before and after intervention.

Data from Green LW, Kreuter MW (1999). *Health Promotion Planning: An Educational and Ecological Approach* (3rd edition). McGraw-Hill.

place to initiate and sustain behavioral change (step 4: educational and ecological assessment) and identifying policies, resources and other circumstances that may assist or hinder efforts (step 5: administrative and policy assessment).

The implementation and evaluation phase of PROCEED begins with implementation of the strategies developed based on the findings from the PRECEDE phase in step 6. Knowing what works and what does not work is important across all public health interventions; therefore, evaluation is a critical component embedded within this planning model. In step 7, evaluation of the intervention components takes place to determine if the program is functioning the way it was intended, reaching the target population, etc. Step 8 evaluates the impact the intervention has on the factors being targeted. In step 9, outcomes of the intervention are evaluated to determine whether the intervention has affected the overall public health issue it set out to address.

As we have seen, understanding and applying social and behavioral theories are central to population health. Expect to see new theories emerge and existing theories be modified as we gain greater understanding of social and individual behaviors. Social and behavioral sciences play an important role in population health. Analyzing the factors that influence health behavior assists in developing targeted interventions to promote healthy behavior and reduce health disparities. Health behavior theories and models are important tools used to explain and predict health behavior, providing useful road maps for the development of health promotion strategies. Additional planning frameworks, such as social marketing and PRECEDE-PROCEED, are also employed throughout the development, implementation, dissemination, and evaluation processes, contributing to sound health behavior interventions aimed at preserving, promoting, and protecting the health of populations.

KEY WORDS

- Social justice
- Socioeconomic status
- Socioeconimic gradient
- Gini index
- Social determinants of health
- Food desert
- Health disparities
- Healthcare disparity
- Health equity
- Health inequity
- Health inequality
- Mental health
- Downstream factors
- Mainstream factors
- Upstream factors
- Theory
- Model
- Health Belief Model
- Transtheoretical Model (or Stages of Change Model)
- Theory of Planned Behavior
- Social Cognitive Theory
- Reciprocal determinism
- Diffusion of Innovation
- Social marketing
- Product
- Price
- Place
- Promotion
- Branding
- PRECEDE-PROCEED

Discussion Questions

Take a look at the questions posed in the following scenarios, which were presented at the beginning of this chapter. See now whether you can answer these questions.

1. You travel to a country in Asia and find that this nation's culture affects most parts of life. From the food the people eat and their method of cooking, to their attitudes toward medical care, to their beliefs about the cause of disease and the ability to alter it through public health and medical interventions, this country is profoundly different from the United States. You ask: How does culture affect health?

2. You are working in a country with strict Islamic practices and find that religion, like culture, can have major impacts on health. Religious practices differ widely—from beliefs about food and alcohol; to sexual practices, such as male circumcision and female sexual behavior; to acceptance or rejection of interventions aimed at women's health. You ask: How does religion affect health?

3. You are trying to help your spouse quit smoking cigarettes and prevent your kids from starting. You know that gentle encouragement and support on a one-on-one basis are essential, but often not enough because cigarette smoking is an addiction that produces withdrawal and long-term cravings. You wonder what other factors in the social system influence behavior and how they can be addressed.

4. Your efforts to convince your friends to avoid smoking (or stop smoking) focus on giving them the facts about how cigarettes cause lung cancer, throat cancer, and serious heart disease. You are frustrated by how little impact you have on your friends. You wonder what tools are available to better explain and predict health behavior.

5. Your classmate, who is first in her family to attend college, received word that her father lost his job at the local factory and she needs to take a leave from school because her family can no longer afford tuition. You wonder how this will affect her and her family.

6. Your town board just approved extending public transportation services to a wider geographic area. Although there are several opponents to the plan, you learn that a group of public health professionals supports this extension of services. You wonder what this transportation plan has to do with health.

7. You are in the checkout line at the grocery store, and a pregnant mother is ahead of you. You glance at the sugary cereals, snacks, and sodas she is purchasing and happen to notice that she is using an EBT card from the Supplemental Nutrition Assistance Program (SNAP), formerly known as the Food Stamp program. You wonder what could be done to encourage the consumption of healthy food options.

8. One of your friends asked for your assistance in helping his aunt move from her farm in the rural part of the state into the city center. He explained that his aunt was recently diagnosed with cancer and required regular chemotherapy treatments. You wonder why this diagnosis necessitates a move from a rural to urban area.

9. Every day on your way to work, you pass the same homeless man on the same corner. He does not look very old—you guess he is about

25 years of age. You notice that over the past few weeks, he has been coughing, and you figure he must have a cold. Today when you walk by his usual place on the corner, he is not there, but someone has left a sign that reads, "Rest in peace, Ramón." You are surprised, especially because he was so young. You wonder whether there was anything that could have been done to prevent his death.

10. As a new parent, you hear from your pediatrician, nurses in the hospital, and even the makers of your brand of diapers that babies should sleep on their backs. They call it "Back-to-Sleep." You are surprised to find that it is part of the class on baby-sitting given by the local community center and a required part of the training for those who work in registered day care centers. You find out that it is all part of a social marketing campaign that has halved the number of deaths from sudden infant death syndrome. You ask: Why has the Back-to-Sleep campaign been so successful?

REFERENCES

1. Edberg M. *Essentials of Health Behavior: Social and Behavioral Theory in Public Health.* Sudbury, MA: Jones and Bartlett Publishers; 2007.

2. Berkman LF, Kawachi I, eds. *Social Epidemiology.* New York, NY: Oxford University Press; 2000.

3. Commission on Social Determinants of Health. Closing the gap in a generation: health equity through action on the social determinants of health. *Final Report of the Commission on Social Determinants of Health.* Geneva, Switzerland: World Health Organization; 2008.

4. Marmot M. *The Status Syndrome: How Social Standing Affects Our Health and Longevity.* New York, NY: Henry Holt and Company; 2004.

5. Wilkinson R, Marmot M, eds. *Social Determinants of Health: The Solid Facts.* 2nd ed. Copenhagen, Denmark: World Health Organization; 2003.

6. Central Intelligence Agency. Country comparison: distribution of family income—Gini index. The world factbook. https://www.cia.gov/library/publications/the-world-factbook/rankorder/2172rank.html. Accessed August 5, 2013.

7. Braveman P, Egerter S. *Overcoming Obstacles to Health.* Washington, DC: Robert Wood Johnson Foundation Commission to Build a Healthier America; 2008.

8. Murray CJL, Michaud CM, McKenna M, et al. *U.S. Country Patterns of Mortality by County and Race: 1965–1994.* Cambridge, MA: Harvard Center for Population and Development Studies; 1998.

9. Marmot M. *The Status Syndrome: How Social Standing Affects Our Health and Longevity.* New York, NY: Henry Holt and Company; 2004.

10. The World Health Organization. Social determinants of health. http://www.who.int/social_determinants/en. Accessed August 5, 2013.

11. *Healthy People 2020.* Social determinants of health. http://www.healthypeople.gov/2020/topicsobjectives2020/overview.aspx?topicid=39. Accessed August 5, 2013.

12. Wilkinson R, Marmot M, eds. *Social Determinants of Health: The Solid Facts.* 2nd ed. Copenhagen, Denmark: World Health Organization; 2003.

13. The World Health Organization. Social determinants of health. Themes. http://www.who.int/social_determinants/themes/en. Accessed August 5, 2013.

14. *Healthy People 2020.* Mental health and mental disorders. http://www.healthypeople.gov/2020/topicsobjectives2020/overview.aspx?topicid=28. Accessed August 5, 2013.

15. *Healthy People 2020.* Mental health and mental disorders. National spotlight. http://www.healthypeople.gov/2020/topicsobjectives2020/national snapshot.aspx?topicId=28. Accessed August 5, 2013.

16. National Cancer Institute. U.S. Department of Health and Human Services. *Theory at a Glance: A Guide for Health Promotion Practice.* 2nd ed. http://www.cancer.gov/cancertopics/cancerlibrary/theory.pdf. Accessed August 5, 2013.

17. Prochaska JO, DiClemente CC. Stages and processes of self-change of smoking: toward an integrative model of change. *Journal of Consulting and Clinical Psychology.* 1983;51(3):390–395.

18. Azjen I, Drive BL. Prediction of leisure participation from behavioral, normative, and control beliefs: an application of the theory of planned behavior. *Leisure Science.* 1991;13:185–204.

19. Bandura A. *Social Foundations of Thought and Action: A Social Cognitive Theory.* Englewood Cliffs, NJ: Prentice Hall; 1986.

20. National Institute on Drug Abuse. Drug facts: nationwide trends. http://www.drugabuse.gov/publications/drugfacts/nationwide-trends. Accessed August 5, 2013.

21. Centers for Disease Control and Prevention. Faststats alcohol use. http://www.cdc.gov/nchs/fastats/alcohol.htm. Accessed August 5, 2013.

22. Rogers EM. *Diffusion of Innovations, 5th edition.* New York, NY: Free Press; 2003.

23. Hayden J. *Introduction to Health Behavior Theory.* Sudbury, MA: Jones and Bartlett; 2009:135.

24. Weinreich NK. What is social marketing? http://www.social-marketing.com/Whatis.html. Accessed August 5, 2013.

25. Wong F, Huhman M, Asbury L, et al. VERB™—a social marketing campaign to increase physical activity among youth. *Prev Chronic Disease.* 2004;3(1):1–7.

26. Green LW, Kreuter MW. *Health Promotion Planning: An Educational and Ecological Approach.* 4th ed. New York, NY: McGraw-Hill; 2005.

CHAPTER 5

Health Law, Policy, and Ethics

LEARNING OBJECTIVES

By the end of this chapter, the student will be able to:

- explain the scope of health law, policy, and ethics.
- identify key legal principles that form the basis for public health law.
- identify four types of law.
- discuss the role played by *Healthy People* in setting public health priorities.
- explain the differences between market and social justice.
- illustrate the potential tensions between individual rights and the needs of society using public health examples.
- discuss key principles that underlie the ethics of human research.
- identify principles of public health ethics.

A new statute and subsequent administrative regulations give only a temporary license to newly licensed drivers, prohibiting late night driving and the use of cell phones and limiting the number of passengers. You ask: Should elderly drivers be subject to these same types of regulations, such as being required to take a driver's test?

The CDC reports that the country is facing an unprecedented epidemic of obesity in all regions. It indicates that it is doing everything within its legal authority to address the epidemic. Unfortunately, it concludes there is little more that the federal government can do to fight obesity. Why, you wonder, is the federal authority to address health problems so limited?

You hear that a neighbor has TB and refuses treatment. You wonder: What if he has the type of TB that can't be cured with drugs? You ask: Can't they make him take his medicine or at least get him out of the neighborhood?

A friend of yours experienced a grand mal seizure in which she totally lost consciousness. Fortunately, cancer is ruled out and she is tolerating the medications without serious side effects and without another seizure. It is two months later and your friend tells you her driver's license was taken away by the motor vehicle administration and she does not know when she will get it back. You ask: What types of issues are involved in deciding if and when she can drive again?

You receive an email encouraging your participation in a new research study. It sounds like you are eligible, so you check into it. You are surprised to find that even if you participate, you may not receive the new drug, and you will not even be told which treatment you are receiving. Despite your willingness to take your chances, you are told that you are not eligible for the study due to conditions that put you at increased risk of developing side effects. You ask: Why am I barred from participating if I am willing to take the risks?

© Africa Studio/ShutterStock, Inc.

These are the types of issues that are part of health law, policy, and ethics. Let us begin by examining the scope of these issues.

WHAT IS THE SCOPE OF HEALTH LAW, POLICY, AND ETHICS?

Health law, policy, and ethics reflect a wide range of tools that society uses to encourage and discourage behaviors by individuals and groups. These tools apply to health care, as well as to traditional public health. In addition, in recent years, a field called **bioethics** has been defined, which includes elements of both health care and public health and focuses on applying morals or values to areas of potential conflict.[1]

Health law, policy, and ethics affect the full range of issues that confront us in population health. They address such things as the access to and the quality and cost of health care. They also address the organizational and professional structures designed to deliver health care. Health law, policy, and ethics are key tools for accomplishing the goals of traditional public health, ranging from occupational safety to drug and highway safety, and from control of communicable diseases to noncommunicable and environmental diseases. Bioethics lies at the intersection of health law and policy and attempts to apply individual and group values and morals to controversial issues, such as abortion, stem cell research, and end-of-life care. **Table 5-1** outlines a range of issues that are addressed by health law, policy, and ethics.

The scope of health law, policy, and ethics is so vast that we will focus on first defining key principles and philosophies that underlie our society's approach to these issues. Then we will focus on three examples that illustrate key issues confronted in the healthcare, public health, and bioethics arenas. These are:

1. Is there a right to health care?
2. How does public health attempt to balance the rights of individuals and the needs of society?
3. What bioethical principles are used to address public health issues?

TABLE 5-1 Components of Health Law, Policy, and Ethics

Component	Scope	Examples of issues
Health care	Access, quality, and cost of health care Organizational and professional structures for the delivery of care	Rules governing Medicare and Medicaid, as well as laws governing private insurance Hospital governance and professional licensure
Public health	Population health and safety, including governmental efforts to provide services to entire populations, as well as vulnerable groups	Food and drug laws and procedures, environmental laws and procedures, regulations for control of communicable diseases
Bioethics	Application of individual and group values and morals to controversial areas	End-of-life care, stem cell research, abortion, protection of research subjects

Let us start by taking a look at key legal principles that underlie the approach to public health and health care in the United States.

WHAT LEGAL PRINCIPLES UNDERLIE PUBLIC HEALTH AND HEALTH CARE?

In order to better appreciate the issue of health policy and law, it is important to understand some key legal principles that underlie both public health and healthcare law in the United States.[1] First, the U.S. Constitution is a fundamental document that governs the issues of public health and healthcare law. However, the U.S. Constitution does not mention health. As a result, public health and health care are among those issues that are left primarily to the authority of the states, unless delegated by the state to local jurisdictions, such as cities or counties. The use of this authority, known as **police power**, allows states to pass legislation and take actions to protect the common good. The authority to protect the common good may justify a wide range of state actions, including the regulation of healthcare professionals and facilities; the establishment of health and safety standards in retail and other occupational settings; and the control of hazards ranging from requiring the use of car restraint systems, to vaccinations, to restricting the sale of tobacco products.[1, 2]

The use of state police power is limited by the protections afforded to individuals. These protections are known as **rights** and are created either through the U.S. Constitution, through a state's constitution, or through laws passed at the federal or state levels. The U.S. Constitution allows, but does not require, governments to act to protect public health or to provide healthcare services. This has been referred to as the **negative constitution**. Thus, while governments often have the authority to act, they are not required to do so. For instance, the Supreme Court has not found an obligation on the part of states to act to prevent child or spousal abuse even when the state is fully aware of specific circumstances or a court has issued a restraining order.[1]

Second, the Interstate Commerce Clause of the U.S. Constitution is the major source of federal authority in public health and health care. It provides the federal government with the authority to tax, spend, and regulate interstate commerce.[2] This authority has been used to justify a wide range of federal involvement in health care and public health. Federal authority is often exerted through incentives to the states. For instance, states may be offered federal funding or matching funding if they enact specific types of legislation, such as the rules governing Medicaid or definitions of blood-alcohol levels for driving under the influence.[3] The U.S. Constitution's supremacy clause declares that legitimate federal laws are the supreme laws of the land and they preempt or overrule state laws that conflict with them.[a] This provision has been used by federal public health agencies, such as the Food and Drug Administration and the Environmental Protection Agency, to justify national standards that overrule and limit state rules and regulations ranging from quality controls on drugs to levels of permissible exposures to toxic substances.[1, 2]

Third, the U.S. Constitution grants individual rights. Some of them, such as freedom of speech, religion, and assembly and the right to bear arms, are explicit in the document. Others have been inferred by the U.S. Supreme Court, such as the right to procreation, privacy, bodily integrity, and travel. These inferred rights are often the basis for individual protections in public health and health care, including the right to utilize contraception, have an abortion, and limit the state and federal authority to use quarantine and other travel restrictions.[1,2] Unless the U.S. Constitution explicitly includes a right or one has been "found" by the Supreme Court of the United States, no right exists. However, federal and state legislatures may create rights through legislation ranging from access to education to access to medical care. The existence of a right implies that state and/or federal courts are expected to uphold and enforce the right.[b]

Health law is based upon these rules governing the authority of federal and state governments and also the rights of individuals. It is derived from four sources that are summarized in **Box 5-1**.[1]

Thus, health law refers to a vast array of legal issues that influence much of what goes on in public health and health care. However, the influence of health policy often extends beyond that of the formal legal system. Let us take a look at what we mean by "health policy."

---

[a] Another implication of constitutional law is the supremacy of the U.S. Constitution even over international law. Human rights and standards incorporated into international documents are not directly enforceable in the United States. These rights and standards are only enforceable in the United States through enactment of federal or state laws.[1]

[b] Enforcement is required by law to occur based on due process. Due process includes **substantive due process**, which refers to the grounds for depriving an individual of a right, as well as **procedural due process**, which refers to the processes that must be undertaken to deprive an individual of a right. The former implies that state and federal governments must justify depriving an individual of life, liberty, and property. When fundamental rights are involved or laws are based on suspect classifications, such as gender or race, the court applies strict criteria that place difficult burdens of proof on the government to justify these types of actions. Procedural due process implies that when a right exists, governments may not deny individuals the right in an arbitrary or unfair way. This process requires that acceptable legal processes be followed before an individual can be deprived of a right. The Supreme Court has considered a fundamental right as one that is explicit in the U.S. Constitution, that has been "found" in the U.S. Constitution by the Supreme Court, or that is rooted in the nation's history and traditions.[1,2]

BOX 5-1 Types of Law

To appreciate the complex relationship between the law and public health and health care, it is important to appreciate that there are four sources of law. These may be classified as **constitutional law**, **legislative statutes**, **administrative regulations**, and **judicial law** (also called **case law** or **common law**).

Constitutional law includes not only the U.S. Constitution, but also the constitutions of the 50 states. The provisions of state constitutions are important because the responsibilities for health lie with the states unless the federal Constitution grants authority to the federal government. As we have seen, the commerce clause and the due process clauses of the Constitution have been the basis for extensions of federal authority into areas of health. State constitutions are often easier to amend than the federal Constitution, and thus can and do change more frequently. Constitutions often limit the role of government and define its processes. Constitutional law, however, does not usually directly mandate roles for government in the area of health.

Legislative law, or statutes, is written by legislative bodies at local, state, and federal levels. Federal statutes preempt, or overrule, conflicting state statutes, as long as they are consistent with the limitation placed on the federal government by the U.S. Constitution. Statutes often directly address health issues. Legislative law may place requirements or prohibition on future activities. Statutes may authorize governmental regulation, such as professional or institutional licensure; require specific activities, such a restaurant inspections; prohibit other activities, such as smoking in public places; or provide funding to pay for governmental services or reimburse those who provide the services, such as health care.

Administrative law is produced by executive agencies of the federal, state, and local governments in order to implement legislative statutes, which are often written in quite general language. Executive agencies must follow legally defined processes and stay within what is called the legislative intent of the statute. Administrative law can be seen as operationalizing statutes passed by legislative bodies. These types of laws may define who is eligible for services, how these services may be provided, the levels of reimbursement received, and a large number of other important details that affect the day-to-day operations of government services and programs. Administrative law affects public health in many ways, from the regulation of septic tanks to requirements for immunization to enroll in public education. Executive agencies often set up quasi-judicial processes to review contested cases. These judicial processes usually provide for limited access to the court system to contest their decisions.

Judicial, case, or common law is law made by courts when applying constitutional, statutory, or administrative law to specific cases. In addition, common law may fill in the holes when statutory law does not provide guidance. For instance, case law may be the basis for addressing environmental health issues, which the law defines as "nuisances" ranging from excess noise to disposal of garbage. Judges' primary responsibility is to apply previous rulings or precedence to new cases that come before them; however, they may take into account existing traditions and customs of society when applying the law to specific cases. Higher courts including appellate courts, and ultimately the U.S. Supreme Court, and in some instances, state Supreme Courts may decide that a statute violates the relevant constitutions. That is, they can rule a statute unconstitutional.

WHAT DO WE MEAN BY "HEALTH POLICY"?

Within the constraints set by law, there is considerable latitude for governments, as well as private groups, to develop policies that affect the ways that public health and health care are conducted. The main distinction between a law and a policy is defined by who can create each and how they can be enforced. Essentially any organization can create a policy and subsequently enforce the policy it created. A range of governmental organizations create the law that is enforced through the legal system.

Health policy is a subset of the larger arena of public policy. According to Teitelbaum and Wilensky, "when deciding on whether something is a public policy decision, the focus is not only on who is making the decision, but also on what kind of decision is being made."[4] They define individuals or groups that make public policy based on the ability of the individual or group to make an **authoritative decision**. An authoritative decision is a decision made by an individual or group that has the power to implement the decision. A range of governmental and private groups make public policy decisions in areas such as cigarette smoking. In government, authoritative decisions may be made by an executive branch official, such as the president or a governor, or administrative officials, such as federal, state, or local health officers. These may range from policies that discourage the growing of tobacco, to policies that encourage the sale of tobacco products abroad, to policies that restrict smoking in public places or tax tobacco sales. These policies may or may not be incorporated into laws or statutes.

At times, health policy may be made by private groups, including professional societies, such as the American Public Health Association, or commercial trade associations representing hospitals, the drug industry, the insurance industry, etc. Policies that affect large numbers of people, such as those that restrict smoking in hospitals, encourage clinicians to incorporate smoking prevention and cessation programs, compensate clinicians' efforts through insurance, and encourage the development of new drugs to assist with smoking cessation, are all examples of health policies that may be set by groups outside of government. Thus, the "public" in public policies does not necessarily imply that the policies were developed or implemented by government.

Health policy is a rapidly expanding field because there is growing recognition that collaboration is necessary across sectors in order to successfully address the varied and complex health issues facing our society. A **health in all policies approach** has been proposed in which private and public entities work toward common goals to achieve improved health for all while reducing health inequities.

Policies adopted by different sectors must reinforce one another. For instance, a health in all policies approach targeting health and development in early childhood may include education policies that provide opportunities for women of childbearing age among all income-levels to attain a college education; employment policies that allow mothers to take maternity leave while maintaining their salary and health benefits; and housing policies that require landlords to maintain safe structures free of hazards for young children, such as lead poisoning and asthma triggers.

According to Teitelbaum and Wilensky, in addition to being authoritative, a public policy decision must be one that "goes beyond the individual sphere and affects the greater community."[4] Decisions to seek vaccinations or screenings, to smoke cigarettes at home, or to purchase health insurance are individual decisions. Public policy issues revolve around incentives or requirements to encourage or discourage these actions by groups of individuals or the society as a whole.

HOW ARE PUBLIC HEALTH POLICY PRIORITIES ESTABLISHED?

The United States is faced with multiple, complex, and evolving issues that affect the health of the population. Prioritizing these issues has been the task of an initiative known as *Healthy People*. The initiative, organized by the U.S. Department of Health and Human Services, is a collaborative effort of a multitude of private and public organizations that sets evidence-based national objectives aimed at improving the health of the population. Since the decade beginning in 1980, a revised set of objectives has been established for the nation each subsequent decade. *Healthy People 2020* tracks approximately 1,200 objectives organized into 42 topic areas. These objectives, which are supported with data and need to be measurable, assist in identifying issues in need of program and policy development, implementation, and evaluation. They serve as a way to monitor progress toward achieving healthy people and healthy populations. A smaller set of these objectives has been identified as Leading Health Indicators, highlighting high-priority health issues and actions for the nation throughout the decade. **Table 5-2** lists the Leading Health Indicators and measurements that are recommended to monitor progress.[5]

HOW DO PHILOSOPHIES TOWARD THE ROLE OF GOVERNMENT AFFECT HEALTH POLICIES?

The types of health policies favored depend greatly on one's philosophies about the role that public and private institutions should play in public health and health care. Specifically, the appropriate role of government is often a controversial subject.

One of the most fundamental differences within our society is the attitude or philosophy about the roles that government and the economic market should play in advancing health. To appreciate this issue, it is useful to look at two contrasting philosophies regarding the government's role in health care and public health. These philosophies are called **social justice** and **market justice**. A social justice approach views the equitable distribution of health as a social responsibility, in contrast to a market justice approach, which emphasizes individual, rather than collective, responsibility for health.

Understanding these quite different approaches is helpful because our current system of health care and public health borrows from both of these basic approaches to varying degrees. **Table 5-3** outlines the contrasting characteristics of market justice and social justice. **Table 5-4** examines many of the implications of the two different philosophies.[6]

We have now looked at key principles of health law and health policy that underlie our approach to health care and public health. To see how these principles operate in practice, let us review the three questions introduced earlier:

1. Is there a right to health care?
2. How does public health attempt to balance the rights of individuals and the needs of society?
3. What bioethical principles are used to address public health issues?

TABLE 5-2 *Healthy People 2020* Leading Health Indicators

Topic	Indicators
Access to health services	• Persons with medical insurance • Persons with a usual primary care provider
Clinical preventive services	• Adults who receive a colorectal cancer screening based on the most recent guidelines • Adults with hypertension whose blood pressure is under control • Adult diabetic population with an A1c value greater than 9% • Children aged 19 to 35 months who receive the recommended doses of DTaP, polio, MMR, Hib, hepatitis B, varicella, and PCV vaccines
Environmental quality	• Air Quality Index (AQI) exceeding 100 • Children aged 3 to 11 years exposed to secondhand smoke
Injury and violence	• Fatal injuries • Homicides
Maternal, child, and infant health	• Infant deaths • Preterm births
Mental health	• Suicides • Adolescents who experience major depressive episodes (MDE)
Nutrition, physical activity, and obesity	• Adults who meet current federal physical activity guidelines for aerobic physical activity and for muscle-strengthening activity • Adults who are obese • Children and adolescents who are considered obese • Total vegetable intake for persons aged 2 years and older
Oral health	• Persons aged 2 years and older who used the oral health care system in the past 12 months
Reproductive and sexual health	• Sexually active females aged 15 to 44 years who received reproductive health services in the past 12 months • Persons living with HIV who know their serostatus
Social determinants	• Students who graduate with a regular diploma 4 years after starting 9th grade
Substance abuse	• Adolescents using alcohol or any illicit drugs during the past 30 days • Adults engaging in binge drinking during the past 30 days
Tobacco	• Adults who are current cigarette smokers • Adolescents who smoked cigarettes in the past 30 days

Data from Healthy People 2020. Leading Health Indicators. U.S. Department of Health and Human Services. Available at: http://www.healthypeople.gov/2020/LHI /default.aspx. Accessed July 16, 2013.

TABLE 5-3 Characteristics of Market and Social Justice

Market justice	Social justice
Views health care as an economic good	Views health care as a social resource
Assumes free market conditions for health services delivery	Requires active government involvement in health services delivery
Assumes that markets are more efficient in allocating resources equitably	Assumes that the government is more efficient in allocating health resources equitably
Production and distribution of health care determined by market-based demand	Medical resource allocation determined by central planning
Medical care distribution based on people's ability to pay	Ability to pay inconsequential for receiving medical care
Access to medical care viewed as an economic reward for personal effort and achievement	Equal access to medical services viewed as a basic right

Reproduced from Shi L, Singh D. *Delivering Health Care in America*. 3rd ed. Sudbury, MA: Jones and Bartlett Publishers; 2004:59.

TABLE 5-4 Implications of Market and Social Justice

Market justice	Social justice
Individual responsibility for health	Collective responsibility for health
Benefits based on individual purchasing power	Everyone is entitled to a basic package of services
Limited obligation to the collective good	Strong obligation to the collective good
Emphasis on individual well-being	Community well-being supersedes that of the individual
Private solutions to social problems	Public solutions to social problems
Rationing based on ability to pay	Planned rationing of health care

Reproduced from Shi L, Singh D. *Delivering Health Care in America*. 3rd ed. Sudbury, MA: Jones and Bartlett Publishers; 2004:59.

IS THERE A RIGHT TO HEALTH CARE?

In 1948, a right to health care was incorporated into the Universal Declaration of Human Rights and the Constitution of the World Health Organization. The former states that "everyone has the right to a standard of living adequate for the health and well-being of himself and his family, including…medical care…and the right to security in the event of…sickness…."[7] Most developed countries have incorporated a right to health care in their constitution or have created rights to health care as part of the legislative process, usually as part of a healthcare system that provides universal coverage. This internationally recognized right to health care cannot be enforced in the United States unless it is found to be recognized by the U.S. Constitution or a state constitution or has been incorporated into federal, state, or local statutes. Therefore, we need to examine what has happened within the legal system of the United States.

As we have discussed, the U.S. Constitution does not mention the word "health." Rights, however, can be "found" or created by the Supreme Court through its interpretation of the Constitution. Rights to travel and privacy, for example, have been "found" by the Supreme Court, while a right to health care has not been. State courts, such as the Supreme Court of Indiana, have addressed the meaning of a license to practice medicine (the Indiana Supreme Court tackled this in *Hurley v. Eddingfield*). In the case, a licensed physician refused services to a pregnant woman despite being offered prepayment and despite the fact that the physician knew that no other qualified physician was available. As a result, the woman did not receive medical care and both she and her unborn child died.[1] The court established what has been called the **no-duty principle**. This principle holds that healthcare providers (whether they are individuals or institutions) do not have an obligation to provide health services. A right to health care can be created within a state via its constitution. It can also be created in the United States or within a state by legislative action.[1]

Limited rights to health care have been established by legislative action. For instance, federal law includes the 1986 Treatment for Emergency Medical Conditions and Women in Labor Act, which provides a right to emergency medical care usually provided through hospital emergency departments.[c] This act establishes a right to health care by those seeking emergency services and establishes a duty on the part of hospital emergency departments to provide these services.

This right and the corresponding duty, however, are quite limited. Patients have the right to receive care and the hospital has a duty to provide an "appropriate" examination. The institution also has the duty to stabilize an emergency situation by providing as much treatment as possible within its capacity. When a hospital does not have the capacity to treat the emergency condition, it is required to transfer the patient to another facility in a medically appropriate fashion. These rights and duties are limited to emergency conditions in hospital emergency departments and do not provide more general rights to health care.[d]

Thus, a right to health care in the United States has not been generally established. As with health law and policies in general, this issue has not been definitively settled. As the state and federal governments struggle with the problems of providing health care for everyone, the right to health care is again emerging as an issue for debate and consideration. Let us now take a look at another fundamental issue that is at the core of public health law and policy—the balance between the rights of the individual and the needs of society.

---

[c] This act is often referred to as EMTALA, which is an acronym for the law's original name—the Emergency Medical Treatment and Active Labor Act.

[d] Another example of legislation that has established rights to health care is the Medicaid program. Medicaid establishes defined criteria for eligibility to enroll that are partially governed by federal law and partially by state law. During the time that an individual is qualified for Medicaid, they have certain rights to health care that can be enforced by individuals in the courts.

HOW DOES PUBLIC HEALTH ATTEMPT TO BALANCE THE RIGHTS OF INDIVIDUALS AND THE NEEDS OF SOCIETY?

Public health interventions often create a level of tension between the concerns of individuals and the needs of society. This is the situation even when individual rights are not involved. For instance, the courts have been clear that a driver's license is a privilege and not a right. Thus, it can be regulated by states without having to justify that individuals who are denied a driver's license are being denied a right. The regulation of driver's licenses is a state responsibility, and as such, there is enormous variation in factors such as age requirement, the length of time and requirement for learning permits, the type of examination required, the rules for suspension of a driver's license, and requirements for renewal of a driver's license.

Motor vehicle injuries remain a major cause of death and disability. It is widely accepted that there are two age groups at highest risk of death and disability from motor vehicles. The first are adolescents during their initial years of driving and the second are elderly individuals. Until recently, most states imposed minimum or no barriers to either group once an initial driver's license had been issued. In many states, limitations have now been imposed for one or both age groups. Possible public health interventions include raising the driving age; requiring stricter standards for licensure; and placing initial limitations on new drivers, including restricting nighttime driving, the number of passengers, and the use of cell phones. Common restrictions on older drivers include vision and hearing tests and reexamination including road testing. The type of risk also plays a role in determining how we balance individual rights and the needs of society. **Self-imposed risk** is risk an individual knowingly and willingly takes on through his or her own actions, such

as choosing not to wear a motorcycle helmet while riding a motorcycle. Even though helmet laws are intended to protect motorcyclists, the laws could be viewed as infringing on an individual's desire not to wear a helmet. If a motorcyclist decides to forego wearing a helmet, he or she is putting himself or herself at risk for injury.

However, not all risks to health can be attributed to individual behavior, blurring the line between individual rights and societal needs. **Imposed risk** refers to risk to individuals and populations that is out of their direct control. An example of an imposed risk would be exposure to environmental toxins from a local factory. The imposed risk itself may therefore be viewed as infringing on an individual's desire for clean air in his or her town. Because the factory's emissions are out of the direct control of the individual, interventions aimed to address imposed risk require actions external to the individual, perhaps in the form of governmental intervention to enforce environmental emissions regulations. As can be seen, the focus of responsibility differs depending on whether the risk is self-imposed or imposed.

The tension level between the individual and society is even greater when fundamental rights are denied, as is the case with the use of quarantine. **Box 5-2** examines the historical and current uses of quarantine.[8]

Now let us turn our attention to our third question and see how ethical and bioethical principles are being applied to public health.

WHAT BIOETHICAL PRINCIPLES ARE USED TO ADDRESS PUBLIC HEALTH ISSUES?

A code of ethics has been prepared through the Public Health Leadership Society to guide public health practitioners. **Table 5-5** lists the Principles of the Ethical Practice of Public Health.[9]

BOX 5-2 Quarantine as a Public Health Authority

Quarantine, the compulsory physical separation of those with a disease—or at high risk of developing a disease—from the rest of the population goes back to ancient times, when it was used to restrict entry of ships into ports where epidemic diseases threatened. Attempts to control epidemics of yellow fever, smallpox, and other infectious disease by quarantine were very much a part of the early history of the United States.

In the 1800s, tuberculosis (TB) sanatoriums often isolated those afflicted on a voluntary basis. Laws existed and were occasionally used that allowed quarantine of patients who felt well though were thought to be carriers of TB and other contagious diseases, such as typhoid. In the early years of the 1900s, "Typhoid Mary," who was infected with typhoid but had no symptoms, was quarantined on an island in New York after she refused to voluntarily refrain from working as a food handler.

BOX 5-2 Quarantine as a Public Health Authority (*continued*)

Quarantine was only occasionally used to control disease in the 1900s. However, in the early 2000s, it again became a public health issue precipitated by the recognition of SARS and the fear of rapid global spread of SARS and other communicable diseases. The spread of drug-resistant tuberculosis has again made the use of quarantine for TB an ongoing important public health issue.

Quarantine laws are in the process of revision. The issues of quarantine reflect many of the tensions between the right of the individual and the rights of society. For instance, a *New England Journal of Medicine* article on the use of quarantine for control of extremely resistant TB states:

> In recent decades, courts have clarified the legal rights of patients with tuberculosis who are subject to compulsory isolation. Drawing an analogy between isolation orders and civil commitment for mental

illness, courts have affirmed that patients who are isolated by law have many procedural due-process rights, including the right to counsel and a hearing before an independent decision maker. States must also provide "clear and convincing" evidence that isolation is necessary to prevent a significant risk of harm to others. Most important, some courts have held that isolation must be the least restrictive alternative for preventing such a risk. If the government can protect public health without relying on involuntary detention, it must and should do so.[8]

The use of quarantine is thus likely to be restricted and used very infrequently in the future. Increasingly, the emphasis on the rights of the individual outweighs any value that quarantine may have in protecting the public's health.

TABLE 5-5 Principles of the Ethical Practice of Public Health

1. Public health should address principally the fundamental causes of disease and requirements for health, aiming to prevent adverse health outcomes.
2. Public health should achieve community health in a way that respects the rights of individuals in the community.
3. Public health policies, programs, and priorities should be developed and evaluated through processes that ensure an opportunity for input from community members.
4. Public health should advocate and work for the empowerment of disenfranchised community members, aiming to ensure that the basic resources and conditions necessary for health are accessible to all.
5. Public health should seek the information needed to implement effective policies and programs that protect and promote health.
6. Public health institutions should provide communities with the information they have that is needed for decisions on policies or programs and should obtain the community's consent for their implementation.
7. Public health institutions should act in a timely manner on the information they have within the resources and the mandate given to them by the public.
8. Public health programs and policies should incorporate a variety of approaches that anticipate and respect diverse values, beliefs, and cultures in the community.
9. Public health programs and policies should be implemented in a manner that most enhances the physical and social environment.
10. Public health institutions should protect the confidentiality of information that can bring harm to an individual or community if made public. Exceptions must be justified on the basis of the high likelihood of significant harm to the individual or others.
11. Public health institutions should ensure the professional competence of their employees.
12. Public health institutions and their employees should engage in collaborations and affiliations in ways that build the public's trust and the institution's effectiveness.

Modified from Public Health Leadership Society. Principles of the ethical practice of public health. Version 2.2. 2002. http://phls.org/CMSuploads/Principles-of-the-Ethical-Practice-of-PH-Version-2.2-68496.pdf. Accessed July 17, 2013.

Public health officials face the need to make decisions and take action. Therefore, a set of ethical principles to guide action is very important. Bernheim and Childress[10] have outlined a set of principles for guiding public health action as follows:

- Producing benefits
- Avoiding, preventing, and reducing harms
- Producing the maximal balance of benefits over harms and other costs
- Distributing benefits and burdens fairly and ensuring public participation, including the participation of affected parties
- Respecting autonomous choices and actions, including liberty of action
- Protecting privacy and confidentiality
- Keeping promises and commitments
- Disclosing information as well as speaking honestly and truthfully
- Building and maintaining trust

When considering whether action is justified, the following conditions should be met[10]:

- Effectiveness: Is the action likely to accomplish the public health goal?
- Necessity: Is the action necessary to override the conflicting ethical claims to achieve the public health goal?
- Least infringement: Is the action the least restrictive and least intrusive?
- Proportionality: Will the probable benefits of the action outweigh the infringed moral norms and any negative effects?
- Impartiality: Are all potentially affected stakeholders treated impartially?
- Public justification: Can public health officials offer public justification that citizens, and in particular those most affected, could find acceptable in principle?

In addition to applying general ethical principles to public health practice, public health is frequently involved in the development and applications of ethical principles to public health and clinical research. In fact, the modern field of bioethics grew out of the efforts to protect participants in research, while ensuring that society can benefit from the results of ethical human research. Let us look at how these standards developed and how research subjects are protected today.

HOW CAN BIOETHICAL PRINCIPLES BE APPLIED TO PROTECTING INDIVIDUALS WHO PARTICIPATE IN RESEARCH?

Ethical issues pervade nearly every aspect of public health and medical practice. However, ethical considerations have had an especially strong impact on the conduct of research. The modern field of bioethics in general and research ethics in particular grew out of the Nuremberg trials of German physicians who performed experiments on prisoners in Nazi concentration camps. These crimes included exposure to extremes of temperature, mutilating surgery, and deliberate infection with a variety of lethal germs. The report of the Nuremberg trials established internationally accepted principles known as the Nuremberg Code shown in **Box 5-3**.[11]

Abuse of individuals participating in research has not been limited to victims of Nazi concentration camps. In the United States from the late 1930s through the early 1970s, the Tuskegee Syphilis Study used disadvantaged, rural black men to study the untreated course of syphilis. These men were recruited to a study of "bad blood" and were misled into believing that they were receiving effective treatment; in addition, they were provided deceptive information in order to retain them in the study. These subjects were deprived of penicillin treatment in order not to interrupt the research, long after such treatment became generally available for syphilis. The Tuskegee Study was a major reason for the creation of The National Commission for the Protection of Human Subjects of Biomedical and Behavioral Research, which produced what has come to be called the **Belmont Report**. The Belmont Report focused on the key issues of defining informed consent and the selection of participants and led to the development of **institutional review boards (IRBs)**, which now must approve most human research. The report remains a vital part of the framework for defining the rights of research subjects.[12] The following excerpts outline three basic ethical principles:

1. **Respect for persons**—Respect for persons incorporates at least two ethical convictions: first, individuals should be treated as autonomous agents, and second, that persons with diminished autonomy are entitled to protection. The principle of respect for persons thus divides into two separate moral requirements: the requirement to acknowledge autonomy and the requirement to protect those with diminished autonomy.
2. **Beneficence**—Persons are treated in an ethical manner not only by respecting their decisions and protecting them from harm, but also by making efforts to secure

BOX 5-3 The Ten Principles Contained in the Nuremberg Code

1. The voluntary consent of the human subject is absolutely essential.
2. The experiment should be such as to yield fruitful results for the good of society, unprocurable by other methods or means of study, and not random and unnecessary in nature.
3. The experiment should be so designed and based on the results of animal experimentation and knowledge of the natural history of the disease or other problem under study that the anticipated results will justify the performance of the experiment.
4. The experiment should be so conducted as to avoid all unnecessary physical and mental suffering and injury.
5. No experiment should be conducted where there is an a priori reason to believe that death or disabling injury will occur, except, perhaps, in those experiments where the experimental physicians also serve as subjects.
6. The degree of risk to be taken should never exceed that determined by the humanitarian importance of the problem to be solved by the experiment.
7. Proper preparations should be made and adequate facilities provided to protect the experimental subject against even remote possibilities of injury, disability, or death.
8. The experiment should be conducted only by scientifically qualified persons. The highest degree of skill and care should be required through all stages of the experiment of those who conduct or engage in the experiment.
9. During the course of the experiment, the human subject should be at liberty to bring the experiment to an end if he has reached the physical or mental state where continuation of the experiment seems to him to be impossible.
10. During the course of the experiment, the scientist in charge must be prepared to terminate the experiment at any stage, if he has probable cause to believe, in the exercise of the good faith, superior skill, and careful judgment required of him, that a continuation of the experiment is likely to result in injury, disability, or death to the experimental subject.

United States Government. *Trials of War Criminals before the Nuremberg Military Tribunals under Control Council Law*. No. 10, Vol. 2. Washington, DC: U.S. Government Printing Office; 1949:181–182.

---

their well-being. Such treatment falls under the principle of beneficence. . . . Two general rules have been formulated as complementary expressions of beneficent actions in this sense: (1) do no harm and (2) maximize possible benefits and minimize possible harms.

3. Justice—Who ought to receive the benefits of research and bear its burdens? This is a question of justice, in the sense of fairness in distribution or what is deserved. An injustice occurs when some benefit to which a person is entitled is denied without good reason or when some burden is imposed unduly. Another way of conceiving the principle of justice is that equals ought to be treated equally.

Institutional review boards were created to ensure the ethical conduct of research. The code of federal regulations outlines the following key roles that the institutional review board is expected to play. In order to approve research, the IRB shall determine that all of the following requirements are satisfied:[13]

1. Risks to subjects are minimized.
2. Risks to subjects are reasonable in relation to anticipated benefits.
3. Selection of subjects is equitable.
4. Informed consent will be sought from each prospective subject or the subject's legally authorized representative.
5. The research plan makes adequate provision for monitoring the data collected to ensure the safety of subjects.
6. When appropriate, there are adequate provisions to protect the privacy of subjects and to maintain the confidentiality of data.
7. When some or all of the subjects are likely to be vulnerable to coercion or undue influence, such as children, prisoners, pregnant women, mentally disabled persons, or economically or educationally disadvantaged persons, additional safeguards have been included in the study to protect the rights and welfare of these subjects.

We have come a long way from the days when human research was conducted without informed consent on individuals who could be coerced to participate. The standards of research, however, continue to evolve and will most likely continue to change through the identification of ethical limitations of current studies.[e]

We have now examined key principles of health law, policy, and ethics and their applications to issues in health care, public health, and bioethics. These principles are basic tools, along with public health data, health communications and the social and behavioral sciences, and can be considered options for implementation when striving to achieve the goals of public health. They are especially powerful tools because they often carry with them the compulsory authority of government. The police powers of public health are increasingly being used cautiously and with careful consideration of the rights of individuals. In many ways, the use of laws is seen as a last resort when the provision of information and incentives for change have not been successful. Now that we have examined key tools of population health, let

us turn our attention to efforts to prevent disease, disability, and death for noncommunicable diseases, communicable disease, and environmental health and safety.

KEY WORDS

- **Bioethics**
- **Police power**
- **Rights**
- **Negative constitution**
- **Substantive due process**
- **Procedural due process**
- **Constitutional law**
- **Legislative statutes**
- **Administrative regulations**
- **Judicial law or case law or common law**
- **Authoritative decision**
- **Health in all policies approach**
- **Social justice**
- **Market justice**
- **No-duty principle**
- **Self-imposed risk**
- **Imposed risk**
- **Quarantine**
- **Belmont Report**
- **Institutional review boards (IRBs)**
- **Respect for Person**
- **Beneficence**
- **Justice**

[e] Bioethics is continuing to evolve. Recent changes in research ethics include limitations on the use of placebos and requirements to register randomized controlled trials before they begin. Placebos are now considered ethical only when no effective active intervention is accepted as the standard of care. The requirement to register randomized clinical trials before they begin was put into effect after randomized controlled trials came to public attention that were never submitted for publication because the results were in conflict with the interests of the trial's sponsor.

Discussion Questions

Take a look at the questions posed in the following scenarios, which were presented at the beginning of this chapter. See now whether you can answer them.

1. A new statute and subsequent administrative regulations give only a temporary license to newly licensed drivers, prohibiting late night driving and the use of cell phones and limiting the number of passengers. You ask: Should elderly drivers be subject to these same types of regulations, such as being required to take a driver's test?

2. The CDC reports that the country is facing an unprecedented epidemic of obesity in all regions. It indicates that it is doing everything within its legal authority to address the epidemic. Unfortunately it concludes there is little more that the federal government can do to fight obesity. Why, you wonder, is the federal authority to address health problems so limited?

3. You hear that a neighbor has TB and refuses treatment. You wonder: What if he has the type of TB that can't be cured with drugs? You ask: Can't they make him take his medicine or at least get him out of the neighborhood?

4. A friend of yours experienced a grand mal seizure in which she totally lost consciousness. Fortunately, cancer is ruled out and she is tolerating the medications without serious side effects and without another seizure. It is two months later and your friend tells you her driver's license was taken away by the motor vehicle administration and she does not know when she will get it back. You ask: What types of issues are involved in deciding if and when she can drive again?

5. You receive an email encouraging your participation in a new research study. It sounds like you are eligible, so you check into it. You are surprised to find that even if you participate, you may not receive the new drug, and you will not even be told which treatment you are receiving. Despite your willingness to take your chances, you are told that you are not eligible for the study due to conditions that put you at increased risk of developing side effects. You ask: Why am I barred from participating if I am willing to take the risks?

REFERENCES

1. Teitelbaum JB, Wilensky SE. *Essentials of Health Policy and Law.* Burlington, MA: Jones & Bartlett Learning; 2012.

2. Gostin LA. *Public Health Law: Power, Duty, Restraint.* Berkeley, CA, and New York, NY: University of California Press and Milbank Memorial Fund; 2000.

3. Turnock BJ. *Public Health: What It Is and How It Works.* 4th ed. Sudbury, MA: Jones and Bartlett Publishers; 2009.

4. Teitelbaum JB, Wilensky SE. *Essentials of Health Policy and Law.* Sudbury, MA: Jones and Bartlett Publishers; 2007:12.

5. *Healthy People 2020.* U.S. Department of Health and Human Services. Leading health indicators. http://www.healthypeople.gov/2020/LHI/default.aspx. Accessed July 16, 2013.

6. Shi L, Singh D. *Delivering Health Care in America.* 3rd ed. Sudbury, MA: Jones and Bartlett Publishers; 2004.

7. United Nations General Assembly. The universal declaration of human rights. http://www.un.org/Overview/rights.html. Accessed July 19.2013.

8. Parmet WE. Legal power and legal rights—isolation and quarantine in the case of drug-resistant tuberculosis. *New England Journal Medicine.* 2007;357:434.

9. Public Health Leadership Society. Principles of the ethical practice of public health. Version 2.2. 2002. http://phls.org/CMSuploads/Principles-of-the-Ethical-Practice-of-PH-Version-2.2-68496.pdf. Accessed July 17, 2013.

10. Bernheim RG, Childress JF, Melnick AL, et al. *Essentials of Public Health Ethics.* Burlington, MA: Jones & Bartlett Learning; 2014.

11. United States Government. *Trials of War Criminals before the Nuremberg Military Tribunals under Control Council Law.* No. 10, Vol. 2. Washington, DC: U.S. Government Printing Office; 1949:181–182.

12. The National Commission for the Protection of Human Subjects of Biomedical and Behavioral Research. The belmont report: ethical principles and guidelines for the protection of human subjects of research. http://www.hhs.gov/ohrp/humansubjects/guidance/belmont.html. Accessed July 19, 2013.

13. United States Department of Health and Human Services. Title 45: public welfare, Department of Health and Human Services, part 46: protection of human subjects. http://www.hhs.gov/ohrp/humansubjects/guidance/45cfr46.html. Accessed July 19, 2013.

SECTION II

Cases and Discussion Questions

DON'S DIABETES

Don had been a diabetic for over a decade and took his insulin pretty much as the doctor ordered. Every morning, after checking his blood sugar levels, he would adjust his insulin dose according to the written instructions. From the beginning, Don's doctor worried about the effect of the diabetes—he ordered tests, adjusted dosages and prescriptions, and sent his patient to the ophthalmologist for assessment and laser treatment to prevent blindness.

It was the amputation of his right foot that really got Don's attention. Don was not exactly athletic, but he did play a round of golf once in a while. He first noticed a little scratch on his foot after a day on the golf course. It was not until a week later that he noticed the swelling and the redness in his foot and an ulceration that was forming. He was surprised that his foot did not hurt, but the doctor informed him that diabetic foot ulcers often do not cause pain. That is part of the problem with diabetes—you lose your sensation in your feet.

After six months of receiving treatment on a weekly basis, a decision had to be made. "There is not any choice," his doctor said. "The foot infection is spreading, and if we do not amputate the foot, we may have to amputate to the knee or even higher." So after describing the potential benefits and harms of the surgery and asking whether there were any questions, the doctor asked Don to sign a form. The next morning, Don's leg was amputated above the ankle, leaving him with a stump in place of a foot.

The surgeon came to Don's room the day after surgery to take a look at his amputation. "Beautiful work," he said with a big smile on his face. *Maybe it is a beautiful stump*, Don thought to himself, *but it does not work like my old foot.* At first, he felt sorry for himself, thinking of what lay ahead to literally get back on his feet.

The physical therapist who visited Don in the hospital told him, "You got off lucky—now, are you going to take control or let diabetes control you?" *But diabetes is already controlling me*, Don thought to himself—daily insulin; blood sugar testing; weekly trips to the doctor; and now, despite it all, an amputated foot.

"Diabetes is a bad disease," his doctor told him. "We are doing everything we can do, and you are still experiencing complications."

Maybe the doctors were doing everything they could, but Don wondered what else was possible. He enrolled in a self-help group for diabetics. They shared stories of medical care, new advances in diabetes management, and their own frustrations with the disease and with their medical care. Don realized he had received good medical care, but he also acknowledged that good care by good doctors is not enough. There needs to be a system that makes the pieces work together, but there also needs to be a patient who takes charge of his care.

So take charge, he did. He worked closely with the practice's physician assistant and nurse practitioner, who were experts in diabetic management. He learned how to interpret his blood tests and how they were useful for day-to-day monitoring of his disease. He also learned about hemoglobin A1c blood tests, which measure how well diabetes is doing over periods of months. After several months, his clinicians taught him how to adjust his dose of insulin to accommodate for changes in his routine or during minor illnesses. They always let him know that care was available and that he did not need to make decisions all by himself. Don also learned to examine his feet and how to prevent minor injuries from turning into major problems. His sporadic eye doctor appointments turned into regular question-and-answer sessions to compare the most recent photographs of his retina to those from the past.

Don found himself keeping his own records to be sure that he had them all in one place, fearing that one doctor would not talk to another and that the records in one office or one hospital would never make their way to the next. Don's fears were well founded: when his kidney function began to deteriorate and his primary care doctor sent him to a kidney specialist, who sent him to a transplant surgeon, and then to a vascular surgeon to prepare him for dialysis, sure enough, the only records the dialysis doctors could rely upon were the ones that Don had kept on his own.

Soon the dialysis doctor told Don that he had a tough decision to make. Did he want to come into the dialysis center for half a day twice a week, where they take care of everything, or did he want to learn home dialysis and take care of this treatment on his own? Don had lots of questions. He needed to understand what each dialysis scenario entailed and the advantages and disadvantages of both options, including the costs and discomforts. He also wanted to know about any other potential treatments. Don asked questions of his doctors, learned as much as he could about dialysis on the Internet, and outlined the pros and cons of home dialysis. After that, it was an easy decision for Don. "Sure, I will learn how to do it myself. I want to be in charge of my own care. I want to stand on my own two feet," he told the doctor without a moment's hesitation.

Discussion Questions

1. What type of decision-making process was going on during the early stages of Don's diabetes? Explain.

2. What type of decision-making process was used to reach the decision to have an amputation? Explain.

3. What type of decision-making process occurred in the decision about dialysis? Explain.

4. In Don's case, what are the advantages and disadvantages of each of these approaches to decision making from both the patient's and the clinician's perspectives? Explain.

A NEW DISEASE CALLED SADS— A DECISION ANALYSIS

Imagine that a new disease called sudden adult disability syndrome (SADS) has become the most common cause of death among previously healthy 18- to 24-year-olds. The etiology of SADS is unknown, but it is thought to be infectious. SADS is a disease of sudden onset that without treatment produces progressive weakness, slow mental deterioration, and death within a year 50% of the time. The other 50% of individuals who develop SADS make a rapid, spontaneous full recovery without any treatment.

There are three known treatments for SADS:

- Ordinary Knowledge (O.K.)—the conventional treatment (in other words, standard treatment)
- Live-Better
- Live-Longer

The probabilities of cure and side effects have been extensively investigated:

- Ordinary Knowledge (O.K.) results in an 80% probability of cure without side effects. The remaining 20% die of SADS.
- Live-Better results in an 85% probability of cure. There are no known side effects. The remaining 15% die from SADS.
- Live-Longer results in an 80% probability of cure. However, 10% of those who take the treatment become totally and permanently blind in both eyes. The remaining 10% die of SADS.

Discussion Questions

1. Prior to conducting a decision analysis, which intervention would you recommend?

2. Draw a decision tree indicating the potential outcomes for each of the three treatments (O.K. therapy, Live-Better, and Live-Longer) and indicate the probability of occurrence of each of the potential outcomes.

3. Assume cure brings your utility to full health, in other words, 1.0, and death's utility is 0. Use a utility of 0.5 for blindness. Can any of the possible interventions be eliminated based on the expected utilities? Explain.

4. Now use a utility of 0.8 for blindness and recalculate the expected utilities. Which intervention is now recommended by the decision analysis?

5. Now use a utility of 0.2 for blindness and recalculate the expected utilities. Which intervention is now recommended by the decision analysis? What can you conclude about the importance of the utility that is placed on blindness?

6. Now use the utility for blindness that indicates the utility that you personally place on blindness. Again recalculate the expected utilities. What intervention is recommended by this decision analysis? How does this recommendation compare to the recommendation you made prior to conducting the decision analysis? If it is different, what other factors did you take into account in reaching your own recommendation?

JOSÉ AND JORGE—IDENTICAL TWINS WITHOUT IDENTICAL LIVES

José and Jorge were identical twins separated at birth. José grew up in a large family in an impoverished slum in the middle of a crime-ridden and polluted district of a major city. Jorge grew up in an upper-middle-class professional family with one other brother in a suburban community in the same city. Despite the fact the José and Jorge were identical twins, their lives and health could not have been more different.

José had few opportunities for medical care or public health services as a child. His nutrition was always marginal and he developed several severe cases of diarrhea before he was 1 year of age. He received a polio vaccine as part of a community vaccination program, but never received vaccinations for measles, mumps, rubella, or other childhood illnesses. At age 4, he developed measles and was so sick, his mother was sure he would not make it.

As a child, José also developed asthma, which seemed to worsen when he played outdoors on hot smoggy days. Dropping out of school at age 14, José went to work in a factory, but quit when he found himself panting for breath at the end of the day.

As a teenager, José was repeatedly exposed to crime and drugs. Once, he was caught in the cross fire of gangs fighting for control of drugs in his community. Experimenting with drugs with his teenage friends, José contracted HIV from use of contaminated needles. José did not know he had HIV until he was nearly 30 years old and developed tuberculosis (TB). He did receive treatment for the TB free of charge from the health department, but once he felt better, he did not follow up with treatment.

By the time the TB returned, José had lost 30 pounds and could barely make it into the emergency room of the public hospital because of his shortness of breath. He was hospitalized for the last two months of his life, mostly to prevent others from being exposed to what was now drug-resistant tuberculosis. No one ever knew how many people José exposed to HIV or TB.

Jorge's life as a child was far less eventful. He received "well child" care from an early age. His family hardly noticed that he rarely developed diarrhea and had few sick days from diseases of childhood. He did well in school, but like José, he developed asthma. With good treatment, Jorge was able to play on sports teams, at least until he began to smoke cigarettes at age 14.

Jorge soon began to gain weight, and by the time he graduated from college, he was rapidly becoming obese. In his 20s, he developed high blood pressure, and in his 30s he had early signs of diabetes. Jorge had a heart attack in his mid-40s and underwent bypass surgery a few years later. The treatments for diabetes, hypertension, and high cholesterol worked well and Jorge was able to lead a productive professional life into his 40s.

By the time that Jorge turned 50, his diabetes began to worsen and he developed progressive kidney disease. Jorge soon needed twice-a-week dialysis, which kept him alive as he awaited a kidney transplant.

Discussion Questions

1. How do social determinants of health contribute to the different disease patterns of José and Jorge?

2. How do factors in the physical environment explain differences in the health of José and Jorge?

3. What role does medical care play in the differences between the health outcomes of José and Jorge?

4. What roles do public health services play in the health outcomes of José and Jorge?

THE OBESITY EPIDEMIC IN THE UNITED STATES—THE TIP OF AN ICEBERG

Before the last half of the 1900s, obesity was often seen as a sign of prosperity. Look at the great art of 18th and 19th century Europe and you will find portraits of the prosperous and portly prominently displayed. In the last half of the 1900s and the early years of the 2000s, obesity has become the province of the poor and the middle class.

Obesity is defined as a BMI over 30. Overweight is defined as a BMI from 25 to 30. The BMI is calculated as the weight in kilograms/height in meters squared. A BMI of 30 for a 5 foot, 8.5 inch male or female is approximately 200 pounds. To determine whether a child aged 2 to 19 years is considered obese, a BMI for age is calculated, but further assessment is needed to determine fat distribution, such as measurement of skinfold thickness. The prevalence of obesity has been steadily rising in the United States over the last 50 years, increasing over 250%. Today, approximately 20% of children aged 2 to 19 are obese, along with approximately 35% of adults.

U.S. data confirm a strong association of obesity with lower socioeconomic levels overall and in most but not all racial and ethnic groups. Overall, children and adolescents 2 to 19 years in families with an income under 130% of the poverty level (about $30,000 for a family of 4) have almost twice the prevalence of obesity as children and adolescents in families with income over 350% of the poverty level. However, these patterns do not apply to non-Hispanic black girls or to Mexican American boys or girls, in whom high levels of obesity occur at all income and educational levels.

A number of factors play important roles in giving the portrait of obesity in the United States a far less prosperous persona. The availability of cheap, high-calorie foods has played an important role in allowing access to abundant quantities of food by lower socioeconomic individuals. Newer technologies using concentrated sugars, such as high fructose corn syrup, and trans fats have reinforced this tendency. Once obesity is established, exercise may be more difficult, setting in motion a vicious circle of sedentary lifestyle and increased weight. Similarly, once obesity is established, the large quantities of food required daily often necessitate the purchase of cheap high-calorie food.

Obesity is strongly associated with a constellation of other health conditions in what has been called a syndemic, or the occurrence together of two or more health conditions. Obesity is the strongest risk factor associated with type 2 diabetes. Abdominal obesity, defined as a waistline of approximately 37 inches for males and 31.5 inches for females, is central to what is called the metabolic syndrome. The metabolic syndrome requires the presence of abdominal obesity and also includes diabetes, high blood pressure, and cholesterol and triglyceride abnormalities, including low good cholesterol. Each of these conditions can and should be treated, but treatment is far more successful and carries fewer side effects if weight can be reduced. Often a 5 or 10% reduction in body weight has a major impact on these conditions. Cigarette smoking, another strong risk factor for heart and vascular disease as well as cancer, actually has a small impact on reducing weight.

A number of approaches have been suggested to address the epidemic of obesity in the United States. An increasing number of drugs are being developed and approved to treat obesity. A surgical approach called gastric bypass surgery or more generally bariatric or weight loss surgery have been demonstrated to have efficacy using randomized controlled trials, including long-term weight loss and reduction in complications especially among those with a BMI greater than 40.

Newer dietary approaches, such as low-carbohydrate diets, have been shown in a randomized controlled trial to increase weight loss over the short run, but like other diets, the low-carb diet has less impressive results over longer periods of time. A variety of sugar substitutes have been investigated and introduced in recent years. It is controversial whether these sugar substitutes have had a substantial impact on obesity or have merely led to increased consumption of other high-calorie foods.

Other approaches attempt to get at the cultural influences on obesity, including the fact that the average portion size in restaurants has increased over the last few decades. Efforts to limit the size of high-calorie soft drinks are one example of this approach. Focusing on children and adolescents by restricting the availability of food with high sugar and carbohydrates in school lunches and offering healthier alternatives is also being tried. Taxing high-calorie, low-nutrition food is another option being debated. Increasing requirements for physical activity in schools is yet another policy change being advocated.

The answers to the weighty question of obesity in the United States remain a great challenge. What do you think we should do about it?

Discussion Questions

1. Identify the contributions of social determinants of health, including cultural factors, to the increased rate of obesity in the United States. Explain.

2. Discuss the relationship between obesity and other health conditions that lead to cardiovascular disease, including the interactions that occur.

3. Which of the interventions discussed in this case would you endorse? Explain why, including considering the positive and negative aspects of each intervention.

4. How would you combine the interventions that you selected in question number 3 to effectively address the national epidemic of obesity?

CHANGING BEHAVIOR—CIGARETTE SMOKING

It was not going to be easy for Steve to stop smoking. He had been at it for 30 years—ever since he took it up on a dare at age 16 and found that it was a good way to socialize. In his 20s, it seemed to make dealing with the work pressure easier, and in those days, you could smoke in your office and did not even need to shut the door—much less deal with those dirty looks he was getting now.

Steve was always confident that he could take cigarettes or leave them. He would quit when he was good and ready, and a few cigarettes could not hurt. But then he talked to some friends who had quit a decade or more ago and said they would go back in a minute if they thought cigarettes were safe. *Maybe for some people, those cravings just never go away,* he worried to himself. However, there was that bout of walking pneumonia, and then the cough that just did not seem to go away. The cough was so bad that he had trouble smoking more than a few cigarettes a day. The physician assistant let him know that these symptoms were early warning signs of things to come; however, Steve just was not ready to stop. So the physician assistant gave him a fact sheet and let Steve know there was help available when he was ready.

It might have been his fears about his 10-year-old son that finally tipped the scales. "Daddy, those cigarettes are bad for you," he said. Or maybe it was when he found cigarette butts in the backyard after his 16-year-old daughter's birthday party. Steve knew enough to believe that a father who smokes has a child who smokes. So this time, he would do it right.

Steve's physician assistant recognized that Steve was finally ready to quit. He let him know in no uncertain terms that it was important to quit totally, completely, and forever. He also informed Steve that he could rely on help—that he was not alone. With the encouragement of his physician assistant, Steve joined a support group, set a quit date, and announced the date to his friends and family. The new medication he was prescribed seemed to relieve the worst cravings and the feeling he called "crawling the walls."

His wife, Dorothy, was supportive. She cleared the cigarette butts and ashtrays out of the house and dealt with the smell by having all the drapes cleaned. She also helped by getting him up after dinner and taking a walk, which kept him from his old habit of having a cigarette with dessert and coffee. It also helped keep him from gaining too much weight, which she confided was her greatest fear. Dorothy's quiet encouragement and subtle reinforcement without nagging worked wonders.

Saving a couple of dollars a day did not hurt. Steve collected those dollars and put them in a special hiding place. On his first year anniversary of quitting, he wrapped up the dollar bills in a box and gave them to Dorothy as a present. The note inside said: "A trip for us for as long as the money lasts." Dorothy was delighted, but feared the worst when Steve began to open up his present to himself. As he unwrapped a box of cigars, he smiled a big smile and said, "I am congratulating myself on quitting smoking."

Discussion Questions

1. How are each of the phases in the stages of change model illustrated in Steve's case?

2. What other theories or models can be applied to the public health issue described in this case? Explain.

3. Which effective public health (or population) approaches does this case illustrate?

4. What is the impact of combining individual clinical approaches with public health (or population) approaches?

THE ELDERLY DRIVER

It was late in the afternoon on a sunny April day. Maybe it was the sun in her eyes, but 82-year-old Janet found herself in her car in a ditch at the side of the road, unsure of how she got there. Once at the hospital, her son and daughter joined her and heard the good news that Janet had escaped with just a broken arm. The police report strongly suggested that she had swerved off the road, but it was not clear why.

This was not Janet's first driving "episode"; in fact, her driving had been a constant worry to her daughter for over two years. Her daughter often offered to take her Mom shopping and insisted that she do the driving when they were together. "Do you not trust me?" was the only thanks the daughter received. When alone, Janet continued to drive herself, staying off the freeway and increasingly driving only during the day. She knew it was not as easy as it used to be, but it was her lifeline to independence.

Then, a few months after the April incident, the form for Janet's license renewal arrived. A vision test and a physical exam were required, along with a doctor's certification that Janet was in good health and capable of driving; however, no road test was required. So Janet made a doctor's appointment, and at the end of it, she left the forms with a note for the doctor saying, "To the best doctor I have ever had. Thanks for filling this out. You know how much driving means to me."

On Janet's way home from the doctor's office, it happened. She was driving down the road when suddenly she was crossing that yellow line and heading toward an oncoming car. The teenage driver might have been going a little fast, but Janet was in the wrong lane and the head-on collision killed the 16-year-old passenger in the front seat who was not wearing a seat belt. The 18-year-old driver walked away from the collision unharmed, thanks to an inflated airbag.

Janet was never the same emotionally. And despite escaping the collision with just a few bruises, the loss of her driver's license symbolized the end for her. Those lost weekly shopping trips and the strangers in the assisted living center were not the same as living in her own home. The young man in the collision screaming for help woke her up almost every night. It was only a year after the collision when Janet died, and it was just like she had said: "Take my license away and it will kill me."

Discussion Questions

1. How does this case reflect the important issue of balancing the legal rights of the individual and the rights of society as a whole?

2. What role do you believe healthcare providers should play in implementing driving laws and regulations?

3. Identify any changes you would make to prevent the types of outcomes that occurred in this case study.

4. How would you communicate the lessons learned in this case to new and inexperienced drivers?

SECTION III

Preventing Disease, Disability, and Death

In public health, we are increasingly identifying disease, disability, and death as being produced by underlying determinants. While these determinants are useful in thinking about basic reasons for disease and disability, it is often difficult to link the underlying determinants with the diseases and disabilities that result.

The concept of **actual causes** is more closely connected with the development of disease. It provides a way of organizing what we know about the prevention of disease and disability into categories that we can measure. Thus, it allows us to ask a key question: How much disease and disability can be prevented?[1] Actual causes of disease can then be linked to three basic categories: noncommunicable diseases, communicable diseases, and environmental diseases and injuries. **Figure S03-1** illustrates the framework we will use in this section to connect determinants of disease, actual causes, and categories of disease and injury.

The concept of actual causes of disease is a relatively new idea that has been successfully applied to the causes of death, though not to disability. **Table S03-1** provides the most recent data on the actual causes of death. It indicates that nearly half of all deaths in the United States are related to nine potentially preventable actual causes.[a]

The concept of actual causes of disease provides us with a framework for thinking about the underlying problems that lead to death. As indicated in the table, nearly half of all deaths can be ascribed to one of these actual causes. Actual causes can help guide us in placing priorities on where we should put our attention and spend our money to prevent disease.

A substantial portion of the actual causes of death are related to the development of noncommunicable diseases, including tobacco, diet and physical inactivity, alcohol consumption, and illicit drug use. Communicable disease remains an important category related not only to microbial agents, but also to sexual behavior. Finally, a broad range of environmental diseases and injuries are related to toxic agents, motor vehicle–related injuries, and firearm-related injuries. In Chapters 6, 7, and 8, we will address noncommunicable and communicable diseases, review environmental health and injury, and examine the public health strategies that have been used to address each of them. We will aim

---

[a] Causes of death on death certificates have traditionally been defined in terms of specific diseases that have been formally incorporated with thousands of listings in the International Classification of Diseases (ICD codes). This coding system includes a wide range of specific diseases, as well as injuries and other conditions. These items are then categorized based upon organ system or another biological framework.

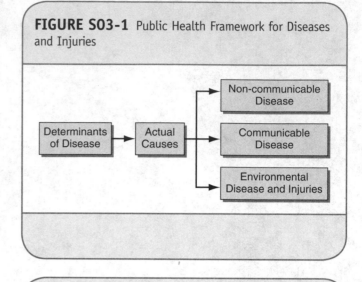

FIGURE S03-1 Public Health Framework for Diseases and Injuries

TABLE S03-1 Actual Causes of Death in the United States

Actual cause	Number of deaths
Tobacco	435,000
Diet and physical inactivity	400,000
Alcohol consumption	85,000
Microbial agents (infections)	75,000
Toxic agents	55,000
Motor vehicles	43,000
Firearms	29,000
Sexual behavior	20,000
Illicit drug use	17,000
Total	1,159,000 (total deaths 2,403,351)

Data from: Mokdad AM, Marks JS, Stroup DF, Gerberding JL. Actual causes of death in the United States 2000. *JAMA*. 2004;291:1,238–1,245.

to better understand the burden of disease and strategies for addressing it. Let us begin with the largest category of disease in the United States today—noncommunicable diseases.

KEY WORDS

- **Actual causes**

REFERENCES

1. Mokdad AM, Marks JS, Stroup DF, Gerberding JL. Actual causes of death in the United States 2000. *JAMA*. 2004;291:1,238–1,245.

CHAPTER **6**

Noncommunicable Diseases

Learning Objectives

By the end of this chapter, the student will be able to:

- describe the burden of noncommunicable diseases on mortality and morbidity in the United States.
- describe the ideal criteria for a screening program.
- explain why two or more tests are nearly always required to screen for asymptomatic disease.
- explain the multiple risk factor intervention approach to control a noncommunicable disease.
- describe the meaning of "cost-effectiveness."
- describe several ways that genetic interventions can affect the burden of noncommunicable diseases.
- describe ways that population interventions can be combined with individual interventions to more effectively reduce the burden of noncommunicable diseases.

Sasha did not want to think about the possibility of breast cancer, but as she turned 50, she agreed to have a mammography, which, as she feared, was positive or "suspicious," as her doctor put it. Waiting for the results of the follow-up biopsy was the worst part, but the relief she felt when the results were negative brought tears of joy to her and her family. Then she wondered: Is it common to have a positive mammography when no cancer is present?

The first sign of Michael's coronary heart disease was his heart attack. Looking back, he had been at high risk for many years because he smoked

and had high blood pressure and high bad cholesterol. His lack of exercise and obesity only made the situation worse. Michael asked: What are the risk factors for coronary heart disease and what can be done to identify and address these factors for me and my family?

John's knee injury from skiing continued to produce swelling and pain, greatly limiting his activities. His physician informed him that the standard procedure today is to look inside with a flexible scope and do any surgery that is needed through the scope. It is simpler and cheaper, and does not even require hospitalization. "We call it 'cost-effective,'" his doctor said. John wondered: What does "cost-effective" really mean?

Jennifer and her husband, George, were tested for the cystic fibrosis gene and both were found to have it. Cystic fibrosis causes chronic lung infections and greatly shortens the length of life. They now ask: What does this mean for our chances of having a child with cystic fibrosis? Can we find out whether our child has cystic fibrosis early in pregnancy?

Fred's condition deteriorated slowly, but persistently. He just could not remember anything and repeated himself endlessly. The medications helped for a short time, but before long, he did not recognize his family and could not take care of himself. The diagnosis was Alzheimer's, and he was not alone. Almost everyone in the nursing home seemed to be affected. No one seems to understand the cause of Alzheimer's disease. The family asked: What else can be done, not only for Fred, but also for those who come after Fred?

Alcohol use is widespread on your campus. You do not see it as a problem as long as you walk home or have a designated driver. Your mind changes one day after you hear about a classmate who nearly died from alcohol poisoning as a result of binge drinking. You ask yourself: What should be done on my campus to address binge drinking?

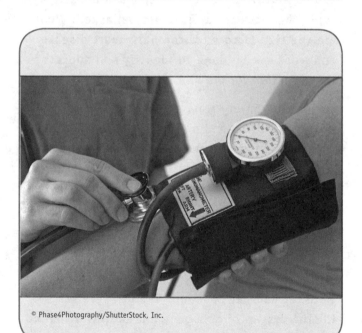

© Phase4Photography/ShutterStock, Inc.

Each of these scenarios represents one of the approaches to noncommunicable diseases that we will examine in this chapter.

WHAT IS THE BURDEN OF NONCOMMUNICABLE DISEASE?

Noncommunicable disease represents a wide range of diseases, from cardiovascular disease, cancers, and depression, to Alzheimer's and chronic arthritis. Together, they represent the majority of causes of death and disability in most developed countries. Today, cardiovascular diseases and cancer alone each represent nearly 25% of the causes of death as reflected on death certificates in the United States.

The impact of noncommunicable diseases on death only reflects part of the influence of these diseases on people's lives. Chronic disabilities, largely due to noncommunicable diseases, are now the most rapidly growing component of morbidity in most developing as well as developed countries. As populations age, noncommunicable diseases increase in frequency. The presence of two or more chronic diseases makes progressive disability particularly likely. The consequences of the rapidly growing pattern of disability due to noncommunicable diseases have enormous economic implications. The great increase in direct costs for health care is in part due to the increased burden of noncommunicable diseases. The impact extends beyond healthcare costs, as it affects the quality of life and may limit the ability of those who wish to work to continue to do so.

Noncommunicable diseases have not always dominated the types of diseases that impact a society. **Box 6-1** discusses the **epidemiological transition**[1] and provides a perspective on where we stand today.

There are a wide range of preventive, curative, and rehabilitative approaches to noncommunicable diseases. However, there are a limited number of basic strategies being used that are part of the population health approach, including:

- Screening for early detection and treatment of disease
- Multiple risk factor interventions
- Identification of cost-effective treatments
- Genetics counseling and intervention
- Research

We will take a look at each of these approaches. Finally, we will see how many of these approaches can be combined using the population health approach. Let us begin with what we call **screening** for disease.

HOW CAN SCREENING FOR DISEASE ADDRESS THE BURDEN OF NONCOMMUNICABLE DISEASES?

Screening for disease implies the use of tests on individuals who do not have symptoms of a specific disease. These individuals are **asymptomatic**. This implies that they do not have symptoms related to the disease being investigated. They may have symptoms of other diseases. Screening for disease can result in detection of disease at an early stage under the assumption that early detection will allow for treatment that will improve outcome. Screening has been successful for a

BOX 6-1 The Epidemiological Transition and Noncommunicable Diseases

Disease patterns have not always been the same, and they will continue to evolve. To gain a big picture understanding of this process of change, it is useful to understand the concept known as the epidemiological or **public health transition**.

The epidemiological transition describes the changing pattern of disease that has been seen in many countries as they have experienced social and economic development. Its central message is that prior to social and economic development, communicable diseases—or microbial agents, using the term from actual causes—represent the dominant cause of disease and disability. In countries in early stages of development, infections are a key cause of mortality, either directly or indirectly. For instance, in undeveloped countries, maternal and perinatal conditions, as well as nutritional disorders, are often identified as the causes of death. Microbial agents play a key role in maternal and perinatal deaths, as well as deaths ascribed to nutrition. Most maternal deaths are due to infection not necessarily transmitted from others, but related to exposure to microbial agents at the time of birth and in the early postpartum period.

Similarly, most deaths among young children in undeveloped countries are related directly or indirectly to infection. Inadequate nutrition predisposes children to infection and interferes with their ability to fight off infection when it does occur. Many of the deaths among children with malnutrition are related to acute infections, especially acute infectious diarrhea and acute respiratory infections.

As social and economic development progresses, noncommunicable diseases—including cardiovascular diseases, diabetes, cancers, chronic respiratory ailments, and neuropsychiatric diseases, such as depression and Alzheimer's—predominate as the causes of disability and death. Depression is rapidly becoming one of the major causes of disability, and the World Health Organization (WHO) estimates that it will produce more disability than any other single condition in coming years. In addition, illicit drug use has become a major cause of death among the young and includes not only illegal use of drugs, but also abuse of prescription drugs.

In much of the developing world, the same basic patterns are occurring in the developing regions within these countries. Often, earlier distributions of disease dominated by communicable diseases coexist with patterns of noncommunicable diseases typical of developed countries. Thus, is it not unusual to find that malnutrition and obesity are often present side-by-side in the same developing country.

The epidemiologic transition does not imply that once countries reach the stage where noncommunicable diseases dominate that this pattern will persist indefinitely. Newly emerging diseases, such as HIV/AIDS, pandemic flu, and drug-resistant bacterial infections, raise the possibility that communicable diseases will once again dominate the pattern of disease and death in developed countries.

---

range of noncommunicable diseases, including breast cancer and colon cancer, as well as childhood conditions, including vision and hearing impairments. In all of these conditions, screening has resulted in reduced disability and/or deaths. Not all noncommunicable diseases, however, are good candidates for screening, and in some cases, screening programs have yet to be devised and studied for some noncommunicable diseases for which early detection could be useful.

Four criteria need to be fulfilled for an ideal screening program.[2] While few, if any, health conditions completely fulfill all four requirements, these criteria provide a standard against which to judge the potential of a screening program. These criteria are:

1. The disease produces substantial death and/or disability.
2. Early detection is possible and improves outcome.

3. There is a feasible testing strategy for screening.
4. Screening is acceptable in terms of harms, costs, and patient acceptance.

The first criterion is perhaps the easiest to evaluate. Conditions such as breast and colon cancer result in substantial death and disability rates. Breast cancer is the second most common cancer in terms of causes of death and is the most common cancer-related cause of death among women in their 50s. Colon cancer is among the most common causes of cancer death in both men and women. Childhood conditions, such as hearing loss and visual impairment, are not always obvious; however, they cause considerable disability.

Determining whether early detection is possible and will improve outcomes is not as easy as it may appear. Screening may result in early detection, but if effective treatment is not available, it may merely alert the clinician and the patient to the disease at an earlier point in time without offering hope of an improved outcome. Screening cigarette smokers for lung cancer using X-rays would seem reasonable because lung cancer is the number one cancer killer of both men and women. However, X-ray screening of smokers has been beneficial only in terms of early detection. By the time lung cancer can be seen via chest X-ray, it is already too late to cure. This early detection without improved outcome is called **lead-time bias**.[a]

As indicated in the third criterion, in order to implement a successful screening program, there must be a feasible testing strategy.[b] This usually requires identification of a high-risk population. It also requires a strategy for using two or more tests to distinguish what are called **false positives** and **false negatives** from those who truly have and do not have the disease. False positives are individuals who have positive results on a screening test but do not turn out to have the disease. Similarly, false negatives are those who have negative results on the screening test but turn out to have the disease.

Screening for asymptomatic disease usually identifies more false positives than **true positives**. True positives are individuals who have a positive test and also have the disease. This is true for most screening tests, as discussed in **Box 6-2** on **Bayes' theorem**.

How can we develop feasible testing strategies?[3] To understand the need for and use of feasible testing strategies, it is important to recognize that screening for diseases is usually conducted on groups that are at an increased risk for the condition. For instance, screening men and women for colon cancer and women for breast cancer is often conducted on people aged 50 years and older. This type of group is considered high risk, usually with a chance or risk of having the disease of 1% or more. Use of high-risk groups like

these allows tests that are less than perfect to serve as initial screening tests.

As we have seen, screening for diseases such as breast cancer almost always requires two or more tests. These tests need to be combined using a testing strategy. The most commonly used testing strategy is called **sequential testing**, or **consecutive testing**. This approach implies that an initial screening test is followed by one or more definitive or diagnostic tests. Sequential testing is used in breast cancer, hearing, and vision testing, and most other forms of screening for noncommunicable diseases. It is generally the most cost-effective form of screening because only one negative test is needed to rule out the disease.

Sequential testing by definition misses those who have false negative results because when a negative test occurs, the testing process is over, at least for the immediate future. Thus, a testing strategy needs to consider how to detect those missed by screening. We need to ask: Is there a need for repeat screening, and if so, when should it occur?[c]

Finally, an ideal screening test should be acceptable in terms of harms, costs, and patient acceptance. Harms must be judged by looking at the entire testing strategy—not just the initial test. Physical examination, blood tests, and urine tests often are used as initial screening tests. These tests are virtually harmless. The real question is: What needs to be done if the initial test is positive? If a large number of invasive tests, such as catheterization or surgery, are required, the overall testing strategy may present substantial potential harms.

Screenings and diagnostic tests themselves can be quite costly. In addition, costs are related to the length of time between testing. Testing every year will be far more costly than testing every five or ten years. The frequency of testing depends on the speed at which the disease develops and progresses, as well as the number of people who can be expected to be missed on the initial test. Mammographic screening is traditionally conducted every year because breast cancer can

---

[a] The concept of lead time implies that screening produces an earlier diagnosis that may be effectively used to intervene prior to diagnosis without screening. If there is little that can be done to improve outcomes, the extra lead time may result in lead-time bias.

[b] A prerequisite to the use of tests in screening and other situations is establishing the cutoff line that differentiates a positive test and a negative test. Often this is done by using what is called a reference interval. The range of the reference interval is often established by utilizing populations that are believed to be free of a disease. The central 95% of the range of values (or the mean plus or minus 2 standard deviations) for this population is then used as the reference interval, or range of normal. This approach has a number of limitations, including equating existing levels on a test with desirable levels. When data is available on the desirable levels, it is preferable to utilize these levels to establish a reference interval and to define a positive and negative test result. Establishing the desirable level for a test result requires long term follow-up. For such measurements as blood pressure, cholesterol, and fasting blood sugar, desirable levels are now available.

[c] A sequential testing strategy also requires a decision on the order of administering the tests. Issues of cost and safety are often the overriding considerations in determining which test to use first and which to use to confirm an initial positive test. At times, a testing strategy known as **simultaneous testing**, or **parallel testing**, is used. In this scenario, two tests are used initially if one test can be expected to detect one type of disease and the other test can be expected to detect a different type of disease. Traditionally, flexible sigmoidoscopy, which examines the lower approximately 35 cm of the colon, has been used along with tests for occult blood in the stool. Tests for occult blood attempt to screen for cancer in the large section of colon proximal to the sigmoid region. Using both of these tests has been shown to be more accurate for screening than use of either test alone because each attempts to find cancer in different anatomical sites.

BOX 6-2 Bayes' Theorem

Bayes' theorem is a mathematical formula that has very practical applications to interpreting the meaning of diagnostic and screening tests. Bayes' theorem provides the connection between the probability of disease before a test is conducted, or the **pretest probability of disease**, and the probability of disease after knowing whether the test result is positive or negative, or the **posttest probability of disease**. To understand Bayes' theorem, we need to appreciate its three elements:

- The meaning of the pretest probability of the disease
- The measures used to summarize the information provided by the results of a test
- The meaning of the posttest probability of the disease when the test is positive and when the test is negative

Pretest probability of disease: The pretest probability of a disease is an estimate based on combining information about the prevalence of the disease and risk factors for the disease.[a]

Measure to summarize information provided by the test: The measures used to summarize the information provided by a test are called **sensitivity** and **specificity**. Sensitivity is the probability that the test will be positive in the presence of the disease (positive-in-disease). Specificity is the probability that the test will be negative in the absence of the disease (negative-in-health). Ideally, tests have 100% sensitivity and 100% specificity, in which case the test results are always correct. Unfortunately, most tests have a lower sensitivity and specificity, more in the range of 90%, as is the situation with use of mammography for screening for breast cancer.

Posttest probability of disease: The posttest probability of disease is the probability of disease after taking into account the pretest probability of disease as well as the sensitivity and specificity of the test. If a test is positive, the posttest probability of disease is called the **predictive value of a**

positive. If the test result is negative, the posttest probability that the disease is absent is called the **predictive value of a negative**.

Let us look at how this process works using the example of screening for breast cancer using mammography among women 50 years of age and older. We will assume that the pretest probability of breast cancer among women 50 years of age and older is 1%.

We begin by creating what we call a 2x2 box. In the 2x2 box, the mammography results positive (+) or negative (−) appear on the left, while the actual presence or absence of breast cancer, as established by a definitive or gold standard test, appears across the top. For illustration purposes, we are assuming that there are 1,000 women 50 years and older in this population. Because we are assuming that the pretest probability of disease is 1%, we can conclude that 10 of the 1,000 women actually have breast cancer, as is indicated along the bottom row.

	Breast cancer present	Breast cancer absent	
Mammography (+)			
Mammography (−)			
	10	990	1000

Now let us include the information provided by the test. We are assuming that mammography has a 90% sensitivity and a 90% specificity. The following boxes illustrate what happens when we apply a test with 90% sensitivity and 90% specificity to a group with a 1% pretest probability of a disease.

	Breast cancer present	Breast cancer absent	
Mammography (+)	9	99	108
Mammography (−)	1	891	892
	10	990	1000

Because the sensitivity of mammography is assumed to be 90%, among the 10 women with breast cancer, 9 will be detected by the test, allowing us to fill in the 9 and 1 in

[a] When signs or symptoms of a disease are present, the pretest probability of disease also takes these into account. When screening a population or group of people, we include only individuals who are asymptomatic; that is, they do not have any signs or symptoms of the disease for which screening is being conducted. Often when screening for disease, the pretest probability is low—that is, 1% or even less. For instance, the recommendations for screening women over 50 years of age for breast cancer and screening men and women over 50 for colon cancer are based on data showing that the prevalence of the disease in these risk groups is in the range of 1%.

(continues)

BOX 6-2 Bayes' Theorem (continued)

the left-hand column. Similarly, because we are assuming that the specificity of mammography is also 90%, there are 891 women without breast cancer (0.9 x 990) who will have a negative mammography. That leaves 99 women without breast cancer who will have a positive mammography.

This 2x2 box form of Bayes' theorem lets us calculate the probability of breast cancer if the mammography is positive. Note that there are 108 positive mammography tests out of 1,000 tests, but only 9 reflect breast cancer. The positive mammographies that reflect breast cancer are called true positives. The positive mammographies that do not reflect breast cancer are called false positives. Therefore, only 9 out of 108, or less than 9% of the positive tests, are true positives. This implies that if a mammography is positive, the chance, or probability, of breast cancer is still less than 9%.

As we have seen in this illustration, the pretest probability of breast cancer was 1%, while the posttest probability of breast cancer after obtaining a positive mammography was less than 9%. The bottom line of this illustration is that the pretest probability of the disease is a major factor in determining the posttest probability of the disease unless the test is nearly perfect—that is, unless its sensitivity and specificity are nearly 100%.

One key implication of Bayes' theorem for screening for disease is that most screening tests cannot do the job on their own. Follow-up testing, which provides more definitive evidence of disease, is almost always needed. For instance, with breast cancer, a biopsy is often done to make the diagnosis. Most of the time, the biopsy will be negative after a positive mammography, so it is important not to jump to conclusions based on a screening test.

develop and spread rapidly. In the case of colon cancer, however, longer periods between testing are acceptable because the disease is much slower to develop. Thus, cost considerations may be taken into account when choosing between technologies and when setting the interval between screenings.[d]

Finally, patient acceptance is key to successful screening. Many screening strategies present little problem with patient acceptance. However, colon cancer screening has had its challenges with patience acceptance because many consider it an invasive and uncomfortable procedure. Fewer than half the people who qualify for screening based upon current recommendations currently pursue and receive colon cancer screening. This contrasts dramatically with mammography, where a substantial majority of women over 50 now receive the recommended screening.

The screening tests that completely fulfill these ideal criteria are few, and many more are successfully used despite not fulfilling all these criteria. Screening may still be useful as long as we are aware of its limitations and prepared to accept

its inherent problems. **Table 6-1** illustrates how commonly used screening tests for risk factors for cardiovascular disease and common cancers perform based upon the four criteria we have outlined.

These criteria also help identify types of screening that should not be done. In general, we do not screen for disease when early detection does not improve outcome. We do not screen for rare diseases, such as many types of cancers, especially when the available tests are only moderately accurate. Finally, we do not screen for disease when the testing strategy produces substantial harms. Screening for disease is not the only population health approach that can be used to address the burden of noncommunicable disease. Multiple risk factor reduction is a second strategy that we will examine.

HOW CAN IDENTIFICATION AND TREATMENT OF MULTIPLE RISK FACTORS BE USED TO ADDRESS THE BURDEN OF NONCOMMUNICABLE DISEASE?

As we have seen, the concept of risk factors is fundamental to the work of public health. Risk factors ranging from high levels of blood pressure and LDL cholesterol to multiple sexual partners and anal intercourse help us identify groups that are most likely to develop a disease. Evidence-based recommendations often focus on addressing risk factors, and implementation efforts often address the best way(s) to target high-risk groups. Thus, identifying and reducing risk

---

[d] Today, there is a wide range of methods for screening for colon cancer, including colonoscopy, which examines the entire colon, and virtual colonoscopy, which does not require an internal examination. These newer tests are much more costly than sigmoidoscopy and occult stool testing. Which is the most accurate and cost-effective test remains controversial. However, the need for and benefits of screening for colon cancer are widely accepted.

TABLE 6-1 Examples of Screening Tests for Heart Disease and Cancer and Ideal Criteria

	Substantial mortality and/or morbidity	Early detection is possible and alters outcome	Screening is feasible (can identify a high-risk population and a testing strategy)	Screening is acceptable in terms of harms, costs, and patient acceptance
Hypertension	Contributory cause of strokes, myocardial infarctions, kidney disease	High blood pressure precedes bad outcomes often by decades and effective treatment is available	Test everyone—desirable range has been established	Screening itself is free of harms, low cost, and acceptable to patients Treatments, however, may be complicated and have harms, costs, and side effects
LDL cholesterol	Contributory cause of strokes, myocardial infarctions, and other vascular diseases	Precedes the development of disease by decades and treatment is effective in altering outcome	Test everyone—desirable range has been established	Screening itself is free of harm, low cost, and acceptable to patients Treatment has rare side effects, which can be detected by symptoms and low-cost blood tests
Breast cancer	2nd most common fatal cancer among women and most common for women under 70	Early detection improves outcome	For those 50 and over, combination of mammography and follow-up biopsy shown to be feasible	Harm may occur due to false positives, low risk of harm from radiation, patient acceptance good, but test can be somewhat painful Screening younger women increases costs and false positives
Cervical cancer	If undetected and untreated—may be fatal	Early treatment dramatically reduces the risk of death	Pap smear and follow-up testing have been extremely successful	Pap results in substantial number of false positives New DNA testing may be used to separate true and false positives
Colon cancer	Second most common fatal cancer in men and third in women	Early detection of polyps reduces development of cancer, and early detection of cancer improves chances of survival	Men and women 50 and older, plus those with high-risk types of colon disease Options for screening include: fecal occult blood testing, plus flexible sigmoidoscopy, colonoscopy, and virtual colonoscopy	Patient acceptance has been major barrier, small probability of harm from procedure, substantial cost for colonoscopy and virtual colonoscopy

factors is an inherent part of the population health approach to noncommunicable diseases.

A special form of intervention aimed at risk factors is called **multiple risk factor reduction**. As the name implies, this strategy intervenes simultaneously in a series of risk factors, all of which contribute to a particular outcome, such as cardiovascular disease or lung cancer. Multiple risk factor reduction is most effective when there are constellations, or groups of risk factors that cluster together in definable groups of people. It may also be useful when the presence of

BOX 6-3   Coronary Artery Disease and Multiple Risk Factor Reduction

An epidemic of coronary artery disease and subsequent heart attacks spread widely through the United States in the mid-1900s. Sudden death, especially among men in their 50s and even younger, became commonplace in nearly every neighborhood in the suburban United States. To better understand this epidemic, which caused nearly half of all deaths in Americans in the 1940s and 1950s, the National Institutes of Health began the Framingham Heart Study in the late 1940s.[4]

In those days, there were only suggestions that cholesterol and hypertension contributed to heart disease, and little, if any, recognition that cigarettes played a role. The Framingham Heart Study enrolled a cohort of over 7,000 individuals in Framingham, Massachusetts, questioning, examining, and taking blood samples from them every other year to explore a large number of conceivable connections with coronary artery disease—the cause of heart attacks. Now well into its second half century, after thousands of publications and hundreds of thousands of examinations, the Framingham Heart Study continues to follow the children and grandchildren of the original Framingham cohort.

The study has provided us with extensive long-term data on a cohort of individuals. These form the basis for many of the numbers we use to estimate the strength of risk factors for coronary artery disease. It has helped demonstrate not only the risk factors for the disease, but also the protective, or resilience, factors. The use of aspirin, regular exercise, and modest alcohol consumption have been suggested as protective factors despite the fact that no one ever thought of them in the 1940s.[a]

The Framingham Heart Study demonstrated that high blood pressure precedes strokes and heart attacks by years and often decades. It took the Veterans Administration's randomized controlled trials of the early 1970s to convince the medical and public health communities that high blood pressure needs and benefits from aggressive detection and treatment. Through a truly joint effort by public health and medicine, high blood pressure detection and treatment came to public and professional recognition as a major priority in the 1970s.

The impact of elevated levels of low-density lipoprotein (LDL), the bad cholesterol, was likewise suggested by the Framingham Heart Study, but it was not until the development of a new class of medications called statins in the mid-1980s that treatment of high levels of LDL cholesterol took off. These drugs have been able to achieve remarkable reductions in LDL and equally remarkable reductions in coronary artery disease with only rare side effects. These

---

[a] The data developed for the surgeon general's reports on smoking and health in the 1960s and beyond strongly pointed to substantial effects of cigarettes not only on lung disease, but on coronary artery disease as well. In fact, given the large number of deaths from coronary artery disease compared to lung disease, it became evident that in terms of number of deaths, the biggest impact of cigarette smoking is on heart disease, not lung disease.

---

two or more risk factors increases the risk more than would be expected by adding together the impact of each risk factor.

The success in the last half century in addressing coronary artery disease exemplifies multiple risk factor reduction. **Box 6-3** discusses the impact of this strategy on coronary artery disease. Multiple risk factor reduction strategies are being attempted for a range of diseases, from asthma to diabetes.

Multiple risk factor reduction is most successful when a number of risk factors are at work in the same individual. As we have seen with asthma, factors like indoor and outdoor air pollution, cockroaches and other allergens, and a lack of adherence to medications tend to occur together and may be most effectively addressed together. Similarly, obesity and lack of exercise tend to reinforce each other, often requiring a comprehensive multiple risk factor reduction approach.[e]

---

[e] In some situations, the existence of multiple risk factors does more than add together to produce disease. At times, the existence of two or more factors multiplies the risk. In these situations, addressing even one of the factors can have a major impact on disease. For instance, it is now well established that asbestos exposure and cigarette smoking multiply the risks of lung cancer. Thus, if the relative risk for cigarettes is 10 and the relative risk for asbestos exposure is 5, then the relative risk if both factors are present is approximately 50. If an individual who has previously been exposed to both risk factors stops smoking cigarettes and the effects of cigarette smoking are immediately and completely reversible, we can expect the relative risk of lung cancer to decline from approximately a fifty-fold increase to a five-fold increase. This type of interaction is increasingly central to addressing complex public health issues.

BOX 6-3 Coronary Artery Disease and Multiple Risk Factor Reduction (*continued*)

drugs have been so successful that some countries have made them available over the counter. Clinicians are using them more and more aggressively to achieve levels of LDL cholesterol that are less than half those sought a generation ago.[b]

Although diabetes has been treated with insulin since the 1920s and with oral treatments beginning after World War II, the treatment of diabetes to prevent its consequences—including coronary artery disease—was not definitely established as effective until the 1990s. Our current understanding of diabetes has come from a series of randomized controlled trials and long-term follow-ups that demonstrate the key role that diabetes can play in diseases of the heart and blood vessels and the impressive role that aggressive treatment can play in reducing the risks of these diseases.

---

[b] Recent data even suggests that for individuals with levels of LDL cholesterol within the currently accepted range of normal, statins may be beneficial in the presence of evidence of inflammation as measured by a test called C-reactive protein.[5]

Efforts aimed at early detection and treatment of heart attacks and prevention of second heart attacks through the use of medications have become routine parts of medical practice. Medical procedures, including angioplasty and surgical bypass of diseased coronary arteries, have also been widely used. Widespread availability of defibrillators in public areas is one of the most recent efforts to prevent the fatal consequences of coronary artery disease.

Between the 1950s and the early years of the 2000s, the death rate from coronary artery disease has declined by over 50%. The impact is even greater among those in their 50s and 60s. Sudden death from coronary artery disease among men in their 50s is now a relatively rare event.

For years, medicine and public health professionals debated whether public health and clinical preventive interventions or medical and surgical interventions deserved the lion's share of the credit for these achievements. The evidence suggests that both prevention and treatment have had important impacts.[6] When medicine and public health work together, the public's health is the winner.

Screening for disease and multiple risk factor reduction are key approaches to using testing as part of secondary intervention.[f] The enormous burden of noncommunicable disease cannot be totally prevented, even by maximizing the use of these strategies. It is important to couple them with cost-effective treatment. Thus, a third population health strategy for addressing the burden of noncommunicable disease is to develop cost-effective interventions to treat common diseases.

HOW CAN COST-EFFECTIVE INTERVENTIONS HELP US ADDRESS THE BURDEN OF NONCOMMUNICABLE DISEASES?

Clinicians today have a wide range of interventions to treat disease. Many of these interventions have some impact on the course of a disease. The proliferation of interventions means

---

[f] The principles of testing discussed here are not limited to screening for disease and identification of risk factors. They are also useful as part of a cost-effective approach to diagnosis of symptomatic diseases. In addition, testing is often used for a range of applications in medicine and public health, including monitoring response to treatment, identifying side effects, identifying genetic predictors of disease, and establishing baseline levels for future testing. Public health applications include the use of environmental testing and testing for disease prevalence.

that it is especially important to identify which provide the greatest benefits at the lowest cost. In order to understand how cost-effective interventions can help address the burden of noncommunicable disease, we need to understand what we mean by "cost-effective."

Cost-effectiveness is a concept that combines issues of benefits and harms with issues of financial costs. It starts by considering the benefits and harms of an intervention to determine its **net-effectiveness** or **net benefit**. Net-effectiveness implies that the benefits are substantially greater than the harms, even after the value (or utility), as well as the timing of the harms and benefits, are taken into account. Only after establishing net-effectiveness do we take into account the financial costs.

Cost-effectiveness compares a new intervention to the current or standard intervention. It usually asks: Is the additional net-effectiveness of an intervention worth the additional cost? At times, it may also require us to ask: Is a small loss of net-effectiveness worth the considerable savings in cost? **Figure 6-1** is a tool for categorizing interventions in order to analyze their costs and net-effectiveness. **Box 6-4** provides more details on the use of cost-effectiveness analysis.[7]

Preventive interventions often undergo cost-effectiveness analysis. Many interventions, ranging from mammography

FIGURE 6-1 The Four Quadrants of Cost and Net-Effectiveness

to most childhood vaccinations to cigarette cessation programs, get high or at least passing grades on cost-effectiveness. However, many widely used treatment interventions do not or would not meet the current standards of cost-effectiveness. The application of cost-effectiveness criteria to common clinical interventions is considered a population health intervention aimed at getting maximum value for the dollars spent.

The results of cost-effectiveness analysis have already had an impact on a number of common clinical procedures. For instance, cost-effective treatments include the use of minimally invasive orthopedic surgery, such as knee surgery; the reduced length of intensive care and hospitalization for coronary artery disease; and the use of home health care for intravenous administration of antibiotics and other medications. These efforts to increase the cost-effectiveness of routine healthcare procedures are becoming key to maximizing

BOX 6-4   Cost-Effectiveness and Its Calculations

Cost-effectiveness is often judged by comparing the costs of a new intervention to the cost of the current, standard, or state-of-the-art intervention. A measure known as the **incremental cost-effectiveness** ratio is then obtained. This ratio represents the additional cost relative to the additional net-effectiveness.

Net-effectiveness may measure a diagnosis made, a death prevented, a disability prevented, etc. Operationalizing the concept of net-effectiveness requires us to define, measure, and combine the probabilities and utilities of benefits with the probabilities and utilities of harm and take into account the timing of the benefits and the harms. Thus, the process of calculating net-effectiveness can be quite complex.

Similarly, calculating costs can be challenging. Most economists argue that the costs are not limited to the costs of providing the intervention and the current and future medical care, but should also include the cost of transportation, loss of income, and other expenses associated with obtaining health care and being disabled. Thus, calculating a cost-effectiveness ratio has become a complex undertaking.

The criteria for establishing cost-effectiveness have changed over time. Most experts in cost-effectiveness prefer the use of a measurement called quality-adjusted life years, or QALYs. QALYs ask about the number of life-years, rather than the number of lives, saved by an intervention. Thus, one QALY may be thought of as one year of life at full health compared to immediate death.

In cost-effectiveness analysis, a financial value is usually placed on a QALY, reflecting what a society can afford to pay for the average QALY as measured by its per capita gross domestic product (GDP). In the United States, where the GDP is approximately $50,000, there is a general consensus that a QALY currently should be valued at $50,000. Thus, when you hear that a formal cost-effectiveness analysis has shown that an intervention is cost-effective, it generally implies that the additional cost is less than $50,000 per QALY.[a]

The ideal intervention is one in which the cost goes down and the effectiveness goes up. Cost-saving, quality-increasing interventions have a negative incremental cost-effectiveness ratio. That is, QALYs go up while the costs go down. These cost-reducing, QALY-increasing interventions, while highly desirable, are very rare. Usually, we need to spend more to get additional QALYs. One example of an intervention that reduces costs and at the same time produces additional QALYs is treatment of hypertension in high-risk individuals, such as those with diabetes.[b]

_____

[a] An increase of one QALY may be the result of obtaining small improvements in utility from a large number of people. For instance, if ten people increase their utility from 0.1 to 0.2, the result is an increase of one QALY. Setting the value of a QALY at $50,000 reflects how much we can afford to pay rather than strictly reflecting how much we think a QALY is worth.

[b] Another example is the use of the influenza vaccine among the elderly and those with chronic disease predisposing them to the complications of influenza. It is important to distinguish these types of interventions from those that reduce the costs, but also reduce the QALYs, because at times, both are referred to as cost-saving measures.

the benefits obtained from the vast amount of money spent on health care in the United States.

Applying cost-effectiveness analysis to routine clinical interventions is often coupled with efforts to better predict the outcome of disease and treatment. Improving the ability to predict the outcome of diseases and interventions can help us know when, how, and if to intervene. Improved prediction or prognosis using **prediction rules** developed based on large amounts of clinical data holds out the hope of increased effectiveness, as well as reduced costs by tailoring the treatment to the individual patient.[g]

In addition to screening, multiple risk factor reduction, and cost-effective interventions using prediction rules, the revolution in genetics has opened up another possible strategy for addressing the burden of noncommunicable diseases.

HOW CAN GENETIC COUNSELING AND INTERVENTION BE USED TO ADDRESS THE BURDEN OF CHRONIC DISEASES?

Interventions based upon genetics have been part of medical and public health practice since at least the 1960s, when it was recognized that abnormalities of single genes for such conditions as Tay-Sachs disease (found among Ashkenazi Jews) and sickle-cell anemia (found among African Americans) could be detected by testing potential parents who could then be counseled on the risks associated with childbearing.

It was also recognized that chromosomal abnormalities that produce Down syndrome, the most commonly recognized cause of mental retardation, could be detected at an early stage in pregnancy. In addition, certain genetic defects, such as phenylketonuria (PKU), can be recognized at birth, and in the case of phenylketonuria, relatively simple dietary interventions can prevent the severe retardation of mental development that would otherwise occur.

In light of all this valuable knowledge, today, genetic testing and counseling are often offered to prospective parents. Testing for Down syndrome is a standard part of prenatal care, and testing for a wide range of rare, but serious, disorders is a population health intervention. In fact, in most states, these tests are legally required soon after birth.

The triumph of the human genome project in the early years of the 2000s has sparked interest in expanding the applicability of genetic interventions in medicine and public health. For instance, the gene for cystic fibrosis, the most common genetic disorder among whites in the United States, has been identified, and screening of large numbers of couples is now possible. Even among whites without a history of cystic fibrosis, the chance of carrying the gene is about 3%. If both the mother and the father carry the gene, the chance of having a child with cystic fibrosis is 25% with each pregnancy. The fetus can be tested for the disease early in pregnancy.

There are a wide range of current and developing applications of genetics, including:[8]

- Genetic prevention—This approach incorporates efforts to prevent the occurrence of single genes or multiple gene combinations that are likely to produce disease. This includes expanded use of genetic counseling, prenatal testing, and early abortion or fetal therapies. Knowledge of the human genome holds promise for expanding this approach beyond diseases caused by single-gene defects to diseases that depend on multiple genes. It is important to recognize that diseases that are dependent on multiple genes will be more difficult to predict than those resulting from a single gene.

- Genetic detection prior to disease—This approach includes efforts aimed at the detection of genetic defects and the implementation of early intervention to prevent what is called the **phenotypic expression** of genes. Building on the success of treatment of PKU and other inborn errors of metabolism, risk factors for common diseases, such as high cholesterol, high blood sugar, or obesity, may be detected early and aggressively managed during childhood.

- Gene-environmental protection—Genetic testing holds out the possibility of defining combinations of genes that identify individuals who are especially likely to develop disease when they experience specific environmental exposures, such as those interactions that occur in occupational settings where workers are exposed to specific chemicals often at low doses. Identification of gene-environment interactions may lead to identification of those who are at high risk if they work in certain occupational settings.

- Genotypic-based screening for early disease—Combinations of genes may identify groups that are at high risk of common diseases and that can be targeted for screening. For instance, studies suggest that for certain common cancers, such as those of the breast, prostate, and colon, genetic factors are associated

---

[g] Research designed to develop prediction rules has become a major focus of clinical, as well as public health, research. This challenging type of research may be able to improve evidence-based recommendations by providing different recommendations for groups with different prognoses and/or different responses to treatment. Efforts to improve the effectiveness of breast cancer treatments, for instance, are now focused on testing patients to determine the best type of chemotherapy to use to treat their particular cancer. This approach shows promise of producing greater benefit and less harm at reduced cost.

with 30–40% of these diseases. Finding predisposing genetic patterns early in life may be useful for identifying those who need earlier or more intensive screening for early detection.

Each of these potential uses of genetics in public health present ethical as well as technological issues. Questions to consider include: Should we identify diseases when little can be done to prevent or treat them? How can we identify genetic risk factors without stigmatizing or putting those with the genes at a disadvantage? Will screening programs be improved by identifying groups at genetic risk of disease, or will high-risk groups without genetic risk factors unfairly be passed over for screenings?

These and other approaches based on the rapidly accumulating knowledge of genetics are likely to become routine medical and public health strategies for primary, secondary, and tertiary interventions for noncommunicable disease in the coming years. Their successful adoption, however, will require careful attention by those in the fields of public health and medicine to ensure that benefits are gained and harms minimized. Despite the enormous advances that have occurred in public health and medicine in recent decades, there is still much to be learned. A final strategy for noncommunicable diseases addresses the question: What can we do when highly effective interventions do not exist?

WHAT CAN WE DO WHEN HIGHLY EFFECTIVE INTERVENTIONS DO NOT EXIST?

Alzheimer's is among the most rapidly increasing conditions among those that we classify as noncommunicable diseases. The aging of the population has been and is expected to be associated with many more cases of Alzheimer's, which primarily affects the quality of life with its progressive damage to memory—especially short-term memory.[h]

Today, we have limited treatment options for those afflicted with Alzheimer's. Several drugs are available that have modest positive impacts on memory. Efforts to stimulate mental activity through keeping active mentally and physically have also been shown to have positive, yet modest,

impacts. Public health efforts have encouraged the use of these existing interventions, especially when there is evidence that they allow individuals to function on their own or with limited assistance for longer periods of time.

The population health approach to Alzheimer's disease, however, also stresses the need for additional research. Epidemiological research has helped produce the modest advances in preventing progression and treating the symptoms of the disease. A population health approach, however, needs to acknowledge the need for a basic biological understanding of what causes Alzheimer's. Fortunately, the cause and treatment of Alzheimer's disease is being aggressively researched, and evidence for contributory cause(s) is accumulating, as discussed in **Box 6-5**.

BOX 6-5 Alzheimer's Research

Alzheimer's disease provides an example of the ways that genes affect the development of disease and how knowledge of genetics is helping establish the etiology of diseases. Epidemiological research is increasingly utilizing genetic information to help establish etiology as well as to investigate new interventions.[9]

Pathological studies have demonstrated increases in a protein called amyloid-B deposited in the brains of patients dying with Alzheimer's disease. Case-control studies have demonstrated that individuals with clinical evidence of a genetic form of Alzheimer's disease have increased odds of having a mutation that increases production of amyloid-B. In addition, case-control studies have demonstrated that individuals over 85 who are free of clinical evidence of Alzheimer's disease have over 5 times the odds of having a gene that reduces the production of amyloid-B. Thus, an association at the individual level between amyloid-B and Alzheimer's has been firmly established.

A cohort investigation of patients at increased risk of Alzheimer's due to the presence of the gene mutation has established that amyloid-B precedes the presence of Alzheimer's. In addition, those with increased amyloid-B production have been shown to have biochemical changes in the cerebral spinal fluid consistent with Alzheimer's disease and clinical declines in memory years to decades prior to the diagnosis of Alzheimer's disease. This has established that the "cause" precedes the "effect." Definitive proof that altering the "cause" alters the "effect" is still needed to demonstrate that

---

[h] Not all cases of memory loss or dementia are due to Alzheimer's. Additional causes include strokes and cerebral vascular disease, chronic alcoholism, thyroid disease, specific infectious diseases (such as syphilis and AIDS), as well as the effects of drugs and a long list of rare diseases. Today, however, Alzheimer's is the most common and the most important cause of memory loss and dementia. We tend to classify a disease as noncommunicable unless there is convincing evidence that it can be transmitted or that it is due in large part to environmental exposures or injuries. Despite the fact that we do not yet know the etiology of Alzheimer's disease, it is generally classified as noncommunicable.

BOX 6-5   Alzheimer's Research
(*continued*)

amyloid-B is a contributory cause of Alzheimer's. This will require randomized controlled trials of treatments that reduce amyloid-B production.

Fortunately, an increasingly sophisticated and well-financed effort is being directed at understanding the etiology, prevention, and treatment of Alzheimer's. We now for the first time have hope and increasing confidence that the epidemic being faced by many of your grandparents will be brought under control in the not-too-distant future.

We have now explored the major population health strategies for addressing noncommunicable diseases. These include screening, multiple risk factor reduction, cost-effective treatments, genetic counseling, and more research. A complex problem often requires us to combine many of these approaches.

HOW CAN WE COMBINE STRATEGIES TO ADDRESS COMPLEX PROBLEMS OF NONCOMMUNICABLE DISEASES?

Multiple interventions combining health care, traditional public health approaches, and social interventions are often needed to address the complex problems presented by noncommunicable diseases. The combined and integrated use of multiple interventions is central to the population health approach. **Box 6-6** looks at what we can learn about the population health approach to noncommunicable diseases

BOX 6-6   Alcohol Abuse and the Population Health Approach

Alcohol has been a central feature of U.S. society and U.S. medicine and public health since the early days of the country. It was among the earliest painkillers and was used routinely to allow surgeons to perform amputations during the Civil War and earlier conflicts. The social experiment of alcohol prohibition during the 1920s and early 1930s ended in failure as perceived by a great majority of Americans.

Efforts to control the consequences of alcohol took a new direction after World War II. Americans began to focus on the consequences of alcohol, including liver disease, fetal alcohol syndrome, automobile accidents, and intentional and unintentional violence.

Population health interventions became the focus of alcohol control efforts. For instance, taxation of alcohol based upon 1950s legislation raised the price of alcohol. Restrictions on advertising and higher taxes on hard liquor, with its greater alcohol content, eventually contributed to greater use of beer and wine. Despite the continued growth in alcohol consumption, the number of cases of liver disease and other alcohol-related health problems have declined. In recent years, efforts to alert pregnant women to the health effects of drinking through product labeling and other health communications efforts have had an impact.

The highway safety impacts of alcohol use have led to population health efforts in cooperation with transportation and police departments. Greatly increased police efforts to catch drunk drivers and stripping of the licenses of repeat offenders have become routine and have been attributed to impressive reductions in automotive accidents related to alcohol. Efforts such as the designated driver movement originated by Mothers Against Drunk Driving (MADD) have demonstrated the often-critical role that private citizens can play in implementing population health interventions.

Focusing on high-risk groups, as well as using what we have called "improving-the-average" strategies, has had an important impact. Alcoholics Anonymous (AA) and other peer support groups have focused on encouraging individuals to acknowledge their alcohol problems. These groups often provide important encouragement and support for long-term abstinence.

Medical efforts to control alcohol consumption have been aimed primarily at those with clear evidence of alcohol abuse—often those in need of alcohol withdrawal, or "drying out." Drugs are available that provide modest help in controlling an individual's alcohol consumption. Screening for alcohol abuse has become a widespread part of health care. These interventions have been aimed at those with the highest levels of risk. The combination of individual, group, and population interventions has reduced the overall impact of alcohol use without requiring its prohibition. In fact, modest levels of consumption, up to one drink per day for

(*continues*)

> **BOX 6-6** Alcohol Abuse and the Population Health Approach (*continued*)
>
> women and two for men, may help protect against coronary artery disease.
>
> The issue of alcohol and public health has not gone away. The focus today has returned to identifying high-risk groups and intervening to prevent bad outcomes. A key risk factor today is binge drinking, with its risk of acute alcohol poisoning, as well as unintentional and intentional violence. College students are among the highest risk group. One episode of binge drinking dramatically increases the probability of additional episodes, suggesting that intervention strategies are needed to reduce the risk. We've made a great deal of progress controlling the impacts of alcohol, but we clearly have more to do.

from the long history of alcohol use and abuse, as well as the substantial recent success in addressing disease due to alcohol.[10]

We have now taken a look at strategies to control noncommunicable diseases, which are currently the most common reason for disability and death in most developed countries. Now, let us look at a second category that has been central to the history of public health and threatens to become central to its future: communicable disease.

KEY WORDS

- Epidemiological transition or public health transition
- Screening
- Asymptomatic
- Incremental cost-effectiveness
- Lead-time bias
- False positives
- False negatives
- True positives
- Bayes' theorem
- Pretest probability of disease
- Posttest probability of disease
- Sensitivity
- Specificity
- Predictive value of a positive
- Predictive value of a negative
- Sequential testing (or consecutive testing)
- Simultaneous testing (or parallel testing)
- Multiple risk factor reduction
- Cost-effectiveness
- Net-effectiveness or net benefit
- Prediction rules
- Phenotypic expression

Discussion Questions

Take a look at the questions posed in the following scenarios, which were presented at the beginning of this chapter. See now whether you can answer them.

1. Sasha did not want to think about the possibility of breast cancer, but as she turned 50, she agreed to have a mammography, which, as she feared, was positive or "suspicious," as her doctor put it. Waiting for the results of the follow-up biopsy was the worst part, but the relief she felt when the results were negative brought tears of joy to her and her family. Then she wondered: Is it common to have a positive mammography when no cancer is present?

2. The first sign of Michael's coronary heart disease was his heart attack. Looking back, he had been at high risk for many years because he smoked and had high blood pressure and high bad cholesterol. His lack of exercise and obesity only made the situation worse. Michael asked: What are the risk factors for coronary heart disease and what can be done to identify and address these factors for me and my family?

3. John's knee injury from skiing continued to produce swelling and pain, greatly limiting his activities. His physician informed him that the standard procedure today is to look inside with a flexible scope and do any surgery that is needed through the scope. It is simpler and cheaper, and does not even require hospitalization. "We call it cost-effective," his doctor said. John wondered: What does cost-effective really mean?

4. Jennifer and her husband, George, were tested for the cystic fibrosis gene and both were found to have it. Cystic fibrosis causes chronic lung infections and greatly shortens the length of life. They now ask: What does this mean for our chances of having a child with cystic fibrosis? Can we find out whether our child has cystic fibrosis early in pregnancy?

5. Fred's condition deteriorated slowly, but persistently. He just could not remember anything and repeated himself endlessly. The medications helped for a short time, but before long, he did not recognize his family and could not take care of himself. The diagnosis was Alzheimer's, and he was not alone. Almost everyone in the nursing home seemed to be affected. No one seems to understand the cause of Alzheimer's disease. The family asked: What else can be done, not only for Fred, but also for those who come after Fred?

6. Alcohol use is widespread on your campus. You do not see it as a problem as long as you walk home or have a designated driver. Your mind changes one day after you hear about a classmate who nearly died from alcohol poisoning as a result of binge drinking. You ask yourself: What should be done on my campus to address binge drinking?

REFERENCES

1. Omran AR. The epidemiologic transition: a theory of the epidemiology of population change. *The Milbank Memorial Fund Quarterly.* 1971;49(4):509–538.

2. Riegelman RK. *Studying a Study and Testing a Test: Reading the Evidence-based Health Research.* Philadelphia, PA: Lippincott, Williams & Wilkins; 2012.

3. Gordis L. *Epidemiology.* 4th ed. Philadelphia, PA: Elsevier Saunders; 2009.

4. Framingham Heart Study. History of the Framingham heart study. http://www.framinghamheartstudy.org/about/history.html. Accessed November 11, 2013.

5. Ridker PM, Danielson E, Foneseca FAH, et al. Rosuvastatin to prevent vascular events in men and women with elevated C-reactive protein. *N Engl J Med.* 2008;259(21):2195–2207.

6. Critchley J, Capwell S, Unal B. Life-years gained from coronary heart disease mortality reduction in Scotland—prevention or treatment? *J Clin Epi.* 2003;56(6):583–590.

7. Gold MR, Siegel JE, Russell LB, Weinstein MC. *Cost-Effectiveness in Health and Medicine.* New York, NY: Oxford University Press; 1996.

8. Khoury MJ, Burke W, Thomson EJ. *Genetics and Public Health in the 21st Century: Using Genetic Information to Improve Health and Prevent Disease.* New York, NY: Oxford University Press; 2000.

9. Alzheimer's Association. What we know today about Alzheimer's disease. http://www.alz.org/research/science/alzheimers_disease_causes.asp. Accessed July 19, 2013.

10. Room R, Babor T, Rehm J. Alcohol and public health. *Lancet.* 2005;365(9458):519–530.

CHAPTER 7

Communicable Diseases

LEARNING OBJECTIVES

By the end of this chapter, the student will be able to:

- describe the burden of disease caused by communicable diseases.
- describe the criteria that are used to establish that an organism is a contributory cause of a disease.
- identify factors that affect the transmissibility of a disease.
- identify the roles that barrier protections play in preventing communicable diseases.
- identify the roles that vaccinations can play in preventing communicable diseases.
- identify the roles that screening, case finding, and contact treatment can play in preventing communicable diseases.
- identify the conditions that make eradication of a disease feasible.
- describe a range of options for controlling the HIV/AIDS epidemic.

Your college roommate went to bed not feeling well one night, and early the next morning, you had trouble arousing her. She was rushed to the hospital just in time to be effectively diagnosed and treated for meningococcal meningitis. The health department recommends immediate antibiotic treatment for everyone who was in close contact with your roommate. They set up a process to watch for additional cases to be sure an outbreak is not in progress. Fortunately, no more cases occur. You ask yourself: Should your college require that all freshmen have the meningococcal vaccine before they can register for classes?

As a health advisor to a worldwide HIV/AIDS foundation, you are asked to advise on ways to address the HIV and developing tuberculosis (TB) epidemics. You are asked to do some long-range thinking and to come up with a list of potential approaches to control the epidemics, or at least ways to reduce the development of TB. The first recommendation you make is to forget about eradicating HIV/AIDS. How did you come to that conclusion?

Your hometown of 100,000 is faced with a crisis as an airplane lands containing a passenger thought to have a new form of severe influenza that has recently gained the ability to spread from person to person through airborne transmission. As the mayor of the city, what do you decide to do?

You are a principal at a local high school. One of your top athletes is in the hospital with a spreading bacterial infection due to staphylococcus bacteria resistant to all known antibiotics. The infection occurred after what appeared to be a minor injury during practice. As the principal, what do you decide to do?

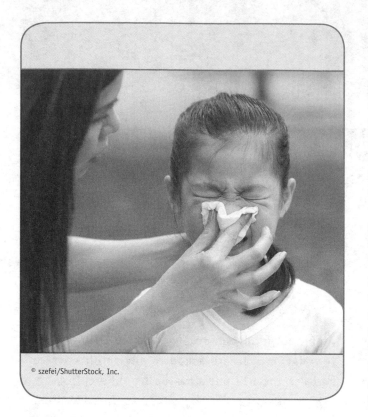

© szefei/ShutterStock, Inc.

Diseases due to infection form a large part of the history of public health and are again a central part of its present and its future. Infections of public health importance are primarily those that are communicable; that is, they can be transmitted from person to person or from animals or the physical environment to humans. **Communicable disease** may be caused by a wide variety of organisms, ranging from bacteria, to viruses, to a spectrum of parasites, including malaria and hookworm. Let us examine the burden of disease due to communicable diseases.[a]

---

[a] The term **infectious disease** is intended to include both communicable disease and disease caused by organisms that are not communicable. The central feature that distinguishes communicable disease from other diseases caused by organisms is its ability to be transmitted from person to person or from animals or the physical environment to humans.. Other **infections** of public health interest are caused by organisms, such as the bacteria pneumococcus (*streptococcus pneumoniae*), which usually coexist with healthy individuals, but are capable of causing disease when relocated to areas of the body with increased susceptibility or when they are provided opportunities to multiply or invade new areas because of an individual's decreased resistance. It is important to note that the distinction between infectious diseases and communicable diseases is not always made, and at times, they are considered synonyms.

WHAT IS THE BURDEN OF DISEASE CAUSED BY COMMUNICABLE DISEASES?

For many centuries, communicable diseases were the leading cause of death and disability among all ages, but especially among the young and the old. Communicable diseases are not only the causes of great epidemics, but they can also become endemic and become routine causes of death.[b] These diseases included a key role in maternal deaths associated with childbirth, infant and early childhood deaths, as well as deaths of malnourished infants and children.

The last half of the 1900s saw a brief respite from deaths and disabilities caused by communicable diseases and other infections. This was due in large part to medical efforts to treat infections with drugs and public health efforts to prevent infections (often with vaccines) and to eradicate or control other infections. Even as these great accomplishments were underway, warning signs of bacteria resistant to antibiotics began to appear. Staphylococcus organisms resistant to current antibiotics began to plague hospitals in the 1950s until new antibiotics were developed. Resistance of gonorrhea and pneumococcus to a range of antibiotics became widespread. World Health Organization (WHO) and U.S. government–sponsored programs, such as those to promote the eradication of malaria and TB, were not able to have sustained impacts, and the goals were trimmed back to control rather than eradicate.

The early 2000s have seen the return of infections that were previously under control, as well as an emergence of new diseases. Tuberculosis, the great epidemic of the 1700s and 1800s, has returned in force, partially as a result of HIV/AIDS. **Box 7-1** looks at the history of TB and the historical and current burden of disease caused by it.[1,2]

Over a dozen previously unknown infections have emerged in recent decades—the majority of which are believed to have originated in animal species. In the United States, the presence of Lyme disease and the West Nile virus were unknown until the late 1900s, but have now spread to extensive areas of the country. Long-established diseases, such as malaria, are extending their geographic range, and farther extension is expected with global warming.

Influenza is anticipated to return again in pandemic form, as has occurred repeatedly in prior centuries. A **pandemic** is an epidemic occurring worldwide, or over a very wide area, crossing international boundaries and affecting

---

[b] **Epidemic** implies that a disease has increased in frequency in a defined geographic area far above its usual rate. **Endemic** implies that a disease is present in a community at all times but at a relatively low frequency.

BOX 7-1 The Burden of TB

"If the importance of a disease for mankind is measured by the number of fatalities it causes, then tuberculosis must be considered much more important than those most feared infectious diseases, plague, cholera and the like. One in seven of all human beings die from tuberculosis. If one only considers the productive middle-age groups, tuberculosis carries away one-third, and often more."[1]

—Robert Koch, March 24, 1882

The history of tuberculosis (TB) goes back to ancient times, but beginning in the 1700s, it took center stage in much of Europe and the United States. It has been estimated that in the two centuries from 1700 to 1900, tuberculosis was responsible for the deaths of approximately one billion human beings. The annual death rate from TB when Koch made his discovery was approximately seven million people.[1] Today, that would be the equivalent of over 30 million people, considering today's population.

Robert Koch's discovery of the association between the tuberculosis bacilli, its culture and isolation, and its transmission to a variety of animal species provided a clear demonstration that the bacilli are a contributory cause of the disease. While the tuberculosis bacilli are clearly a contributory cause of the disease tuberculosis, they are not sufficient alone to produce disease. A large percentage of the world's population harbors tuberculosis. Other factors are needed to produce active disease. These factors include reduced immunity and nutrition, as well as genetic factors.

The discovery of the tuberculosis bacilli actually followed the development of what was called the sanitarium movement, which began in Europe and the United States. Sanitariums isolated tuberculosis victims, while providing good nutrition and clean air. The sanitarium movement was coupled in the early 1900s with the use of the Bacillus Calmette-Guérin (BCG) vaccine, purified protein derivative (PPD) skin tests, and the recently invented chest X ray. These three early and rather crude technologies are still in use today and are designed to prevent and diagnose TB. In addition, the understanding of the epidemiology of the tuberculosis bacteria led to a clear victory for public health, with the near elimination of TB from the milk supply early in the 1900s.

Thus, even before the ability to actively treat tuberculosis, public health interventions were able to dramatically reduce the frequency of the disease, at least in Europe and the United States. A second round of efforts to control TB began in the 1940s with the discovery of streptomycin, the first anti-TB drug, followed over the next decade by para-aminosalicylic acid (PAS) and isoniazid (INH). Combination drug treatments proved highly effective. In addition, INH was found to be effective on its own to prevent skin-test-positive TB from progressing to active disease. Public health and medical efforts to conduct screening for positive skin tests and selectively treating with INH became widespread.

Thus, by the late 1950s and 1960s, TB was brought under control by the combination of medical and public health advances. The success of this effort resulted in the closing of TB sanitariums, gradual cutbacks in screening and treatment programs, and a general loss of interest in TB. Beginning in the mid-1960s, there was little interest in or research on TB. Tuberculosis became a treatable disease usually handled as part of routine medical care. Most medical and public health practitioners regarded it as a disease ready for eradication.

Unfortunately, TB was prematurely pronounced dead. It had never come under control in many parts of the world, and approximately 33% of those living in developing countries today are estimated to harbor the TB bacillus. That is, they carry TB organisms that may multiply and spread in the future.

Soon after the beginning of the AIDS epidemic in the 1980s, active TB came back with a vengeance. AIDS patients with latent TB often developed active TB quite early in their battle with AIDS. They then became contagious to others. Tuberculosis may be more difficult to diagnose and may progress faster in AIDS patients.

Coupled with the return of TB as a public health problem, resistance to TB drugs began to emerge. The problem was successfully combated in the 1990s by the simple public health intervention known as directly observed therapy, or DOT. DOT helped ensure that patients received all the prescribed treatment, thus greatly increasing adherence to effective treatment.

Nonetheless, in the early years of the 2000s, resistance to multiple TB drugs increased all over the world. We were faced with a triple threat of limited recent research, leaving us without modern diagnostic aids or new drugs; a rapidly emerging threat from multiple-drug-resistant tuberculosis; and a spreading epidemic of HIV/AIDS, predisposing patients to active tuberculosis. Each of these can be addressed by coordinated public health and medical actions, which have been occurring in recent years. In the past, TB has been exceptionally responsive to a wide range of public health and medical efforts to control its spread. There is hope that with increased awareness and further research, this will happen again.[2]

a large number of people. A pandemic of influenza is most likely to occur when ongoing mutations produce new strains capable of person-to-person transmission. Whether you live in a dorm, are a public health professional, a clinician, a politician, a high school principal, or are involved in almost any profession, communicable diseases are part of your present and your future.

History suggests that public health and medical interventions have and will continue to have major impacts on the burden of communicable diseases. Let us look at how we establish that an organism is in fact capable of transmitting a communicable disease.

HOW DO WE ESTABLISH THAT AN ORGANISM IS A CONTRIBUTORY CAUSE OF A COMMUNICABLE DISEASE?

Establishing that an organism is a contributory cause of a disease traditionally relied on Koch's postulates. Koch's postulates hold that in order to definitively establish a cause-and-effect relationship, all of the following four conditions must be met:

1. The organism must be shown to be present in every case of the disease by isolation of the organism.
2. The organism must not be found in cases of other disease.
3. Once isolated, the organism must be capable of replicating the disease in an experimental animal.
4. The organism must be recoverable from the animal.

Ironically, TB could not be shown to fulfill Koch's postulates. However, a very useful set of Modern Koch's postulates has been developed by the National Institute of Allergy and Infectious Disease. Modern Koch's postulates require:

1. Evidence of an epidemiological association
2. Isolation
3. Transmissions to establish that an organism is a contributory cause of the disease[3]

At times, researchers have been able to directly isolate and transmit diseases from person to person. For instance, fluid from chicken pox skin was collected and transferred to other individuals, resulting in active cases of chicken pox.

This type of direct evidence of transmission is unusual in humans. Nonetheless, outbreaks of disease can often provide the evidence needed to fulfill Modern Koch's postulates, as illustrated in the case of the bacteria *Neisseria meningitidis,* which has been established as the organism that causes meningococcal meningitis and sepsis.

Meningococcal meningitis, an important cause of meningitis and blood-borne infection, or sepsis, was first recognized

during an epidemic in Geneva, Switzerland, in 1805 and occurred in epidemic form especially during military conflicts throughout the 1800s. The bacteria *Neisseria meningitidis* was first cultured from patients with acute meningitis in 1887. Efforts to fulfill **Koch's postulates** were not successful because transmission to animals was not possible and a large number of humans were carriers without developing the disease.

The ability to culture or isolate the bacteria in sick individuals in the meninges and the blood, areas of the body that should be free of bacteria, was key evidence in establishing the causal role of *Neisseria meningitidis* in the disease. Transmission from person to person has been documented in outbreaks of the disease and has been used to confirm the final criteria of **Modern Koch's postulates.**

Understanding the mechanism of transmission is important for establishing etiology, but it is also important for appreciating the degree of communicability of a disease and in designing interventions to reduce its spread. Let us take a look at the factors that affect the ease with which a communicable disease is transmitted.

WHAT FACTORS AFFECT THE EASE WITH WHICH A COMMUNICABLE DISEASE IS TRANSMITTED?

Three factors have major impacts on the ease of transmission of communicable disease. These are:

- **Route of transmission**—the anatomical and physiological methods for transmission from person to person and from animal species to humans
- **Asymptomatic transmission**—the ability to transmit the disease while humans or animals are free of symptoms of the disease
- **Reproduction ratio (R_0)**—the number of new cases one individual with the disease generates on average over the course of its communicable period

Let us take a closer look at each of these factors.

Route of Transmission

A wide range of possible routes of transmission has been demonstrated for communicable disease. Communicable diseases may be transmitted from person to person or from animal species or the physical environment to humans. **Table 7-1** outlines the major methods of transmission of human disease and provides examples of each of the methods.[4]

Asymptomatic Transmission

Diseases with the potential to create human epidemics are often diseases that can be transmitted from person to person while the individual is free of symptoms. Classic examples include

TABLE 7-1 Methods of Transmission of Human Disease

Method of transmission	Examples
Insects	Malaria, Lyme disease, West Nile virus, yellow fever
Other animals	Rabies, avian flu, anthrax, plague, other zoonotic diseases
Airborne—person-to-person	Influenza, SARS, measles, chicken pox, tuberculosis, common cold
Sexual transmission/open sores	Gonorrhea, syphilis, herpes genitalis, chlamydia, hepatitis B, HIV
Water/food	Hepatitis A, cholera
Fecal/oral	Polio, salmonella
Transfusions/blood/contaminated needles	Hepatitis B and C +
Transplacental	Rubella, HIV
Breastfeeding	HIV
Contaminated articles ("fomites")	Chicken pox, common cold, influenza

Data from Timmreck T.C., An Introduction to Epidemiology 3rd Edition Jones and Bartlett, Sudbury Mass 2002 p. 34.

influenza, chicken pox, measles, and mumps. Transmission often occurs in the days or weeks prior to the development of symptoms, but it can also occur from individuals who never develop signs or symptoms of the disease.

In addition to those who transmit the disease as part of their initial exposure to it, other individuals can transmit the disease after they have recovered from the clinical disease or after they are infected with it but do not develop symptoms. Those individuals without symptoms but with the ability to chronically transmit the disease are called **chronic carriers**. Examples of disease that often lead to chronic carriers are HIV, hepatitis B, and hepatitis C.

Reproduction Ratio

The reproduction ratio, often called R_0, provides a measure of the inherent transmissibility of a disease. It indicates the number of new cases one individual with the disease generates on average over the course of its communicable period. The reproduction ratio depends heavily on the disease's route(s) of transmission as well as the presence or absence of asymptomatic transmission, but the reproduction ratio provides a measure of the potential for an epidemic's development given the patterns of transmission in a particular society.

When R_0 is less than 1, each infected individual results, on average, in less than one new infected individual. Therefore, a communicable disease with an R_0 less than 1 is thought to have a low potential for becoming an epidemic disease. If the R_0 is greater than 1, the infection is likely to become endemic or epidemic in the population. Diseases with high R_0s have great potential for developing into epidemics. While the R_0 is not a perfect predictor of the chances that a disease will

become epidemic, a number of historical epidemic diseases have a high R_0, including measles (R_0 12 to 18), pertussis (R_0 12 to 17), polio (R_0 5 to 7), and mumps (R_0 4 to 7).[5, 6]

Now let us turn our attention to the tools that are available to public health to deal with communicable diseases.

WHAT PUBLIC HEALTH TOOLS ARE AVAILABLE TO ADDRESS THE BURDEN OF COMMUNICABLE DISEASES?

A range of public health tools are available to address the burden of communicable diseases. Some of these are useful in addressing noncommunicable diseases as well, but they have special applications when directed toward infections. These include:

- Barrier protections, including isolation and quarantine
- Immunizations designed to protect individuals as well as populations
- Screening and case finding
- Treatment and contact treatment
- Efforts to maximize effectiveness of treatments and prevent resistance to treatment

Let us look at each of these tools.

HOW CAN BARRIERS AGAINST DISEASE BE USED TO ADDRESS THE BURDEN OF COMMUNICABLE DISEASES?

Examples of barriers to the spread of infections are as old as hand washing and as new as insecticide-impregnated bed nets, which have had a major impact on the rate of malaria transmission. Barrier protection, such as condoms, is believed by many to be the most successful intervention to prevent sexually transmitted diseases. The use of masks may be effective in reducing the spread of disease in healthcare institutions, such as hospitals. The same measures may be preventative in the community at large and are a routine part of winter weather habits in much of Asia.

A special form of barrier protection consists of separating individuals with disease from the healthy population to prevent exposure. As we discussed previously, sanitariums had a major impact in reducing outbreaks of TB in the 1800s and the first half of the 1900s. Today, once again, we are faced with issues of isolation and occasionally have to legally enforce quarantine.

A second traditional public health approach to communicable and noncommunicable infections is the use of immunizations. Let us take a look at a range of ways that immunizations can be used to address the burden of communicable disease.

HOW CAN IMMUNIZATIONS BE USED TO ADDRESS THE BURDEN OF COMMUNICABLE DISEASE?

Immunization refers to the strengthening of the immune system to prevent or control disease. Injections of antibodies may be administered to achieve **passive immunity**, which may provide effective short-term protection. **Inactivated (dead)** and **live vaccines (attenuated live)** can often stimulate the body's own **antibody** production. Live vaccines utilize living organisms that also stimulate **cell-mediated immunity** and produce long-term protection that more closely resemble the body's own response to infection.

Vaccines are now available for a wide range of bacterial and viral diseases and are being developed and increasingly used to prevent infections as varied as malaria and hookworm.[7] Unfortunately, it has been difficult to produce effective vaccines for some diseases, such as HIV/AIDS. Vaccines, like medications, are rarely 100% effective and may produce side effects, including allergic reactions that can be life threatening. Live vaccines have the potential to cause injury to a fetus and can themselves produce disease, particularly in those with reduced immunity. Some vaccines are not effective for the very young and the elderly. Therefore, the use of vaccines requires extensive investigations to define their effectiveness and safety as well as to identify high-risk groups for whom they should be recommended.

For instance, college students and military recruits who tend to live in close quarters represent two high-risk groups for meningococcal disease. This bacterial infection can be rapidly life threatening, and when present, it requires testing and antibiotic treatment of close contacts. Effective vaccination is now a key tool for controlling this disease.

Ideally, vaccination occurs before exposure. However, when an outbreak occurs, vaccination of large numbers of potentially exposed individuals living in the surrounding area may be key to effective control. Thus, public health uses of vaccines need to include consideration of who should receive the vaccine, when it should be administered, and how it should be administered.

Vaccine administration has traditionally been limited to injections as shots or ingestion as pills. New methods of administration, including nasal sprays, are now being developed. In addition, it is often possible to combine vaccines, increasing the ease of administration. Inactivated vaccines may not produce long-term immunity and may require follow-up vaccines or boosters. Thus, the use of vaccinations requires the development of a population health strategy that gives careful attention to "who," "when," and "how."

Some infections, especially those viruses that are highly contagious, can be controlled by vaccinating a substantial proportion of the population, often in the range of 70 to 90%. In this situation, those who are susceptible rarely, if ever, encounter an individual with the disease. This is known as **herd immunity** or **population immunity**. When a population has been vaccinated at these types of levels for diseases—such as chicken pox, measles, and polio—those who have not been vaccinated are often protected. For some vaccines, such as live polio vaccine, herd immunity is facilitated by the fact that the virus in the vaccine can itself be spread from person to person, providing protection for the unvaccinated. Thus, public health authorities are interested in the levels of protection in the community—that is, the level of protection of the unvaccinated as well as the vaccinated.

In addition to tools for preventing disease in individuals and populations, public health efforts are often directed at screening for disease and conducting what is called case finding.

HOW CAN SCREENING AND CASE FINDING BE USED TO ADDRESS THE BURDEN OF COMMUNICABLE DISEASE?

Ideally, screening for communicable diseases fulfills the same criteria for noncommunicable diseases. Screening for communicable diseases has played a role in controlling the spread of a number of infections. For example, screening for tuberculosis and syphilis has been an effective part of the control of these infections even before they could be cured with antibiotics. Today, screening for sexually transmitted diseases, including gonorrhea and chlamydia, are a routine part of clinical care. HIV screening has long been recommended for high-risk individuals and for populations with an estimated prevalence above 1%. Today, universal screening is increasingly being discussed as a basic strategy for controlling HIV/AIDS.

Screening for communicable diseases has often been linked with the public health practice known as **case finding**. Case finding implies confidential interviewing of those diagnosed with a disease and asking for their recent close physical or sexual contacts. Case finding techniques have been key to the control of syphilis and to a large extent TB both before and after the availability of effective treatment. The advent of effective treatment meant that case finding was of benefit both to those diagnosed with the disease and those located through case finding.

Successful case finding aims to maintain confidentiality. However, when following up with sexual contacts, confidentiality is difficult to maintain. The potential for public recognition and the attendant social sigma has inhibited the use of case finding in HIV/AIDS in many parts of the world. The reluctance to utilize case finding may change in coming years, as early diagnosis and perhaps early treatment become more effective in controlling the epidemic.

In addition to the use of barrier protections, vaccination of individuals and populations, as well as the use of screening and case finding, public health tools also encompass treatment of those with disease and their contacts.

HOW CAN TREATMENT OF THOSE DIAGNOSED AND THEIR CONTACTS HELP TO ADDRESS THE BURDEN OF COMMUNICABLE DISEASE?

Treatment of symptomatic disease may in and of itself reduce the risk of transmission. Successful treatment of HIV has been shown to reduce the viral load and thereby reduce the ease of transmission. Similarly, treatment of active TB reduces its **infectivity**. In addition to direct treatment, a public health tool known as **epidemiological treatment**, or treatment of contacts, has been effective in controlling a number of communicable diseases. Sexual partners of those with gonorrhea and chlamydia are routinely treated, even when their infections cannot be detected. This approach presumably works because early and low-level infections caused by these organisms may be difficult to detect. As we saw in the meningococcal scenario, epidemiological treatment may be the most effective way to halt the rapid spread of a disease.

Contact treatment of HIV/AIDS may become a routine part of controlling the disease. It is already recommended and widely used for treatment of needlestick injuries in healthcare settings. Let us look at one additional public health tool being increasingly used to maximize effectiveness of treatment and prevent resistance.

HOW CAN PUBLIC HEALTH EFFORTS MAXIMIZE EFFECTIVENESS OF TREATMENT AND PREVENT RESISTANCE?

In recent years, the impact of antibiotic resistance has become painfully obvious—resistant pneumococcus, gonococcus, and tuberculosis have become widespread. In fact, extensively drug-resistant strains of TB exist in many areas of the world today. Efforts to control resistance have been modest compared to the forces encouraging resistance. Forces encouraging drug resistance include overuse of prescribed antibiotics, over-the-counter sales of antibiotics in many countries, and widespread use of antibiotics to stimulate modest growth in agricultural animals.

As we have seen, one successful effort known as directly observed therapy (DOT) has led to a more effective treatment of TB. As the name implies, DOT aims to ensure complete adherence to TB treatment by observing individuals taking treatment at daily or at less frequent intervals. This effort has been credited with success even in the presence of drug resistance, perhaps on the basis that the body can handle resistant TB if most of the organisms are effectively treated. Efforts are now underway to reduce or eliminate the use of antibiotics for animal growth and to place increased restrictions on the prescribing of highly useful new antibiotics.

The recent emergence of methicillin-resistant staphylococcus aureus (MRSA) outside hospitals has drawn long-overdue attention. It is spreading to communities and beginning to affect otherwise healthy individuals, including athletes and others simply in close physical contact. An effective program to control MRSA will require the use of a range of interventions. This is the situation for many of today's increasingly complex communicable diseases.

Let us now turn our attention to strategies that combine many of the specific public health tools designed to address the problems of communicable diseases. We will look at two basic strategies for combating complex infections: elimination and control.

HOW CAN PUBLIC HEALTH STRATEGIES BE USED TO ELIMINATE SPECIFIC COMMUNICABLE DISEASES?

Smallpox was the first human disease to be eradicated. An international effort is hopefully nearing completion to eradicate polio. These two viral diseases are the only ones that have been successfully targeted for eradication. As we have discussed, programs to eradicate TB and malaria have never come close to meeting their goals. Talk of the end of HIV/AIDS is even more unrealistic. Let us see what it takes to successfully eradicate a disease and why so few diseases are on the short list for potential eradication.

The history of smallpox has a unique place in public health. The disease goes back thousands of years, and it played a prominent role in the colonial United States, where epidemics often killed a quarter or more of their victims, especially children, and left most others, including George Washington, with severe facial scars for life. The concept of vaccination and the first successful vaccination were developed for smallpox. During the 1800s and early 1900s, smallpox was largely eliminated from most developed and developing countries through modest improvement on Jenner's basic approach to vaccination in which fluid from cowpox sores was placed under the skin to protect individuals against smallpox, despite the many side effects of this quite crude treatment.[c]

Despite the control of smallpox in most developed countries, there were still over 10 million cases annually of the disease in over 30 countries during the early 1960s. In 1967, the WHO began a campaign to eliminate smallpox. The success of the campaign over the next decade depended on extraordinary organizational management and cooperation, but the prerequisites for success were the unique epidemiological characteristics of smallpox that made it possible. Let us outline the characteristics of smallpox that made eradication possible:[8]

- *No animal reservoir*—Smallpox is an exclusively human disease. That is, there is no reservoir of the disease in animals. It does not affect other species that can then infect additional humans. This also means that if the disease is eliminated from humans, it has nowhere to hide and later reappear in human populations.
- *Short persistence in environment*—The smallpox virus requires human contact and cannot persist for more

than a brief time in the environment without a human host. Thus, droplets from sneezing or coughing need to find an immediate victim and are not easily transmitted except by human-to-human contact.

- *Absence of a long-term carrier state*—Once an individual recovers from smallpox, he or she no longer carries the virus and cannot transmit it to others. Smallpox contrasts with diseases such as HIV/AIDS and hepatitis B, which can maintain long-term carrier states and be infectious to others for years or decades.
- *The disease produces long-term immunity*—Once an individual recovers from smallpox, very effective immunity is established, preventing a second infection.
- *Vaccination also establishes long-term immunity*—As with the disease itself, the live smallpox vaccine produces very successful long-term immunity. Smallpox has not mutated to become more infectious despite the extensive use of vaccination.
- *Herd immunity protects those who are susceptible*—Long-term immunity from the disease or the vaccine makes it possible to protect large populations. At least 80% of the population needs to be vaccinated to interrupt the spread of the infection to the remaining susceptible people.
- *Easily identified disease*—The classic presentation of smallpox is relatively easy to identify by clinicians with experience observing the disease, as well as by the average person. This makes it possible to quickly diagnose the disease and protect others from being exposed.
- *Effective postexposure vaccination*—The smallpox vaccine is effective even after exposure to smallpox. This enables effective use of what is called **ring vaccination**. Ring vaccination involves identification of a case of smallpox, vaccination of the individual's household and close contacts, followed by vaccination of all those within a mile radius of the smallpox case. In the past, households within ten miles were typically searched for additional cases of smallpox. These public health surveillance and containment efforts were successful even in areas without high levels of vaccination.

The presence of all of these characteristics makes a disease ideal for eradication. While fulfilling all of them may not be necessary for eradication, the absence of a large number of them makes efforts at eradication less likely to succeed. **Table 7-2** outlines these characteristics of smallpox and compares them to polio—the current viral candidate for eradication—as well as to measles. Based upon the content of

---

[c] While the vaccine against smallpox is very effective, it has many side effects. The live virus contained in the vaccine can itself cause disease in those vaccinated, especially if they have widespread skin disease or have a compromised immune system. Today, these side effects may have prevented the widespread use of the smallpox vaccine because it could threaten the lives of the large number of HIV positive individuals, many of whom are unaware of their HIV infection. Allergic reactions to the vaccine are also quite common. Allergic reactions to the smallpox vaccine, including inflammation of the lining of the heart, prompted discontinuation of a campaign to vaccinate first responders and healthcare professionals soon after the 9/11 attack.

TABLE 7-2 Eradication of Human Diseases—What Makes It Possible?

	Smallpox	Polio	Measles
Disease is limited to humans, i.e., no animal reservoir?	Yes	Yes	Yes
Limited persistence in the environment?	Yes	Yes	Yes
Absence of long-term carrier state?	Yes	Yes—Absent, but may occur in immune-compromised individuals	Yes—Absent, but may occur in immune-compromised individuals
Long-term immunity results from infection?	Yes	Yes—But may not be sustained in immune-compromised individuals	Yes—But may not be sustained in immune-compromised individuals
Vaccination confers long-term immunity?	Yes	Yes—But may not be sustained in immune-compromised individuals Virus used for production of the live vaccine can produce poliolike illness and has potential to revert back to "wild type infection"	Yes—But may not be sustained in immune-compromised individuals
Herd immunity prevents perpetuation of an epidemic?	Yes	Yes	Yes
Easily diagnosed disease?	Yes	Yes/No—Disease relatively easy to identify, but large number of asymptomatic infections	No—Disease may be confused with other diseases by those unfamiliar with measles
Vaccination effective postexposure?	Yes	No	No

the table, you should not be surprised to learn that the polio campaign has been much more difficult and has taken much longer than that of smallpox. The potential for a successful measles eradication campaign is still being debated.[d]

Finally, take a look at **Table 7-3**, which applies these characteristics to HIV infection. It demonstrates why the eradication of HIV/AIDS is not on the horizon.

Unfortunately, eradication of most diseases is not a viable strategy. Thus, public health measures are usually focused on control of infections. In order to understand the range of strategies that are available and useful for controlling communicable diseases, we will take a look at three important and quite different diseases—HIV, influenza A, and rabies.

---

[d] Efforts are underway for the eradication of Guinea worm, which exhibits a number of favorable characteristics for eradication.

WHAT OPTIONS ARE AVAILABLE FOR THE CONTROL OF HIV/AIDS?

HIV/AIDS has been a uniquely difficult epidemic to control. An understanding of the biology of the HIV virus helps us understand many of the reasons for this. The HIV virus attacks the very cells designed to control it. The virus can avoid exposure to treatments by residing inside cells and temporarily not replicating. Many treatments work by interrupting the process of replication and thus are not effective when replication stops. The virus establishes a chronic carrier state, enabling long-term infectivity. High mutation rates reduce the effectiveness of drugs, as well as the effectiveness of the body's own immune system to fight the disease.

Despite these monumental challenges, considerable progress has been made by reducing the load of virus through drug treatment and preventing the transmission of

TABLE 7-3 Potential for Eradication of HIV/AIDS

	HIV/AIDS
Disease is limited to humans, i.e., no animal reservoir?	No—Animal reservoirs exist
Limited persistence in the environment?	No—May persist on contaminated needles long enough for transmission
Absence of long-term carrier state?	No—Carrier state is routine
Long-term immunity results from infection?	No—Effective long-term immunity does not usually occur
Vaccination confers long-term immunity?	No—None currently available and will be difficult to achieve
Herd immunity prevents perpetuation of an epidemic?	No—Large number of previously infected individuals increases the risk to the uninfected
Easily diagnosed disease?	No—Requires testing
Vaccination effective postexposure?	No—None currently available

the disease through a variety of public health interventions. To appreciate the efforts to control transmission of HIV/AIDS, it is important to understand the large number of ways that it can be transmitted.

HIV is most infectious when transmitted directly by blood. Blood transfusions were an early source of the spread of the virus. The introduction of HIV virus testing in the mid-1980s led to a dramatic improvement in the safety of the blood supply. Nonetheless, the safest blood transfusions are those that come from an individual's own blood. Thus, donation of one's own blood for later transfusion when needed has become a routine part of elective surgery preparation in many parts of the world. The most dangerous forms of transfusions are those that come from blood or blood products pooled from large numbers of individuals. Hemophiliacs in many developed countries used pooled blood products to control their bleeding in the 1980s. They suffered perhaps the world's highest rate of HIV infection before this hazard was recognized and addressed. A more recent pooling of blood products occurred in China and contributed to a surge of the disease.

Unprotected anal intercourse is a highly infectious way to transmit HIV. This may help to explain the early spread of the disease among male homosexuals. Today, however, heterosexual transmission is the most common route of infection; additionally, there is a higher risk of transmission from male to female than from female to male. A series of public health interventions has now been shown to be effective: properly used latex condoms, male circumcision, and abstinence are being promoted in efforts to control the disease throughout the world. Additional interventions to provide protection before, during, and after intercourse are being

investigated. Aggressive treatment of AIDS at an early stage reduces the viral load and the ease of transmission to others.[e]

Maternal-to-child transmission of HIV was a common, but not universal, event before the advent of effective drug treatment. The use of treatment during pregnancy and at the time of delivery has dramatically reduced the maternal-to-child transmission of the infection. Today, this route of transmission is close to being eliminated, which is an important public health achievement. Breastfeeding represents an ongoing and more controversial route of transmission. Up to 25% of HIV-positive breastfeeding women may transmit HIV to their children. In countries where breastfeeding provides an essential defense against a wide range of infections, the issue of whether or not to breastfeed has been very controversial. Fortunately, drug treatment of HIV infections during breastfeeding has been shown to greatly reduce, but not eliminate, transmission.

Finally, HIV can be transmitted through contaminated needles. Thus, the risk of HIV transmission needs to be addressed in two very different populations—healthcare workers and those who abuse intravenous drugs. New needle technologies and better disposal methods have reduced the likelihood of needlestick injuries in healthcare settings. Postexposure treatment with drugs has been quite successful in reducing healthcare-related HIV infections. Reductions in HIV transmission through intravenous drug use have also occurred in areas where public health efforts have focused

---

[e] It has been suggested that serial monogamy reduces the risk of HIV transmission in populations compared to having two or more concurrent partners. Serial monogamy contributes to only one chain of transmission at a time and thus may slow, if not halt, the speed or spread of the epidemic in a population.

attention on this method of transmission. Needle exchange programs have met resistance and remain controversial, but most likely contribute to transmission reductions when the programs are carefully designed and administered.

Thus, a range of existing interventions linked to the method of transmission of HIV have been moderately successful in controlling the disease. New methods of control are needed and are being investigated and increasingly applied. Unfortunately, vaccination is not yet a successful intervention. In fact, early randomized controlled trials demonstrated no substantial degree of protection from vaccinations and raised the concern that vaccination may actually increase the probability of acquiring HIV. More recent studies combining two or more types of vaccines have again provided hope for at least a partially effective vaccine in the years to come.

The recognition that highly effective vaccinations are not likely in the foreseeable future has brought forth a wide array of ideas on how to control the spread of infection. Antiviral creams, postcoital treatments, and early testing and case finding may become effective interventions. Antiviral creams may become both an adjunct to condom use, as well as a substitute in those situations where condom use is not acceptable. The success of postneedlestick interventions in the healthcare setting has raised the possibility that postexposure treatment may also be effective after high-risk sexual contact.

Finally, new diagnostic tests for HIV that allow for detection of the disease in the most contagious early weeks of the infection are being investigated for widespread use. To be effective, testing for early disease would need to be coupled with rapid case finding to identify and ideally treat contacts.

It is encouraging to know that existing and emerging interventions for HIV hold out the possibility of effective control. Public health and medical interventions complement each other and are both needed if we are to effectively address the most widespread epidemic of the 2000s. **Table 7-4** summarizes the routes of transmission and the estimated transmission rates per exposure.[9] Finally, it outlines the potential interventions that we have discussed.

TABLE 7-4 Mode and Chances of Transmission of HIV and Existing Interventions

Route of transmission	Estimated transmission rate per exposure	Potential interventions
Blood transfusion Blood and blood products, such as pooled blood products previously used in United States by hemophiliacs	Contaminated blood over 90% chance of transmission with infected blood; pooling of blood dramatically increases infection risk	Screening of blood to detect HIV early Use of individual's own blood for surgery
Sexual contact—anal higher than vaginal, which is much higher than oral	Range from 0.1% to 10% per contact, with unprotected receptive anal intercourse posing highest risk Vaginal male to female greater than female to male Circumcision reduces risk by half Other sexually transmitted diseases may increase risk	Latex condom Circumcision Abstinence Serial monogamy reduces spread compared to two or more concurrent partners
Mother-to-child transmission	15% to 40% higher in developing countries Highest rate of transmission at time of vaginal delivery	Cesarean delivery Drug treatment during pregnancy and at time of delivery for mother and child
Breastfeeding	Very low per exposure, but up to 25% over year or more of breastfeeding	Continuation of drug treatment reduces, but does not eliminate, transmission
Needlestick exposures Healthcare occupational risk	Less than 0.5% of HIV-positive needlesticks result in transmission	Postexposure treatment with drugs established as effective prevention
Injection drug use	Less than 1% per episode of needle sharing	Needle exchange programs

Data from Population Reference Bureau. Facing the HIV/AIDS Pandemic. Population Bulletin 2002: 57(3).

BOX 7-2   The Influenza Pandemic of 1918

The history of the influenza pandemic of 1918 is summarized by the United States National Archives and Records Administration as follows:[10]

> World War I claimed an estimated 16 million lives. The influenza epidemic that swept the world in 1918 killed an estimated 50 million people. One fifth of the world's population was attacked by this deadly virus. Within months, it had killed more people than any other illness in recorded history.
>
> The plague emerged in two phases. In late spring of 1918, the first phase, known as the "three-day fever," appeared without warning. Few deaths were reported. Victims recovered after a few days. When the disease surfaced again that fall, it was far more severe. Scientists, doctors, and health officials could not identify this disease which was striking so fast and so viciously, eluding treatment and defying control. Some victims died within hours of their first symptoms. Others succumbed after a few days; their lungs filled with fluid and they suffocated to death.
>
> The plague did not discriminate. It was rampant in urban and rural areas, from the densely populated East coast to the remotest parts of Alaska. Young adults, usually unaffected by these types of infectious diseases, were among the hardest hit groups along with the elderly and young children. The flu afflicted over 25 percent of the U.S. population. In one year, the average life expectancy in the United States dropped by 12 years.

WHAT OPTIONS ARE AVAILABLE FOR THE CONTROL OF INFLUENZA?

Pandemic influenza is not a new problem. The influenza epidemic of 1918 is estimated to have killed 50 million people in a world populated with 2 billion people. Today, that would translate to over 150 million deaths. The history of the 1918 influenza pandemic is briefly summarized in **Box 7-2**.[10] The 1958 pandemic of Asian flu caused a similar, if less deadly, pandemic. Thus, we should not be surprised if pandemic flu returns in the coming years.

Influenza A is a viral infection that has long been capable of pandemic or worldwide spread.[f] Its ability to be rapidly transmitted through the air from person to person and its short incubation period have made it an ongoing public health problem. It often kills the very young, the very old, and those with chronic illnesses, particularly those with respiratory diseases and suppressed immune systems. In addition, the disease continues to mutate, creating new types against which previous infections and previous vaccinations have little or no impact. Thus, new vaccines are required every flu season. Seasonal influenza kills over 30,000 people in the United States alone in the average year despite the increasingly widespread use of vaccinations.

A variety of public health and medical interventions have been and continue to be used to address the current and potential threat posed by influenza. They may well all be needed to address future threats. Let us take a look at a number of these interventions.

Inactivated or dead vaccines have been the mainstay of immunization against influenza. Unfortunately, current technology requires approximately six months lead time to produce large quantities of the vaccine. Thus, influenza experts need to make educated guesses about next year's dominant strains of influenza. In some years, they have been wrong and the deaths and disability from seasonal influenza have increased. New technologies for vaccine production are now available and should be able to help with this issue in the future.

In recent years, live vaccines administered through nasal spray have been developed and increasingly used. These vaccines are more acceptable than shots to most patients and are now considered safe for a wide range of age groups. They raise the hope of greater acceptance and wider use of influenza vaccinations in coming years.

Medications to treat influenza and modestly shorten the course of the disease have also been developed. Influenza experts view these drugs as most useful to temporarily slow the spread of new strains, providing additional time for the development of vaccines to specifically target the new strain. Widespread use of influenza drugs has already resulted in resistance, raising concerns that these drugs will not be

---

[f] Influenza B can also cause epidemics of influenza; however, it is not thought to pose the same hazard of pandemic disease that is possible with influenza A.

effective when we need them the most. Efforts are underway to develop new drugs and reserve their use solely for potential pandemic conditions.

Despite our best efforts, influenza is expected to continue its annual seasonal epidemic and to pose a risk of pandemic spread. The use of barrier protection such as masks, isolation methods, and even quarantine has been considered part of a comprehensive effort to control influenza. It is clear that we have a variety of public health methods to help control the impact of the disease. It is likely that we will need all of these efforts and new ones if we are going to control the potential deaths and disabilities due to influenza in coming years.[11] Now, let us look at our last example of the development of public health strategies to control communicable diseases—that of rabies.

WHAT OPTIONS ARE AVAILABLE FOR THE CONTROL OF RABIES?

Rabies is an ancient disease that has plagued human beings for over 4,000 years. It is caused by a ribonucleic acid (RNA) virus that is transmitted through saliva of infected animals and slowly replicates. It spreads to nerve cells and gradually invades the central nervous system over a 20- to 60-day incubation period. Once the central nervous system is involved, the disease progresses almost inevitably to death within one to two weeks. Any warm-blooded animal can be infected with rabies, but some species are particularly susceptible—most commonly raccoons, skunks, and bats. Cats and dogs can also be infected and transmit the virus.

A multicomponent vaccination strategy has been very successful in preventing the development of rabies in humans. In most recent years, there have been between one and five fatal cases of rabies per year in the United States despite the persistence and periodic increase in rabies among wildlife populations. Let us take a look at how this quite remarkable control effort has occurred.

The ability to successfully vaccinate humans against rabies after the occurrence of a rabies-prone bite has long been a component of the success of rabies reduction among humans. The use of postexposure vaccination was first demonstrated by Louis Pasteur in 1887 and was used to dramatically save the life of a young victim. Early live vaccines had frequent and severe side effects. They were sequentially replaced by inactivated vaccines grown in animal nerve tissue. These replacement vaccines still led to occasional acute neurological complications and gave the treatment a reputation of being dangerous. The development of a vaccine grown in human cell cultures in the 1970s led to safety records comparable to those of other commonly used

vaccines. Today, over 30,000 rabies vaccination series are administered annually in the United States.

The success of rabies control is a result of a series of coordinated efforts to utilize vaccinations in different settings. Vaccines are administered to individuals who are bitten by suspicious species of wild animals, including raccoons, bats, skunks, foxes, and coyotes. Victims of suspected rabies bites by dogs and cats may await the results of quarantine of the animal and observation over a 10-day period. When substantial doubt still exists after this time frame, vaccination is recommended. Laws requiring rabies vaccination of dogs and cats have been enforced in the United States for decades and have greatly reduced the number of reported infections in these animals. Today, only 10% or less of suspect rabies-prone bites come from dogs and cats.

Wildlife remains the greatest source of rabies—wildlife epidemics occur with regularity. Rabies-prone bites still occur especially from raccoons, which regularly feed from garbage cans in rural, suburban, and occasionally urban parts of the United States. The recent development of effective oral vaccinations that can be administered to wildlife through baits has been credited with reducing the number of infected animals, especially those residing in close proximity to humans.

Rabies illustrates the variety of ways that a key intervention—vaccination—can be used to address a disease. As with many complex diseases of public health importance, a carefully designed and coordinated strategy is required to maximize the benefit of available technology. In addition, ongoing research is needed to continue to develop new and improved approaches to the control of communicable diseases.[12]

HIV/AIDS, influenza A, and rabies represent three very different communicable diseases. However, they all require the use of multiple interventions, close collaboration between the public health and healthcare systems, and continuing efforts to find new and more effective methods for their control.

Efforts to control communicable diseases have increased in recent years along with the increase in emerging and reemerging infectious diseases. Technological advances have provided encouragement for the future but at times have raised concerns about the safety of our interventions.[g] New

---

[g] In recent decades, the number of vaccinations used in children has increased dramatically. The potential for new side effects from multiple vaccinations has been of recent concern, especially the previous use of a mercury-containing compound designed to help preserve vaccines. Concerns have been raised that multiple vaccines have increased the risk of autism. Despite investigations that did not support an association, these concerns persisted. However, it has now been recognized that the initial reports of an association of vaccinations with autism were based on fraudulent data.

technology, new strategies for applying technology, and new ways to effectively organize our efforts are needed to ensure the effectiveness and safety of our efforts to prevent, eradicate, and control communicable diseases.

Now let us turn our attention to our third category of disease: that of environmental diseases and injuries.

KEY WORDS

- Communicable disease
- Infectious disease
- Infections
- Epidemic
- Endemic
- Pandemic
- Koch's postulates
- Modern Koch's postulates
- Route of transmission
- Asymptomatic transmission
- Reproduction ratio (R_0)
- Chronic carriers
- Immunization
- Passive immunity
- Inactivated vaccine or dead vaccine
- Live vaccines (attenuated live)
- Antibody
- Cell-mediated immunity
- Herd immunity or population immunity
- Case finding
- Infectivity
- Epidemiological treatment
- Ring vaccination

Discussion Questions

Take a look at the questions posed in the following scenarios, which were presented at the beginning of this chapter. See now whether you can answer them.

1. Your college roommate went to bed not feeling well one night, and early the next morning, you had trouble arousing her. She was rushed to the hospital just in time to be effectively diagnosed and treated for meningococcal meningitis. The health department recommends immediate antibiotic treatment for everyone who was in close contact with your roommate. They set up a process to watch for additional cases to be sure an outbreak is not in progress. Fortunately, no more cases occur. You ask yourself: Should your college require that all freshmen have the meningococcal vaccine before they can register for classes?

2. As a health advisor to a worldwide HIV/AIDS foundation, you are asked to advise on ways to address the HIV and developing tuberculosis (TB) epidemics. You are asked to do some long-range thinking and to come up with a list of potential approaches to control the epidemics, or at least ways to reduce the development of TB. The first recommendation you make is to forget about eradicating HIV/AIDS. How did you come to that conclusion?

3. Your hometown of 100,000 is faced with a crisis as an airplane lands containing a passenger thought to have a new form of severe influenza that has recently gained the ability to spread from person to person through airborne transmission. As the mayor of the city, what do you decide to do?

4. You are a principal at a local high school. One of your top athletes is in the hospital with a spreading bacterial infection due to staphylococcus bacteria resistant to all known antibiotics. The infection occurred after what appeared to be a minor injury during practice. As the principal, what do you decide to do?

REFERENCES

1. Nobelprize.org. Robert Koch and tuberculosis. http://www.nobelprize.org/educational/medicine/tuberculosis/readmore.html. Accessed July 21, 2013.

2. New Jersey Medical School Global Tuberculosis Institute. History of TB. http://www.umdnj.edu/ntbcweb/tbhistory.htm. Accessed July 21, 2013.

3. National Institute of Allergy and Infectious Diseases. The evidence that HIV causes AIDS. http://www.niaid.nih.gov/topics/hivaids/understanding/howhivcausesaids/pages/hivcausesaids.aspx. Accessed July 21, 2013.

4. Timmreck TC. *An Introduction to Epidemiology*. 3rd ed. Sudbury, MA: Jones and Bartlett Learning; 2002:34.

5. Diekmann O, Heesterbeek JAP, Metz JAJ. On the definition and the computation of the basic reproduction ratio R0 in models for infectious diseases in heterogeneous populations. *J Math Biol*. 1990;28:365–382.

6. Centers for Disease Control and Prevention. History and epidemiology of global smallpox eradication. http://www.bt.cdc.gov/agent/smallpox/training/overview/pdf/eradicationhistory.pdf. Accessed July 20, 2013.

7. Centers for Disease Control and Prevention. Vaccines. http://www.cdc.gov/vaccines. Accessed July 21, 2013.

8. Sompayrac L. *How Pathogenic Viruses Work*. Sudbury, MA: Jones and Bartlett Learning; 2002.

9. Lamptey P, Wigley M, Carr D, Collymore Y. Facing the HIV/AIDS pandemic. *Population Bulletin*. 2002;57(3):1–3.

10. National Archives and Records Administration. The deadly vines: the influenza epidemic of 1918. http://www.archives.gov/exhibits/influenza-epidemic. Accessed July 21, 2013.

11. World Health Organization. Global agenda for influenza surveillance and control. http://apps.who.int/csr/disease/influenza/globalagenda/en. Accessed July 21, 2013.

12. Centers for Disease Control and Prevention. Rabies home. http://www.cdc.gov/rabies. Accessed July 21, 2013.

CHAPTER 8

Environmental Health and Safety

LEARNING OBJECTIVES

By the end of this chapter, the student will be able to:

- define the scope of morbidity and mortality caused by the physical environment.
- identify the range of interactions that occur between human beings and the physical environment.
- identify the components of environmental risk assessment and apply them to an environmental hazard, such as lead.
- distinguish between a risk assessment, a public health assessment, and an ecological assessment.
- discuss the meaning of interactions and how they may impact the size of risks.
- describe how intentional and unintentional injuries can be addressed to prevent their occurrence and diminish their consequences.
- identify successes of outbreak investigations.

Joe grew up in an industrial district of town. His family lived in an old apartment building, and he played in a playground near a major intersection. By the age of 6, Joe was found to have high lead levels in his blood and was not doing well in school. Where could all that lead come from? his mother wondered.

Jill is pregnant and loves fish, which she has eaten almost daily for years as part of her effort to stay healthy. She hears that fish should not be eaten regularly during pregnancy. Why, she wonders, should I cut down on eating something as healthy as fish?

Ralph and Sonya, a prosperous professional couple, and their two children live in an older suburban home. They feel secure that their environment is safe. They were surprised to find when they wanted to put their house up for sale that it did not pass the safety tests for radon. Where did the radon come from, they wondered, and what can be done about it?

Sandra worked for an international agency that had successfully addressed the danger of radiation due to the hole in the ozone layer. She was shocked when she was told that she had a life-threatening skin cancer called melanoma. She asked: What could cause melanoma? Could years of sun exposure have played a role?

You set out on your commute to work, and as you approach the subway station, you see police cars, ambulances, and dozens of emergency responders in hazmat suits. You are told the entire subway system will be shut down indefinitely, as there has been a suspected case of bioterrorism. You wonder how authorities were alerted to this situation and what precautions are being taken to protect the health of those living in the city.

Alex suffered a traumatic brain injury when he was thrown from his motorcycle after colliding with a car in which the driver had an elevated blood alcohol concentration. Alex was not wearing a helmet. His family members wonder what is being done to prevent this from happening to others.

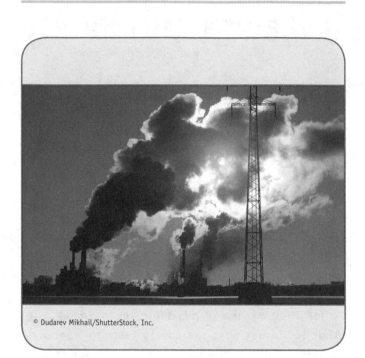

© Dudarev Mikhail/ShutterStock, Inc.

All of these situations are part of what we mean by the burden of environmental disease and injury. In order to understand the impact of the environment on health, we need to define what we mean by "environment" and appreciate the many ways that we interact with it.

WHAT IS MEANT BY "ENVIRONMENT"?

"Environment" is an ambiguous term. It is sometimes used to imply all influences other than genetic influences, including social, economic, and cultural influences. We will define the environment as the physical environment. The physical environment can be thought of in three categories: unaltered ("natural"), altered, and the built environment.[a] **Figure 8-1** diagrams the scope of environmental diseases and injuries.

---

[a] The term "natural" is used in quotations because it can be a misleading term. We often think that the term "natural disasters" implies that human actions had nothing to do with the events. Increasingly, human actions precipitate, worsen, and even cause "natural disasters." Construction on vulnerable lands increases the damage from storms, fires, earthquakes, and even volcanoes. Global warming caused by human activities is also beginning to have its impacts. Our planet has been altered in so many ways that the unaltered environment is becoming difficult to find.

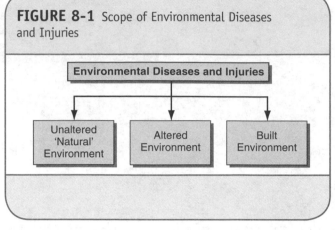

FIGURE 8-1 Scope of Environmental Diseases and Injuries

The health of human beings was affected by the physical environment long before we had the capacity to substantially alter the environment. Floods, earthquakes, and volcanoes have always been a part of the physical environment. In addition to these intermittent and often isolated impacts, daily exposures to communicable diseases in water and food have always been a part of the unaltered environment.

In recent years, we have recognized more subtle impacts of the **unaltered environment**. Radon, a common naturally occurring breakdown product of uranium, increases the risk of lung cancer. Exposure to naturally occurring sunlight increases the chances of skin cancer, including melanoma—a potentially lethal skin cancer—especially among light-skinned individuals.

Human activity has altered nearly every aspect of our physical environment. Some alterations to our environment may improve human health—from water treatment, to waste management, to mosquito and flood control. Nonetheless, we need to consider the overall impacts that these changes have on the physical environment. The sheer growth in the number of human beings—the planet's population has exceeded 7 billion—is likely to magnify our impact on all aspects of our physical environment in the future. This population growth and increasing human activity are believed to be contributing to a range of environmental issues, from deforestation to global warming. The observed changes occurring in the climate will likely impact the health of everyone. **Box 8-1** outlines some possible health effects of climate change.

We often think of the **altered environment** as reflecting the impact of chemicals, radiation, and biological products that we introduce into the environment. The list of intentional or unintentional introductions is in fact very long. It ranges from industrial chemicals, such as pesticides,

BOX 8-1 Climate Change

Global warming, or climate change, as it is being increasingly referred to, is likely to have expected and unexpected impacts on human health. The most predictable changes are those associated with expanded territory for currently existing communicable diseases. For instance, cases of malaria, dengue fever, and insect-borne encephalitis are likely to increase in the United States. Malaria existed for many years in the country as far north as the mid-Atlantic states. The mosquitoes that transmit malaria are present in the United States, and the disease could readily reestablish itself as a major pathogen. Dengue fever, or "breakbone fever," is a mosquito-borne disease related to yellow fever. One strain of the disease, hemorrhagic dengue fever, has a high case-fatality rate. The geographic range of the mosquito that carries dengue fever is currently limited because frost kills both the adult insects and their larvae. Rising temperatures are expected to allow the disease to move steadily northward in future decades. Outbreaks of acute encephalitis (inflammation of the brain) transmitted by mosquitoes are already on the rise. We can expect to see more frequent and severe outbreaks in the future.

In addition, more frequent and intense heat waves are likely to occur, especially in currently temperate climates covering much of the United States. Deaths among the very young and the very old can be expected during heat waves. Additional possible impacts of climate change on health are those associated with hurricanes, flooding, forest fires, and drought—all of which are likely to occur with increased frequency and severity in specific areas of the world. The potential for hurricane damage is not just from the acute storm. As demonstrated by Hurricane Katrina, there can be long-lasting impacts on the safety and availability of housing, as well as destruction of the healthcare and public health infrastructure. Rising ocean levels in and of themselves may displace hundreds of millions of people who currently live in low-lying river delta areas throughout the world.

The exact impacts of climate change remain uncertain and controversial. Alterations in ocean currents could potentially lower temperatures in Europe and other highly populated areas. Despite the great uncertainties ahead, it is clear that climate change will affect not only the lives of today's college students but also people's lives for centuries to come.

benzene, and chlorofluorocarbons (CFCs), to elements mined from the earth, such as mercury and lead. It also includes radiation from nuclear energy and medical wastes. Biological impacts encompass the introduction of invasive species and the management of biological wastes.

The concept of the **built environment** is relatively new and includes all the impacts of the physical environment as a result of human construction. The impacts of human construction include injuries and exposures in the home, the transportation system, and where we work and play. They also include factors ranging from the way we build and heat our buildings and cook our food, to the way we travel from place to place. The built environment influences our safety through its impact on injuries and hazardous exposures. It also influences our activity levels and our social interactions, which impact our health.[2]

The impact of the built environment is wide ranging throughout the world, but differs greatly by geography and stage of social and economic development. Indoor air pollution from cooking is the most prominent source of air pollution in much of the developing world. Motor vehicle injuries

are the most deadly consequences of the built environment in most developed countries. The built environment has subtle impacts as well. The way we build our cities affects the amount of exercise we get and the quantity of noise pollution we experience. Construction methods affect air systems in buildings and can increase our exposure to "sick buildings." Let us take a look at the burden of disease that results from the physical environment.

WHAT IS THE BURDEN OF DISEASE DUE TO THE PHYSICAL ENVIRONMENT?

Measuring the impact of the physical environment on health is difficult because of the many types of impacts and the often subtle effects that occur. The impacts we experience today may pale in comparison to what we can expect in the future. Nonetheless, it is useful to appreciate the current estimates of the magnitude of the direct and indirect burden.

Motor vehicle injuries and exposure to toxic substances are two important actual causes of death that represent the largest known impact of the physical environment. Together, these incidents are estimated to cause nearly 100,000 deaths per year, representing about 20% of preventable deaths in the United States and approximately 10% of all deaths in the United States, according to the Centers for Disease Control and Prevention's (CDC) calculations.[3] Motor vehicle injuries and other unintentional injuries have especially heavy impacts on the young; in fact, they are the number one cause of death in the United States among those 1 to 24 years of age.[4] As a cause of disability, injuries also rank high especially considering their disproportionate impact on the young.

The impact of toxic substances on population health extends beyond acute symptoms such as skin and respiratory irritation to chronic conditions. The impact on death and disability is difficult to measure due to the length of time the substances may take to affect the body. It may be years after an exposure before an individual experiences negative health effects on their kidneys, liver, nerves, and other organs. **Box 8-2** describes the impact of small particle air pollution on health, including the recent recognition of its long-term effects on the development of coronary artery disease. This link substantially increases the estimated impact the environment has on health outcomes.

Many toxic exposures occur in occupational settings. Approximately 5,000 deaths due to injuries occur in the occupational setting per year. Certain occupations are particularly vulnerable to injuries, including mining, construction, and agriculture. Occupational exposures that result in morbidity and mortality include lung diseases caused by exposures to hazardous dusts, hearing loss from loud noises, and back pain from excessive lifting, as well as a wide range of other mechanical problems, including carpal tunnel syndrome, which is often caused by repetitive motion of the hand and wrist. Occupational injuries have been declining in recent years, but they remain an important cause of death and disability.[6] Cancer caused by occupational exposures has been of particular concern. As much as 5% of cancer deaths in males have been estimated to be due to occupational exposures.[7] Cancers of the lung, bladder, and white blood cells (leukemia) are particularly likely to result from chronic exposures to chemicals, such as formaldehyde, benzene, and organic dyes. Reductions in occupational exposures in the last 30 years have resulted in a declining burden of disease from these exposures in the United States. The opposite is being seen in many newly industrializing countries, where current exposures are increasing and may result in more cases of cancer and other diseases in the not-too-distant future.

Finally, we cannot evaluate the impact of toxic exposures solely by tracing them to human deaths and disabilities. The altered environment has impacts on entire ecosystems of plants and animals. The ecological impact of environmental factors can have long-term and largely

BOX 8-2 Impact of Small Particle Air Pollution on Health[5]

Air pollution occurs when particulate matter, a mix of tiny solid and liquid particles, is suspended in the air. The particles can be comprised of a number of components, including acids, organic chemicals, metals, dust, and pollen and mold spores. The size of the particles makes a difference on their impact on health. Our body's natural defense mechanisms, such as coughing and sneezing, can dislodge larger particles. However, small particles, less than 10 micrometers in diameter, can be inhaled into the lungs and enter the bloodstream; therefore, they have potential to pose a great risk to health. The smallest of these particles are referred to as fine particles. Fine particles measure less than 2.5 micrometers in diameter and, therefore, can only be seen with an electron microscope. When millions of these particles are suspended in the air, a haze forms, referred to as smog and often seen in cities due to exhaust from motor vehicles.

Everyone's health is at risk from small particle pollution; however, certain groups are at greater risk. Because children spend more active time outside, their lungs are still developing, and they are more likely to have asthma and acute respiratory disease, they face greater risk. Older adults also have an increased risk for health issues due to small particles because they are more likely to have heart or lung disease, which can be aggravated by inhalation of the particles. People of any age with heart or lung disease are also at increased risk for this reason.

Health effects from short-term exposure can include eye, nose, and throat irritation; shortness of breath; asthma attacks; and bronchitis. Long-term exposure to small particle pollution can contribute to reduced lung function, chronic bronchitis, and premature death.

A number of recent studies demonstrate a link between small particle air pollution and coronary artery disease. It is believed that exposure to fine particulate air pollution leads to thickening of the arteries, disrupting blood flow, which can lead to heart attacks and strokes. Attributing a portion of

BOX 8-2 Impact of Small Particle Air Pollution on Health[5] (continued)

the many deaths from coronary artery disease to air pollution substantially increases the estimates of the environmental burden of disease.

In an effort to alert individuals to the air quality in their region, the Environmental Protection Agency created an Air Quality Index, which is provided in **Figure 8-2**:

FIGURE 8-2 Air Quality Index for Particle Pollution

AIR QUALITY INDEX FOR PARTICLE POLLUTION

Air Quality Index	Air Quality	Health Advisory
0 to 50	Good	None.
51 to 100	Moderate	Unusually sensitive people should consider reducing prolonged or heavy exertion.
101 to 150	Unhealthy for Sensitive Groups	People with heart or lung disease, older adults, and children should reduce prolonged or heavy exertion.
151 to 200	Unhealthy	People with heart or lung disease, older adults, and children should avoid prolonged or heavy exertion. Everyone else should reduce prolonged or heavy exertion.
201 to 300	Very Unhealthy	People with heart or lung disease, older adults, and children should avoid all physical activity outdoors. Everyone else should avoid prolonged or heavy exertion.

Reproduced from United States Environmental Protection Agency. Particulate Matter. Available at: http://www.epa.gov/airquality/particlepollution/index.html. Accessed July 23, 2013.

irreversible consequences. Once chemicals, radiation, and biological products are released into the environment, the process cannot generally be easily reversed. Thus, we need to take a broad and long-term perspective when we address environmental health.

HOW DO WE INTERACT WITH OUR PHYSICAL ENVIRONMENT?

To understand how the physical environment—be it the unaltered, altered, or built environment—affects health, we need to explore the myriad ways that we interact with it. **Box 8-3** illustrates this concept.

Because of the complexity of the interactions between human beings and the physical environment, a range of approaches has been developed for addressing these issues. We will categorize and examine these approaches as follows:

- **Risk assessment**
- **Public health assessment**
- **Ecological assessment**
- **Interaction analysis**

We can think of these strategies as a progression of approaches of increasing complexity. We will organize our approach to environmental diseases and injuries starting with

BOX 8-3 How We Interact with Our Environment

We are exposed to the physical environment every minute of our lives through multiple routes. For each of these routes of exposure, the body has mechanisms for protection. We are primarily exposed to the environment via the skin; the respiratory tract (from the nose to the lungs); the alimentary, or digestive, tract (from the mouth to the anus); and the genital-urinary tract.

Each bodily surface that is directly exposed to the physical environment has developed a form of barrier protection. The skin provides direct protection against radiation, organisms, and physical contact, as well as providing some protections against heat and cold. The respiratory tract is guarded by mucous production and by small hairlike structures called cilia, whose motion in conjunction with coughing removes materials that we breathe into our lungs. Cells called phagocytes literally consume organisms and large particles. Antibodies, along with cell-mediated immunity, also protect against access of harmful particles and organisms through the lungs. The alimentary, or digestive, tract is protected by saliva, mucous membranes, and antibodies, as well as strong acidity in the stomach. The genital-urinary tract is protected by mucous membrane barriers, antibody and cell-mediated immunity, and at times by an acid environment.[a]

---

[a] The effectiveness of our bodily defenses depends on a number of factors—for instance, genetic factors. Dark skin pigmentation reduces the penetration of radiation and reduces the risk of skin cancers, including melanoma, the most serious of skin cancers. Other diseases affect how well our defenses operate—for instance, chronic obstructive lung disease and cystic fibrosis can alter the ability of the cilia in the lungs to operate effectively. Age can affect the ability of our skin to serve as an effective barrier as well as the ability of the immune system to respond. The elderly are especially prone to the effects of heat and cold. They are also more susceptible to a range of infections and cancers. Our defense mechanisms can overreact to environmental stimuli and themselves produce ailments, including allergies and autoimmune disease. The impacts of certain environmental exposures may be limited to a small number of susceptible individuals whose immune systems react especially strongly to specific environmental

Therefore, we need to recognize that the impacts of the environment on health are very complex.[7] We should expect to find that the following issues affect the risk:

- Route of exposure—The consequences of exposures to heavy metals including mercury, lead, and cadmium, for instance, depend on whether the exposure is via the skin or the respiratory or gastrointestinal tracts.
- Timing of exposure—Short-term high-dose impacts often will not be the same as long-term low-dose impacts, even if the total exposure and the routes of exposure are the same. For instance, a small number of severe episodes of sunburn during childhood have been found to greatly increase the risk of skin cancers far more than multiple milder adult sunburns. Chronic low-dose exposures may produce different and more subtle impacts.
- Stage of life—The impact on the very young and the very old is likely to be different than the impact on people at other stages of life. We need to be especially concerned about exposures during pregnancy, early childhood, and the later years of life.
- Other diseases—The presence of other diseases will affect how the body is impacted by an environmental exposure. We need to be especially concerned about environmental exposures for those with chronic lung diseases and those with suppressed immune systems, such as those living with AIDS.
- Special sensitivities—A few individuals will be hypersensitive to specific environmental exposures that have no measurable impact on the vast majority of individuals. We need to be concerned about how to identify and protect these individuals without depriving them of rights or opportunities.

---

exposures. For instance, allergies to peanuts or household or industrial chemicals can produce unusual, but severe, reactions in a small number of susceptible individuals.

---

risk assessment and proceeding in order to examine each of these strategies.

HOW DOES RISK ASSESSMENT ADDRESS THE IMPACTS OF THE PHYSICAL ENVIRONMENT?

Risk assessment is a formal process that aims to measure the potential impact of known **hazards**. A hazard indicates the inherent danger of an exposure, while a risk assessment aims

to take into account not only the inherent danger, but also the quantity, route, and timing of the exposure.[8] The risk assessment approach to environmental hazards represents the mainstay of our current approach. The underlying principles have a long history in public health, often resulting from the investigation of specific occupational exposures.

One of the earliest occupational investigations occurred among chimney sweeps in England during the 1700s. Their

BOX 8-4 Benzene and Risk Assessment

Benzene is an organic chemical that is used as a solvent in the chemical and pharmaceutical industries. Because it readily becomes a gas at room temperature, airborne exposure is an important concern. Benzene is one of the most widely used organic chemicals. It is estimated that over 250,000 U.S. workers are exposed to benzene, particularly in the chemical, printing, paint, and petroleum industries.[a]

A range of toxic effects has been documented from benzene over the last 150 years. These include neurological effects of acute and chronic exposure, as well as life-threatening suppression of the production of red blood cells called aplastic anemia.

In the 1960s and 1970s, it was increasingly recognized that benzene causes cancer, particularly leukemia. Early studies of benzene and leukemia were conducted by Muzaffer Aksoy, a Turkish physician, who observed leukemia among many shoemakers in Turkey where benzene was being used as a solvent in the manufacturing of leather products. His large cohort study helped establish the chemical as a presumed cause of leukemia.

Based on a series of studies that documented the risk of leukemia, in 1978, the federal government established

a standard for exposure to benzene in the air of 1 part per million (1 ppm), as opposed to the former approach of limiting the exposure to 10 parts per million (10 ppm). One part per million is approximately the equivalent of 1 drop in 40 gallons of liquid. In 1980, the U.S. Supreme Court overturned the new standard based upon the argument that the Occupational Safety and Health Administration (OSHA) had not documented the impact of the new 1 ppm standard in terms of the number of lives saved or compared it to the 10 ppm level. The Supreme Court concluded that "safe" did not mean risk-free, giving the analogies of driving a car and breathing city air. The Supreme Court insisted that standards be set based upon the preponderance of evidence from a formal risk assessment. As a result of this Supreme Court decision, a risk-assessment approach was developed that grew into the current risk-assessment process. The 1 part per million standard was supported by quantitative measures of the impact: the federal government estimated that there would be 14 to 17 excess deaths per 1,000 workers exposed to 10 ppm of benzene for a working lifetime, compared to being exposed to the new 1 ppm standard.

Thus, risk assessment today is a highly technical and quantitative activity designed to establish a maximum level of allowed exposure to one particular hazard. The goal is to protect workers and the public from the most important risks to health.

---

[a] Benzene is also a component of gasoline; therefore, the entire population has some exposure to benzene. This discussion focuses on the hazard assessment of benzene in the occupational setting.

Data from: Feitshans IL, Law and Regulation of Benzene. *Environmental Health Perspectives.* 1989; 82:299–307.

---

high-dose exposure to carbon residues in smokestacks led to early and frequent testicular cancer. In the 1800s, industrializing countries also provided ample opportunities to study the impacts of work-related exposures. For instance, the dangers of radiation came to light after high levels of cancer were detected in workers who painted watches with radiation-containing paint for the purposes of nighttime illumination. The dangers of asbestos became evident after high-dose exposures among ship workers during World War II resulted in cases of lung cancer many years later. The dangers of exposure to polyvinyl chloride (PVC), a common industrial compound, were recognized after five workers from the same manufacturing plant came down with a rare liver tumor in the 1970s.

Risk assessment today has become a complex technical effort requiring quantitative measures of the magnitude of the risk. The history of risk assessment in the United States is

closely tied to the investigations and regulations surrounding benzene. **Box 8-4** provides an overview of the history of the study and regulation of this chemical hazard.[9, 10]

The formal process of risk assessment represents the current approach to environmental hazards in the United States.[10,11] **Figure 8-3** illustrates the four-step risk assessment process as used by the U.S. Environmental Protection Agency (EPA).

Risk assessment attempts to evaluate the impact of environmental exposures one at a time and to measure the types and magnitudes of the impacts. If a substantial risk is found to exist, the process then reviews options to protect, detect, and react to the risk to minimize the burden of disease on humans.

The risk assessment process builds in a margin of error designed to provide extra protection for especially vulnerable individuals or populations. Thus, those exposed to levels above the recommended maximum levels of exposure will

FIGURE 8-3 The 4-Step Risk Assessment Process

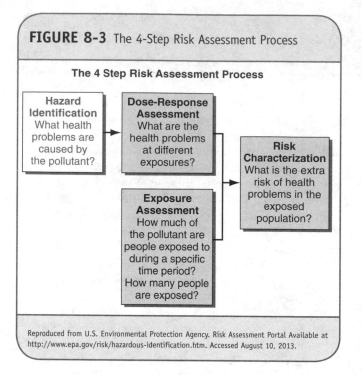

Reproduced from U.S. Environmental Protection Agency. Risk Assessment Portal Available at http://www.epa.gov/risk/hazardous-identification.htm. Accessed August 10, 2013.

WHAT IS A PUBLIC HEALTH ASSESSMENT?

Risk assessment is distinguished from what is called a public health assessment. A public health assessment goes beyond a risk assessment by including data on actual exposure in a community.

Public health assessments have the potential for major impacts on large numbers of people because they address not just the risks in a specific location, such as in an occupational setting, but also the risks to large numbers of individuals and often to the population as a whole. These types of risk assessments have been very controversial and have taken years—often decades—to complete. A classic example of the importance and potential impacts of the public health assessment process and its ongoing challenges is discussed in **Box 8-5**, which looks at the health risks due to lead.[12, 13]

Risk assessments and public health assessments both focus exclusively on the health impacts on human beings. Let us take a look at an additional type of assessment conducted by the EPA that looks at the impact of an exposure on plants and animals.

WHAT IS AN ECOLOGICAL RISK ASSESSMENT?

Environmental health cannot be viewed solely on the basis of current impacts on human health. The impacts of environmental contamination or pollution on plants and animals and the ecosystems in which they exist often have important long-term consequences.

The modern environmental movement in the United States was ignited in large part by Rachel Carson's book,

not necessarily experience adverse effects. **Table 8-1** outlines the four steps in the risk assessment process and uses a simplified example of how airborne exposure to benzene in occupational settings may be presented in this framework.

Now let us take a look at what is meant by "public health assessment."

TABLE 8-1 Four-Step Risk Assessment and Simplified Example—Benzene

Components	Simplified example—benzene
Hazard identification What health effects are caused by the pollutant?	Benzene causes leukemia Strong evidence from cohort studies and supportive animal data exist
Dose-response relationship What are the health problems at different exposures?	Strong dose-response relationship among occupational workers with level of 1 ppm over a working lifetime The impact of exposure at 1 ppm is indistinguishable from unexposed, with rapid increase in rates of leukemia above that level
Exposure assessment How much of the pollutant are people exposed to during a specific time period? How many people are exposed?	Industrial exposures above 1 ppm are common in a range of industries at the time the standard was set Over 250,000 workers exposed to benzene
Risk characterization What is the extra risk of health problems in the exposed population?	14–17 excess cases of leukemia per 1,000 workers exposed to 10 ppm throughout a working lifetime

Data from United States Environmental Protection Agency. Human Health Risk Assessment. Available at http://www.epa.gov/risk_assessment/health-risk.htm. Accessed August 10, 2013.

BOX 8-5 Health Risks Due to Lead

Knowledge of the potential for lead poisoning goes back to ancient civilizations, when the metal was widely used—for example, it was a component of water pipes and part of the process of making wine. In Rome, lead was used as a method of abortion, and high-dose exposures led to a range of mental effects. It is said the Roman emperors were affected by the high levels of lead in Roman wine.

Benjamin Franklin listed every known profession for which lead posed a health hazard and predicted that many years would pass before the public health consequences of lead were addressed. Of course, Benjamin Franklin was right. Things were to get worse before they got better.

In the 1920s, lead was added to gasoline to make for smoother driving. It was highly effective in getting the "knocks" out of early versions of the piston engine, as well as elevating the level of lead in the air. Even today, the lead from gasoline lies in the soil of many playgrounds. High levels of lead also improved the performance of paints. Houses built before the 1970s, and especially before the 1950s, still pose a threat to children who often ingest peeling paint.

It was not until the 1970s that the effect of low-dose lead exposure on the development of intellectual function became clear. The studies of Dr. Herbert Needleman and subsequent investigators documented clear-cut negative effects on the intellectual development of young children even at low levels of exposure. This prompted efforts to remove lead from gasoline, paints, and many other products. In recent years, new sources of lead, including toys, pottery, and water, have been given increased attention. In short, lead is a well-recognized hazard that is still with us.

Efforts to protect the environment have been coupled with efforts to detect and react to elevated lead levels. It is now standard practice in pediatrics and public health to monitor blood levels in high-risk children, investigate their home environments, and treat persistently elevated levels. Lead standards for playgrounds, lead abatement programs for homes, and lead monitoring of consumer products all aim to reduce or eliminate the hazards of lead. The system is by no means foolproof, and in recent years, elevated levels of the metal have been found from such divergent sources as toys manufactured in China and water in Washington, D.C. **Table 8-2** summarizes the potential exposures to lead, including their sources, and offers potential means of reducing or eliminating the hazard.

TABLE 8-2 Where Does Lead in Our Bodies Come From and What Can Be Done About It?

How lead enters our bodies	Where it comes from	Ways to reduce exposure
Inhalation	Workers in many lead-exposure industries, including mining, smelting, metal repair, or foundry work Demolition and renovation activities that generate fumes and dust, including home renovations and hobby activities Addition of lead to gasoline Once inhaled deep into the lungs, it may remain for long periods and be absorbed into blood over time	Occupational controls Phaseout of lead in gasoline in United States from 1976 to 1996
Ingestion	Children—normal ingestion of dirt and dust by infants and young children, with up to 5% of children who ingest large quantities—a condition called "pica" Children absorb greater percentage of ingested lead than adults	Removal of lead paint from older homes—lead levels in paint in the 1950s and earlier were as much as 50% lead Enforce elimination of lead paint from children's toys

(continues)

BOX 8-5   Health Risks Due to Lead (*continued*)

TABLE 8-2 Where Does Lead in Our Bodies Come From and What Can Be Done About It? (*continued*)

How lead enters our bodies	Where it comes from	Ways to reduce exposure
Ingestion	Children's toys and objects that are placed in the mouth are especially important sources Soil near old high traffic areas often contaminated from previous lead in gasoline Glazed pottery often includes lead that can leach into food	Monitoring and control of lead levels in soil in young children's play areas Very high blood levels may require "chelation"—treatment to reduce lead levels in blood
Water	Pipes, especially in older water supplies and homes built before the mid-1980s, often contain lead Lead used in pipes outside and within the home can leach into water—especially warm water—over time	Regulation of levels of lead in public water supply Run home water before use—especially after away for extended period Use cold water for cooking
In utero	Pregnant women absorb higher percentage of ingested lead compared to children, and lead can cross placenta Mother's previous lead exposure stored in her bones can be resorbed into her blood during pregnancy	Special effort to reduce exposure by pregnant women, including special care with home renovations during pregnancy, especially homes built before 1970

Data from Agency for Toxic Substance and Disease Registry. Case Studies in Environmental Medicine-Lead. Available at http://wonder.cdc.gov/wonder/prevguid/p0000017/p0000017.asp. Accessed July 23, 2013.

Silent Spring, which described how the widespread use of DDT had threatened the American Eagle and other birds as it became deposited in and weakened their eggs.[14] Broader concern about the impacts of contaminants on ecological systems ranging from chemicals, to radiation, to genetically altered crops has made clear the importance of ecological risk assessments. Human health consequences remain an important, but not necessarily direct, consequence of the impacts of environmental contamination or pollution as described in **Box 8-6**, which explores the impacts of mercury.[15, 16]

Up to this point, we have addressed the impact of environmental exposures one at a time. Increasingly, we find that the interactions between exposures produce unexpectedly large impacts. Let us now look at a strategy that addresses more than one problem at a time and takes into consideration the interaction between multiple exposures. We will call it an interaction analysis.

WHAT IS AN INTERACTION ANALYSIS APPROACH TO ENVIRONMENTAL DISEASES?

The term **interaction analysis** implies that to understand and control the impacts of environmental exposures, it is necessary to take into account the effect of two or more exposures. **Box 8-7** describes the multiple interacting factors contributing to depletion of the ozone layer.

Risk assessment approaches make the assumption that each exposure stands on its own. Thus, if there is more than one type of exposure, we need to make the assumption that the total impact is the sum of the two impacts. For example, if one exposure has a relative risk of 4 and a second has a relative risk of 6, we assume that exposure to both results in a relative risk of 10. Many times, adding together the relative risks does provide an approximation of the risk of two or more exposures. However, in an increasing number of situations, we are recognizing that there are interactions between exposures themselves so that the

BOX 8-6   Health Risks of Mercury in the Environment

The impact of high-dose mercury on mental function has been recognized since the 1800s. More recently, it was established that much lower levels of mercury pose risks to the fetus. Neurological damage, including learning disabilities and hearing loss, have been documented at low levels of exposure. The human risks of mercury exposure need to be understood as part of the impact of mercury on an entire ecological system.

For much of the late 1800s and the 1900s, mercury was a common product of industry that heavily contaminated the Great Lakes of the United States. The impacts were not appreciated despite the high levels of contamination and the impacts on animal species. Mercury in bodies of water is filtered by fish species and can concentrate in their fat. Thus, certain fish species can and do accumulate high concentrations of mercury. These species may be eaten by fish-eating birds and pose a risk to a number of endangered avian species. There is no technologically feasible method for removing mercury from the Great Lakes or other bodies of water. Your

children's children will most likely be living with mercury contamination.

Recommendations for limiting the consumption of fish, especially by pregnant women, have been the mainstay of efforts to address this problem. These efforts are complicated by the fact that the consumption of fish also carries health benefits. Today, the challenge is how to minimize the amount of mercury consumed by women without losing the benefits of fish consumption. Because some fish have much higher mercury levels than others, the March of Dimes recommends that pregnant women avoid shark, swordfish, king mackerel, and tilefish. They indicate that "it is ok" to eat a limited amount of fish that contain small amounts of mercury, including salmon, pollock, catfish, and canned light tuna.[16] The details of how much fish is safe for pregnant women to eat remains controversial. For today and many years to come, we will be living with the impacts of past environmental contamination on entire ecosystems.

BOX 8-7   Addressing the Problem of the Hole in the Ozone Layer[17]

It was first recognized in 1985 that the layer of ozone above Antarctica was being depleted at an alarming rate. Ozone in the upper atmosphere is known to protect against damaging radiation from the sun. Fears were raised that the hole in the ozone would expand progressively, encompass populated areas in the southern hemisphere, and involve the northern hemisphere as well.

It was quickly recognized that the problem was linked to multiple interacting human and naturally occurring systems. The use of chlorofluorocarbons (CFCs) in such products as refrigerators and air-conditioning equipment was quickly identified as a major contributor. In addition, commonly used aerosol sprays from deodorants and hair sprays contained CFCs. More concerning was the use of CFC in devices to deliver medications.

The timely accumulation of data, the rapid understanding of the multiple contributors to the problem, and a worldwide media campaign soon brought together a remarkably effective response to the problem. By 1987, an international agreement, known as the Montreal Protocol, was developed and quickly implemented by most nations. The agreement and subsequent revisions resulted in the rapid phaseout of most uses of CFC, with more gradual elimination of CFCs in medical devices.

The hole in the ozone layer continues to expand due to the extremely long half-life of CFCs. The projections, however, are for a turnaround in the near future and a resolution of the problem by 2050. The coordinated scientific, public health, health communications, and political responses have encouraged future efforts to recognize and jointly address multifactor environmental health problems.

presence of both exposures results in an overall impact much greater than expected. For instance, we may find that having both exposures results in a relative risk of a bad outcome of 4 times 6, or 24, instead of 10. This type of interaction is called **multiplicative interaction**. **Box 8-8** examines the multiplicative interaction between radon and cigarette smoking.[18]

BOX 8-8 Interaction Between Radon and Cigarettes

Radon is a naturally occurring radioactive gas. It is colorless and odorless. Radon is produced by the decay of uranium in soil, rock, and groundwater. It emits ionizing radiation during its radioactive decay. Radon is found all over the country, though there are areas of the country with substantially higher levels than other areas. Radon gets into the indoor air primarily by entering via the soil under homes and other buildings at the basement or lowest level.

Today, it is recognized that radon is the second most important cause of lung cancer after cigarettes and the most common cause of cancer among nonsmokers. The EPA estimates that radon accounts for over 20,000 cases of lung cancer, as compared with the over 100,000 cases attributed to cigarettes. The average indoor level in the United States is about 1.3pCi/L. The EPA has set a level of 2pCi/L as an attainable level and a level of 4pCi/L as the maximum recommended level. Approximately 15% of homes in the United States have basement radon levels above 4pCi/L.

Cigarette smoking and radon exposure are multiplicative; that is, when both are present, the hazard is multiplied. For instance, using the EPA's figures, the relative risk of lung cancer for the average smoker is approximately 9 times the risk compared to a nonsmoker. The relative risk from radon when the level is 10pCi/L compared to 2pCi/L is over 4.5. When both cigarette smoking and a level of radon exposure of 10pCi/L are present, the relative risk of lung cancer increases over 40 times.

The recognition that radon and also asbestos multiply the impacts of cigarette smoking has had a key impact on the approaches used to address these potential hazards. For smokers with exposure to these hazards, the risk can be greatly reduced by reductions in radon and asbestos, as well as by stopping smoking. Because both radon and asbestos are potentially controllable environmental exposures, there has been a great deal of attention and money given to the control of these hazards. Thus, the recognition of interactions that multiply or greatly increase the risk have become an important tool for setting priorities and developing approaches to risk reduction.

Not all risks for environmental disease require high-level or long-term exposure. In addition to causing lung cancer, asbestos has also been shown to cause a form of cancer called mesothelioma, which originates in the lining of the lung or pleura. Even small and short-term exposures to asbestos may cause mesothelioma, as evidenced by well-documented cases among household members who washed the clothing of those exposed. New technologies, such as nanotechnology, are raising concerns that the risks of low-level exposure need to be investigated as much as those of high-level exposure. Low-dose environmental exposures to estrogen-like substances may pose threats to the reproductive health of animal species and could even affect the human rate of breast cancer. Addressing these types of issues requires us to focus on the interactions between multiple factors.

Now we have taken a look at the basic regulatory approaches we currently use to address the hazards from the physical environment. Let us now take a look at the safety component of environmental health and safety, starting with injuries.

WHAT DO WE MEAN BY "INTENTIONAL AND UNINTENTIONAL INJURIES"?

Injuries can occur in a wide array of settings and circumstances, including actions at work, home, and where we play. They can affect everyone, regardless of age, income, race, or ethnicity. It is estimated that, in the United States, one person dies every three minutes due to violence or injury. Injuries are the leading cause of death among persons aged 1 to 44 years.[20] Injuries do not always result in death and can result in long-term health effects, impacting quality of life.

In public health, we try to avoid the use of the term "accident" because "accident" implies that the reasons for the injury are beyond our control. Injuries can be categorized as intentional and unintentional. **Intentional injuries** are brought about on purpose, that is, by intention, whether the injury is self-inflicted or meant for others. Intentional injuries can impact entire populations, such as bioterrorist actions that lead to fear and fatalities among a population, or can directly impact individuals, such as with suicide. Harms that occur not on purpose—that is, not by intention—are categorized as unintentional injuries. **Unintentional injuries** encompass injuries sustained in motor vehicle collisions, drownings, falls, fires, unintentional poisonings, and many other incidents.

WHAT IS BEING DONE TO KEEP THE POPULATION SAFE?

Safety is approached like many other public health issues: the problem is described; risk and protective factors are identified; and interventions and strategies are developed, implemented, evaluated, and disseminated. The formal steps of the evidence-based public health approach are often used to examine specific issues and interventions.

One of the most visible public health tools used to keep populations safe is outbreak investigations. These investigations conjure images of public health professionals serving as "disease detectives," tracking and responding to outbreaks of acute disease, and these investigations are often viewed as quintessential public health. **Box 8-9** discusses some of the successes health departments and the CDC have had in outbreak investigations.

Public health's role in protecting the health of populations has evolved as new threats have emerged, including bioterrorism. **Box 8-10** reviews the anthrax case that occurred shortly after the September 11, 2001, terrorist attack and describes its impact on public health.

In recent years, public health agencies have been increasingly integrated into a National Incident Management System (NIMS), which is part of the Department of Homeland Security (DHS). A central feature of the NIMS is an incident command system (ICS) widely used by police, fire, and emergency management agencies. The ICS attempts to establish uniform procedures and terminology, and an integrated communications system with established and practiced roles for each agency. The goal is to integrate these approaches into ongoing operations and not reserve them solely for emergency situations.[19]

The DHS has developed what is called an **all-hazards approach**. An all-hazards approach to public health preparedness uses the same approach to preparing for many types of disasters, including use of surveillance systems, communications systems, evacuations, and an organized healthcare response. The all-hazards approach has been widely endorsed by public health agencies and organizations in part at least because it recognizes the need for basic public health infrastructure to respond not only to the dramatic crisis or emergency, but to day-to-day needs as well.

Preparing for and responding to emergencies and disasters is key to addressing the expected and unexpected crises that we will inevitably face in the future. In addition to emergency and disaster preparedness and response, public health sets out to ensure safety of the population in everyday tasks. Let us look at the CDC framework used to prevent intentional and unintentional injury and diminish associated consequences.

BOX 8-9 Outbreak Investigations

Outbreak investigations have been a key component of public health's effort to respond to epidemics and clusters of acute disease. These investigations are often successfully handled by local and state health agencies. The Centers for Disease Control (CDC), however, may be called in to assist with them. The CDC is involved in hundreds of outbreak investigations each year.

Famous investigations include the 1976 outbreak of what came to be called Legionnaires' disease. Hundreds of military veterans, called Legionnaires, gathering in Philadelphia in July to celebrate the nation's bicentennial, were infected and many died from pneumonia. The CDC identified the cause as previously unrecognized bacteria—now called Legionella—that can grow in hot water and can be spread through the air.

In the early 1980s, an outbreak of life-threatening cardiovascular shock, known as toxic shock syndrome (TSS), was traced to a new type of absorbent tampon. It brought to light the need for surveillance of new products, even those not suspected of causing disease.

The most important outbreak of the late 1900s was investigated and brought to professional and public attention in 1981 by the CDC. It came to be called acquired immunodeficiency syndrome (AIDS).

Outbreak investigations are not limited to communicable diseases. In fact, the illnesses may originate, for example, from an environmental toxin, a food additive or supplement, or a drug reaction. For instance, eosinophilia-myalgia syndrome (EMS) is an incurable and sometimes fatal neurological condition that often presents with vague flulike symptoms. It was traced by the CDC to poorly produced L-trytophan, an amino acid widely used as a food supplement. Reye's syndrome, an often fatal acute liver disease of children, was traced to the use of "baby aspirin" for healthy children during acute viral infections.

Thousands of outbreak investigations are conducted in the United States each year and are mostly handled by state and local health departments. These types of investigations can take months or even years to complete. Often the outbreak is over before the investigation can be completed. Outbreak investigations will remain an important part of public health. However, new technologies, new tracking systems, and better communications systems will hopefully make these critical investigations more rapid and efficient.

BOX 8-10   Bioterrorism and Anthrax[20]

Shortly after the terrorist attack on the United States on September 11, 2001, a second attack occurred that greatly altered the course of public health in the country. The attack occurred in the form of letters containing a powdered form of anthrax bacteria delivered through the U.S. mail to Congress and national news networks.

Anthrax is bacteria long known for its occasional spread from cattle to humans by close contact and its potential to cause a life-threatening pneumonia. It is considered a particularly deadly agent for bioterrorism, with the potential to kill tens of thousands of people. When prepared in the form of a weapon and delivered in quantity, it has the potential to widely disperse over an entire city or region. Early detection of the substance and treatment of its effects are key to controlling such an attack, including preventing the pneumonia through the early use of antibiotics.

The anthrax attack in 2001 made headlines for weeks, temporarily shutting down Congress and much of Washington, killing five people, and causing severe illness in 17 others. The episode also brought attention and funding to public health programs. It was soon recognized that even large health departments with extensive responsibilities and expertise were not prepared to address bioterrorism and ensure the availability of public health laboratories to diagnose anthrax-related illness and other potential agents of bioterrorism.

Preparation for bioterrorism also focuses on the unique characteristics of bioterrorism and the specific organisms that may be involved with it. The anthrax episode highlighted how terrorism, in general, and bioterrorism, in particular, differ from the types of emergencies and disasters that have become familiar. First, they may involve the military, as well as law enforcement. Second, they require knowledge of agents that are often very rare. Little expertise exists in either the public health or medical communities about agents such as anthrax, botulism, smallpox, and plague. In addition, bioterrorism may not be easily detected, allowing the agent to spread widely before it is noticed and action can be taken. Finally, there is the potential for multiple simultaneous threats at multiple locations. Thus, bioterrorism requires special preparation above and beyond the evolving preparedness system for emergencies and disasters. Public health agencies, including the CDC and local health departments, were on the front lines of the anthrax attack and will continue to be part of the first response to bioterrorism attacks if they occur in the future.

When approaching violence and injury, the CDC:

- Identifies and monitors the injury problem
- Conducts research to guide decision making
- Empowers states through funding and technical assistance
- Builds partnerships for prevention
- Builds awareness through communication and education
- Collaborates with partners around the globe to prevent violence and injuries globally[21]

This framework has been applied to motor vehicle safety, which has been identified as 1 of the 10 great public health achievements in the 20th century. That trend has continued though the first decade of the 2000s. From 2001 to 2010, the number of vehicle miles traveled in the United States increased by 8.5%; however, the death rate for motor vehicle travel declined from 14.9 per 100,000 population to 11.0, while the injury rate declined from 1,130 to 722 per 100,000 population.[22]

The CDC Injury Center uses comprehensive data systems to track the burden of motor vehicle crashes, studying patterns to understand the problem and identify research, intervention, and policy priorities. This has led to the development of educational tools and resources to raise awareness of the effectiveness of seat belts, supporting efforts to reduce drinking and driving, supporting surveillance and evaluation activities to increase motorcycle helmet use, encouraging state adoption of graduated driver's licensing programs, and collaborating with the United Nations and World Health Organization to improve road safety across the globe.[23]

We have now taken a look at approaches being used to address the issues of environmental disease and injuries. The problems of environmental health and safety require increasingly sophisticated solutions. Lessons learned from these efforts have potential applications to other aspects of public health and health care.

We have now looked at noncommunicable diseases, communicable diseases, and environmental health and safety as ways of organizing the major causes of disability and death. Now, let us turn our attention to the organized systems that have been developed for addressing these problems.

KEY WORDS

- Unaltered environment
- Altered environment
- Built environment
- Risk assessment
- Public health assessment
- Ecological assessment
- Interaction analysis
- Hazards
- Hazard identification
- Dose-response relationship
- Exposure assessment
- Risk characterization
- Interaction analysis
- Multiplicative interaction
- Intentional injuries
- Unintentional injuries
- All-hazards approach

Discussion Questions

Take a look at the questions posed in the following scenarios, which were presented at the beginning of this chapter. See now whether you can answer them.

1. Joe grew up in an industrial district of town. His family lived in an old apartment building, and he played in a playground near a major intersection. By the age of 6, Joe was found to have high lead levels in his blood and was not doing well in school. *Where could all that lead come from?* his mother wondered.

2. Jill is pregnant and loves fish, which she has eaten almost daily for years as part of her effort to stay healthy. She hears that fish should not be eaten regularly during pregnancy. *Why*, she wonders, *should I cut down on eating something as healthy as fish?*

3. Ralph and Sonya, a prosperous professional couple, and their two children live in an older suburban home. They feel secure that their environment is safe. They were surprised to find when they wanted to put their house up for sale that it did not pass the safety tests for radon. *Where did the radon come from*, they wondered, *and what can be done about it?*

4. Sandra worked for an international agency that had successfully addressed the danger of radiation due to the hole in the ozone layer. She was shocked when she was told that she had a life-threatening skin cancer called melanoma. She asked: *What could cause melanoma? Could years of sun exposure have played a role?*

5. You set out on your commute to work, and as you approach the subway station, you see police cars, ambulances, and dozens of emergency responders in hazmat suits. You are told the entire subway system will be shut down indefinitely, as there has been a suspected case of bioterrorism. You wondered how authorities were alerted to this situation and what precautions are being taken to protect the health of those living in the city?

6. Alex suffered a traumatic brain injury when he was thrown from his motorcycle after colliding with a car in which the driver had an elevated blood alcohol concentration. Alex was not wearing a helmet. His family members wonder what is being done to prevent this from happening to others.

REFERENCES

1. Science Daily. Global warming and your health. http://www.science daily.com/releases/2006/10/061023192524.htm. Accessed July 23, 2013.

2. Prevention Institute. The built environment and health. http://www .preventioninstitute.org/builtenv.html. Accessed July 23, 2013.

3. Mokdad AM, Marks JS, Stroup DF, Gerberding JL. Actual causes of death in the United States 2000. *JAMA*. 2004;291:1238–1245.

4. Centers for Disease Control and Prevention. Injury prevention and control.http://www.cdc.gov/injury/wisqars/LeadingCauses.html. Accessed July 23, 2013.

5. United States Environmental Protection Agency. Particulate matter. http://www.epa.gov/airquality/particlepollution/index.html. Accessed July 23, 2013.

6. Friis RH. *Essentials of Environmental Health*. 2nd ed. Sudbury, MA: Jones and Bartlett Publishers; 2012.

7. Oncology Encyclopedia. Occupational exposures and cancer. http://www.answers.com/topic/occupational-exposures-and-cancer. Accessed July 23, 2013.

8. Centers for Disease Control and Prevention. National center for environmental health. http://www.cdc.gov/nceh/ehhe/about.htm. Accessed July 23, 2013.

9. Greenberg MR. *Environmental Policy Analysis and Practice*. Piscataway, NJ: Rutgers University Press; 2008.

10. Rom WN, Markowitz SB. *Environmental and Occupational Medicine*. Philadelphia: Lippincott, Williams & Wilkins; 2006.

11. United States Environmental Protection Agency. Human health risk assessment. http://www.epa.gov/risk_assessment/health-risk.htm. Accessed August 10, 2013.

12. Agency for Toxic Substance and Disease Registry. ToxFAQs™ for lead. http://www.atsdr.cdc.gov/toxfaqs/tf.asp?id=93&tid=22. Accessed July 23, 2013.

13. Agency for Toxic Substance and Disease Registry. Case studies in environmental medicine—lead. http://wonder.cdc.gov/wonder/prevguid /p0000017/p0000017.asp. Accessed July 23, 2013..

14. National Defense Resource Council. The story of *Silent Spring*. http://www.nrdc.org/health/pesticides/hcarson.asp. Accessed July 23, 2013.

15. United States Environmental Protection Agency. Mercury: health effects. http://www.epa.gov/hg/effects.htm. Accessed July 23, 2013.

16. March of Dimes. Pregnancy and newborn health education center. http://www.marchofdimes.com. Accessed July 23, 2013.

17. National Aeronautics and Space Administration. Ozone hole watch. http://ozonewatch.gsfc.nasa.gov/facts/hole.html#nav_bypass. Accessed July 23, 2013.

18. United States Environmental Protection Agency. Radon. http://www .epa.gov/radon. Accessed July 23, 2013.

19. United States Federal Emergency Management Administration. National incident management system. http://www.fema.gov/emergency /nims. Accessed July 23, 2013.

20. Hugh JM, Gerberding JL. Anthrax bioterrorism: lessons learned and future directions. http://www.cdc.gov/ncidod/EID/vol8no10/02-0466.htm. Accessed July 23, 2013.

21. Centers for Disease Control and Prevention. Injury prevention and control. http://www.cdc.gov/injury/overview/index.html. Accessed July 23, 2013.

22. Centers for Disease Control and Prevention. Ten great public health achievements—United States, 2001–2010. http://www.cdc.gov/mmwr /preview/mmwrhtml/mm6019a5.htm. Accessed July 23, 2013.

23. Centers for Disease Control and Prevention. Injury control and prevention. http://www.cdc.gov/injury/about/focus-mvs.html. Accessed July 23, 2013.

SECTION III

Cases and Discussion Questions

HIGH BLOOD PRESSURE: A PUBLIC HEALTH AND HEALTHCARE SUCCESS

Elevated levels of blood pressure, or hypertension, have been observed since the development of blood pressure measurements in the 1800s. It was soon recognized that populations with a high frequency of elevated blood pressure were also populations with a high frequency of strokes, yet the dangers of high blood pressure often went unappreciated until recent years.

High blood pressure is a condition that historically has affected both the privileged and the underprivileged in our society. Presidents Woodrow Wilson and Franklin Delano Roosevelt both had high blood pressure and suffered strokes and heart disease. Today, the condition is disproportionately present among African Americans—15 to 20% have some degree of elevated blood pressure.

For many years, high blood pressure was considered a consequence of disease rather than its cause. Clinicians seeing a patient with a stroke, for instance, often attributed their elevation in blood pressure to the stroke rather than the other way around. Long-term studies, such as the Framingham Heart Study, which followed a large number of individuals for many years, established that the high blood pressure actually preceded strokes and not the other way around. High blood pressure as a contributory cause of strokes, as well as heart and kidney disease, was fully confirmed only after randomized controlled trials in the late 1960s and early 1970s established that lower blood pressure leads to reduced frequency of these diseases. Screening for high blood pressure became widespread in the same period in large part as a result of these investigations.

Elevated levels were initially defined as 140/100 or greater, based upon a range of normal obtained by measuring the blood pressure on large numbers of adult Americans. What were once considered acceptable levels of blood pressure have been redefined as elevated levels in recent years. Today, the desirable level is considered 120/80 or lower. These changing levels are justified by follow-up data from a large number of individuals that demonstrates that even levels of blood pressure only slightly above 120/80 are associated with increased risk of stroke and heart disease.

The fluctuating levels of blood pressure often make it difficult to establish an individual's average level. Electronic monitoring of blood pressure over a 24-hour period has become a feasible and acceptable gold standard for establishing an individual's average level. Early detection and successful treatments have been shown to effectively reduce the consequences of high blood pressure. Weight loss and salt restriction are often prescribed initially, with subsequent introduction of one or more drugs. Most, if not all, individuals with elevated blood pressure respond to drug treatment with tolerable or no side effects, but need to continue treatment for many years—usually for the rest of their lives.

A national public health campaign began in the 1970s to encourage individuals to know their blood pressure and to urge clinicians to treat detected elevated levels. In recent decades, national surveys have indicated that a gradually increasing percentage of patients with elevated blood pressures are being successfully treated and that there has been a substantial reduction in strokes and deaths from strokes. Recent evidence showing that reducing the high salt levels in the U.S. diet can reduce the average level of blood pressure has prompted renewed public health efforts to change eating habits and the contents of commercial foods.

Today, treatment of high blood pressure is recognized as one of the most cost-effective interventions. Its cost per quality adjusted life-year (QALY) saved is only a few thousand dollars a year for the average person. For high-risk groups, such as those with diabetes, it actually saves money to monitor and treat high blood pressure rather than allow it to cause or exacerbate other health problems requiring more expensive treatments.

Discussion Questions

1. How does this history of high blood pressure demonstrate the problem description and etiology components of the P.E.R.I.E. process? What different types of studies were used to establish etiology or contributory cause?

2. How does this history of high blood pressure illustrate the evidence-based recommendations and implementation and evaluation components of the P.E.R.I.E. process?

3. Explain the justification for updating the definition of what is considered a "healthy" blood pressure level.

4. How does this history of high blood pressure demonstrate the application of the four criteria for a successful screening program? Explain.

5. Using the four quadrants of cost and effectiveness, how would you classify treatment of hypertension for the average person? For those with diabetes? Explain.

TESTING AND SCREENING

Ken had just turned 40, and with a little encouragement from his wife, he decided that it was time to have a physical—it would be his first real visit to a doctor since he broke his arm as a kid. Seeing a doctor had not made sense to him before. He was in great shape, felt fine, and did not smoke. Maybe it was his 65-year-old father's sudden death from a heart attack just a few weeks after his retirement that finally convinced Ken to find himself a doctor. He knew that his father had had high cholesterol, but he was told his own cholesterol level and electrocardiogram results were okay when he entered the military at age 18. Besides, Ken was not big on desserts and only ate a Big Mac when he took the kids out after their soccer games.

The examination was quite uneventful and Ken was reassured when the doctor could not find anything of concern. A few recommendations on nutrition and better ways to exercise were about all that came out of the visit. Then he got the call from the doctor's office—could he make a follow-up appointment to discuss his cholesterol?

His low-density lipoprotein (LDL, or "bad" cholesterol) was 165 and his high-density lipoprotein (HDL, or "good" cholesterol) was 40.

"We used to think these levels were okay because they are so common," his doctor began. "However, now we consider your LDL cholesterol too high because it increases your chances of developing heart and other blood vessel diseases. There is no evidence of heart disease at this point, but your cholesterol needs attention."

"What do you mean by 'attention'?" Ken replied. "I exercise, do not smoke, and generally keep my fats down."

Ken soon learned a lot more about cholesterol. He first tried his best at changing his diet—it helped a little, but just did not do the trick.

Ken's doctor told him: "For some people, there is a strong genetic component to high cholesterol levels, and while diet is still important, it just cannot always reduce LDL cholesterol enough by itself. Exercise helps, especially by increasing the good cholesterol, but it does not do much for the bad cholesterol. Medication may be needed and there is now evidence that if taken regularly, it reduces the chances of having a heart attack or at least delays its occurrence."

Taking medication every day was not so easy for Ken, but he stuck with the plan. His doctor asked him to have his cholesterol levels checked every few months for the first year. Ken was amazed at how well the medicine worked. His LDL fell from 165 to less than 100 on only a modest dose. In addition to routine cholesterol checks, Ken had his blood tested for potential side effects from the medication, such as impacts to his liver, and he was told to report any long-lasting muscle aches and pains. The good news was that he could not tell he was taking the medication—he felt just fine.

Now that the cholesterol levels had dropped, he thought maybe he could go off the medication if he just watched his diet closely. His doctor let him try that for a month, but after the 30 days were up, his LDL level was back up to 160.

"Looks like you are hooked on medication for life," his doctor said with a wry smile, adding, "At least the extra cost is worth the extra benefit."

Ken and his wife were told the high cholesterol levels were a genetic condition. Not only did Ken need to take the medication on a permanent basis, but the pediatricians began testing his kids.

The doctors said, "We are beginning to understand the genetics behind this condition and would like to do some genetic testing on the children, including that new baby of yours."

Ken wondered if the information on his children's cholesterol levels would be part of their medical records for the rest of their lives. "You are not planning to put that on the Internet, are you?" Ken joked nervously as they drew blood from his newborn son.

Discussion Questions

1. How are the range of normal and desirable-range approaches to establishing a reference interval and defining a positive and negative test illustrated in this case? Explain.

2. What arguments are presented in this case that fulfill the criteria for screening for high LDL cholesterol? Explain.

3. What definition of cost-effectiveness is being used to justify screening and treatment of elevated LDL cholesterol?

4. What ethical issues need to be considered in screening for conditions such as elevated LDL cholesterol? Explain.

H. PYLORI AND PEPTIC ULCERS

Duodenal ulcers and benign stomach ulcers are frequently referred to as peptic ulcers. Peptic ulcers are among the digestive diseases with the highest incidence. Approximately 10% of the population experience a peptic ulcer at some point in their life, though a substantial proportion, perhaps a majority, are not medically diagnosed. Peptic ulcers generally heal even without prescribed treatment in 4 to 6 weeks. Approximately 1% of those with peptic ulcers experience complications, with potentially life-threatening perforation of the stomach or duodenum being the more serious complications. The disease often recurs, with a probability of recurrence in the range of 50%.

For many years, peptic ulcers were believed to be exclusively the result of excess acid production due to such factors as alcohol, aspirin and other anti-inflammatory medications, spicy foods, and stress. The stomach and duodenum were known to be highly acidic, and it was believed that bacteria were unable to survive in this high-acid environment.

In the early 1980s, investigators observed a spiral-shaped bacterium, which they named Helicobacter pylori, or *H. pylori*, in a number of pathological specimens from patients with disease of the stomach and duodenum. Most scientists doubted the relationship to disease, often concluding that the organism must be a contaminant because of the belief that bacteria could not grow in highly acidic environments.

After many unsuccessful attempts, Australian researchers Barry J. Marshall, MD, and J. Robin Warren, MD, were able to culture the bacteria from the stomach and became convinced that the bacteria were actually the cause of peptic ulcers. They were frustrated in their attempts to demonstrate that *H. pylori* was the cause of the disease because of the absence of good animal models. To attempt to establish causation, Marshall drank a flask of the cultured bacteria. He became ill and developed acute ulceration of the stomach. *H. pylori* was cultured from his ulcerations. This dramatic effort brought attention and extensive investigations to address whether *H. pylori* is a contributory cause of duodenal ulcers.

Subsequent studies in the United States and other countries established that *H. pylori* is a frequently occurring organism that increases with increasing age. Overall, over 20% of people in the United States have *H. pylori*, that is its prevalence is over 20% in the United States, with a higher prevalence beginning at an early age in many developing countries, as well as Japan. In case-control studies, *H. pylori* was found to have a strong association with duodenal ulcer, with over 70% of peptic ulcer patients having *H. pylori* at the time of their diagnosis.

Randomized controlled trials examined the recurrence rates of duodenal ulcers after treatment of the bacteria with antibiotics shown to eliminate *H. pylori*. In one study among those randomized to placebo, the recurrence rate was over 10 times as great as among those randomized to antibiotic treatment directed against *H. pylori*. This research led to a search for biological mechanisms. Extensive research established a greater understanding of the physiology of peptic ulcers, including identifying the production of an enzyme by *H. pylori* that reduces acidity and thus facilitates its growth in an acid environment.

New tests demonstrated that *H. pylori* is associated with the great majority of duodenal ulcers among outpatients. Randomized controlled trials and extensive clinical follow-up established the effectiveness and relative safety of antibiotic treatments of *H. pylori*. These investigations led to evidence-based recommendations for routine testing for *H. pylori* among outpatients diagnosed with peptic ulcers and treatment of *H. pylori* with antibiotics when it was detected.

Discussion Questions

1. Describe the negative and positive roles that biological plausibility played in establishing causation.

2. Discuss what would be required to demonstrate that *H. pylori* is a cause of duodenal ulcers and stomach ulcers using Koch's modern postulates. Were these postulates established for *H. pylori*?

3. Discuss how the evidence linking *H. pylori* and peptic ulcers using randomized controlled trials fulfill the contributory cause criteria of association, prior association, and how altering the "cause" alters the "effect."

4. What grade (A, B, C, D, I) would you give the recommendation to treat *H. pylori* among those diagnosed with peptic ulcers and having a positive test for *H. pylori*? Explain based on the strength of the evidence and the magnitude of the impact.

WHAT TO DO ABOUT LYME DISEASE?

You have just moved into a new subdivision—your first home with your young family. The first week you are there, a neighbor tells you that her son has developed Lyme disease and now has chronic arthritis that requires extensive treatment.

Lyme disease is an increasingly common disease that can cause acute and chronic arthritis if not treated early and correctly. In rare instances, it can cause life-threatening heart disease and temporary paralysis often to one side of the face due to nerve damage. The disease is caused by an organism known as a spirochete, which is spread from deer ticks to humans via tick bites. Lyme disease is especially common in communities with large deer populations, which today includes much of the suburban United States as well as rural areas.

Ticks must remain in place on the human skin at least 12 to 24 hours in order to extract human blood and inject the spirochete organism at the site of the bite. Complete removal of the small but visible tick within 24 hours usually prevents the disease. Deer ticks are most abundant in the late spring and tend to live on tall grasses from which they can easily move to the bare legs of children and adults. The disease frequently first appears as a circular red rash around the site of the bite. At this stage, early diagnosis and treatment with antibiotics is usually successful. Several weeks or months later, the onset of arthritis may occur and can be difficult to diagnose. A missed diagnosis may result in severe arthritis that is difficult to treat. A vaccine has been developed and briefly marketed to prevent the disease, but it was quite expensive and only partially successful.

In your new hometown, the local health department is charged with developing a plan for control or elimination of Lyme disease. As an informed and concerned citizen, you are invited to give input on the plan, identifying possible interventions.

Discussion Questions

1. What primary interventions would you consider? Explain.

2. What secondary interventions would you consider? Explain.

3. What tertiary interventions would you consider? Explain.

4. What educational interventions do you recommend? Explain.

5. Can Lyme disease be eradicated? Can it be controlled? Explain.

SHARMA'S VILLAGE

Sharma lives in a small farming village in south Asia, but she could just as well be living in Haiti, Ethiopia, Ghana, or several dozen other countries classified by the World Bank as low-income economies. Her home is a small hut, and she works daily with her mother to gather firewood for their small indoor fireplace, which acts as the kitchen stove. The smoke often makes her eyes water because there is no chimney or other ventilation. At night, she sleeps with her extended family in a room where mosquitoes bite her regularly. Despite the fact that Sharma lives in a rural community, the villagers live in crowded quarters. The water the family drinks is carried by the women from a well several hundred yards from their home. The water sometimes tastes bad, but it is all they have to drink.

The family farms a small plot of land on the hillside, which had become eroded from years of cutting trees. The last big monsoon to hit the area created a landslide, which left the village underwater for several weeks, creating mold in nearly every home. Most of the adults have goiters from the lack of iodine in the soil. The addition of iodine to salt has prevented goiters in the children. Pesticides are used widely to control mosquitoes and agricultural pests, but the farmers

receive little education on their safe use. Recently, a new road was built, connecting her village with the neighboring towns. Despite the advantages of having the new road, cars and trucks now speed through her village, rarely stopping to let people cross the road.

In Sharma's village, the life expectancy is 49 years. Babies often die of diarrheal diseases in the first year of life and mothers occasionally die in childbirth. Malaria is widespread and hookworm disease is present among those who farm the fields and in children, whose ability to learn is often affected. Malnutrition is also widespread despite the fact that farming is the major occupation in the village. Chronic lung disease among adults and asthma among the young is surprisingly common, even though cigarette smoking is rare. Tuberculosis is widespread and a major cause of death, despite the fact that until recently, there have been few cases of HIV/AIDS in the area. Unexplained neurological diseases among farm workers occur regularly. The most common cause of death among teenagers is motor vehicle injuries along the new road, even though there is only one truck in the village.

Discussion Questions

1. What environmental risk factors contributing to disease and other health conditions are illustrated in this case? Classify each as an unaltered, altered, or built environment factor.

2. Discuss at least two examples of how disease or other conditions found in the village can be explained by the environmental risk factors.

3. Identify at least two interventions that would make a large difference in the health of this village.

4. What changes do you expect to occur in this village as social and economic development take place?

LEGAL DRUGS THAT KILL—DEATH FROM PRESCRIPTION DRUG OVERDOSES

Katie found herself flat on her back in pain after falling off her bicycle as she swerved to avoid a collision with a car. She was taken to the emergency department, where she was examined, X-rayed, and given a five-day supply of a prescription pain-killer along with a note saying, "Make an appointment to see your doctor as soon as possible."

Though no one asked, Katie had a history of regular alcohol use and occasional binge drinking on weekends. Her father died of liver disease after many years of heavy drinking. Katie stayed away from most illegal drugs, though she tried marijuana a few times.

Katie had trouble filling her prescription after she left the emergency room late at night. Her nearest 24-hour pharmacy told her they do not carry narcotic pain medicine because they are a target for robberies. When she finally was able to fill her prescription, the pain was so bad that she took double the prescribed dose of medicine. She was running low before she could get an appointment with her doctor, but she found that if she took it with alcohol, it did the trick.

Her doctor agreed that her injuries were bad enough to require additional narcotic pain medications, which he prescribed for a month followed by a couple of refills. Katie quickly filled the prescription. On her way out of the pharmacy, she was stopped by a young man who offered to buy her medication for twice what she had paid. Katie turned the other way and rushed home to take her medication.

Katie could hardly get out of bed, the pain was so bad. After a few pills and a little alcohol, she was able to get going. Getting her work done was an ordeal and she mostly looked forward to the weekends. Partying took on a new meaning now, as it was an escape from constant pain.

One Saturday night, several months after her injury, Katie's friends planned a party to celebrate her 30th birthday. Katie tried her best to get herself together to go to the party despite the pain. She thought a little extra medication and a few drinks were what she needed. She soon felt so tired that before getting ready for the party, she decided to lie down for a little nap. She never heard the knock on the door by her friends, who wanted to know why she did not show up at the party. By the time they had called the rescue squad and the responders had broken in the door, she was found lying in her bed without a heartbeat, a victim of an unintentional prescription overdose.

Katie's friends were astonished to hear that unintentional prescription overdoses now rival motor vehicle injuries, suicides, and firearms as causes of death among young people, far exceeding deaths from illegal drugs. Traditionally a cause of death among young males, deaths from unintentional drug overdoses are rapidly increasing among females. Drug overdoses often occur from a combination of prescription narcotic pain medicine with alcohol, which together form a common and deadly combination that is widely available.

Discussion Questions

1. What underlying factors led to Katie's death?

2. What educational interventions would you recommend to prevent unintentional overdoses? Explain.

3. What motivational interventions directed toward prescribers or patients would you recommend to prevent unintentional overdoses? Explain.

4. What obligation or legal interventions would you recommend to prevent unintentional overdoses? Explain.

5. What changes in the rates of unintentional overdoses in the United States do you expect in the absence of the types of interventions that you identified in questions two, three, and four? Explain.

© Leah-Anne Thompson/ShutterStock, Inc.

SECTION IV

Health Professionals, Healthcare Institutions, and Healthcare Systems

In this section, we will take a look at healthcare systems, the people, institutions, and organizational structures that deliver health care to individuals. In the United States, the healthcare system consumes approximately $3 trillion in resources.

To understand how the U.S. healthcare system functions and is organized, we will start in Chapter 9 by taking a look at the people who provide health services. There are over 15 million people involved in the delivery of health services. We will focus on three of the largest groups: physicians, nurses, and public health professionals.

In Chapter 10, we will discuss the institutions involved in the delivery of healthcare services and how they interact or do not interact with each other. We will also examine methods for maximizing the quality of health care.

Finally, in Chapter 11, we will examine the health insurance system and the healthcare system as a whole. In this chapter, we will aim to understand how the U.S. system is financed and look at the issues of access to care, quality of care, and the costs of that care. As we do this, we will examine the ongoing impact of the Affordable Care Act (ACA). To provide perspective, we will also examine the characteristics of some other healthcare systems in developed countries.

Figure S04-1 displays the components of a healthcare system that will guide our discussion of this complex subject.

Let us begin in Chapter 9 by turning our attention to the types of clinical and public health professionals who are part of the health workforce.

FIGURE S04-1 An Approach to Examining Healthcare Systems

CHAPTER **9**

Health Professionals and the Health Workforce

LEARNING OBJECTIVES

By the end of this chapter, the student will be able to:

- describe roles that education and credentialing play in the development of health professions, such as medicine and nursing.
- describe the continuum of public health education and identify educational pathways for becoming a public health professional.
- identify recent changes in the education of physicians.
- describe the educational options in nursing.
- identify components of prevention and public health that are recommended for inclusion in clinical education.
- explain the concept of primary care and differentiate it from secondary and tertiary care.
- identify a range of mechanisms used to compensate clinical health professionals and explain their advantages and disadvantages.

Upon your arrival at the hospital, the nurse specialist examines you and consults with the radiologists, the gastroenterologist, and the general surgeon. Your medication is reviewed by the pharmacist and your meals by the clinical nutritionist. Throughout the hospitalization, you are followed by a hospitalist. Once you get back home, the home care team comes to see you regularly for the first two weeks, and the certified physician assistant and the doctor of nursing practice (DNP) see you in the office. You realize that health care is no longer just about doctors and nurses. You ask yourself: What roles do all of these health professionals play in the healthcare system?

Jenna decides that after college, she wants to become a doctor and practice medicine. "I thought there was only one kind of doctor who could diagnose disease and prescribe medicine," she mentions at a career counseling meeting. "Not so, anymore," says her advisor. "There are allopathic and osteopathic physicians. In addition, there are nurse practitioners who are authorized to diagnose and prescribe medications, and there are physician assistants who do the same under a physician's supervision. The universe of 'doctors' now includes doctors of nursing practice, as well as other doctoral degree professionals, such as pharmacists, occupational therapists, and physical therapists." Understanding careers in health care can be as difficult for students as it is for patients, Jenna thinks to herself. Now she understands why her advisor asked: "What do you mean by 'practice'? What do you mean by 'doctor'?"

Sarah was about to begin medical school and was expecting two years of "preclinical" classroom lectures focusing on the basic sciences, followed by the study of clinical diseases. Then, as she had heard from her physician father, she expected two years of clinical hospital "rotations" and electives investigating specialties. She is surprised to find that medical school has changed. There are small-group, problem-based learning sessions where she needs to be able to locate and read the research literature. There is contact with patients and their problems right from the beginning. There is increasingly a four-year approach instead of a preclinical and clinical approach to medical education. She wonders: Are these changes for the better? What else needs to be done to improve medical education?

You are interested in clinical care, as well as public health. I need to make a choice, you think to yourself. "Not necessarily," your advisor says. "There are many ways to combine clinical care with public health." After a little investigation, you find out that undergraduate public health education is increasingly seen as preparation for clinical education, and clinical prevention and population health are increasingly becoming part of clinical care. In addition, many careers, from health administration, to health policy, to health education, to clinical research, combine the individual orientation of clinical care with the population perspective of public health. So what is the best pathway to a public health career for you?

WHAT DO WE MEAN BY A "HEALTH PROFESSIONAL"?

Until the early years of the 1900s, education and practice for the health professions in the United States were an informal process, often without standardized admissions requirements, curricula, or even formal recognition of a profession. Throughout the 1900s and into the 2000s, there has been an ongoing movement to formalize and standardize the education process for health professionals. These formal requirements have come to define what we mean by a "health professional" and include admission prerequisites, coursework requirements, examinations of competency, official recognition of educational achievements, and granting of permission to practice. Today, the list of formal health professions is very long. Clinical health professions include physicians, nurses, dentists, pharmacists, optometrists, psychologists, podiatrists, and chiropractors. They also include nurse practitioners, physician assistants, health services administrators, and allied health practitioners.[1] "Allied health practitioner" is a broad category in its own right, ranging from graduate degree–trained professionals, such as physical therapists, occupational therapists, and medical social workers, to technical specialists often with an associate's degree, such as dental assistants, sonographers, and laboratory technicians.

Education and training are central to the development and definition of most health professions. Education implies that a student is pursuing a degree or certificate from an accredited educational institution. Training is often organized and directed outside of educational institutions. Hospitals, health departments, and large group practices often have the responsibility of training new health professionals.

Before we take a look at specific health professions, let us step back and ask the more general question: How do education and training serve to define health professions?

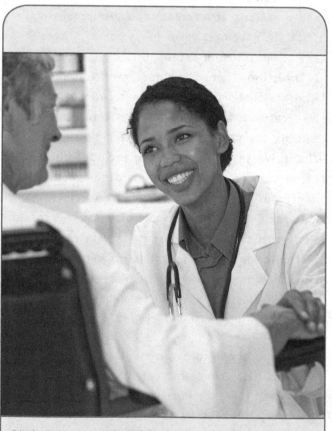

© Monkey Business Images/ShutterStock, Inc.

HOW DO EDUCATION AND TRAINING SERVE TO DEFINE HEALTH PROFESSIONS?

Defining and enforcing educational requirements is central to creating and maintaining a profession. This can be accomplished using two basic approaches: **accreditation** and **credentialing**.

Accreditation implies a process of setting standards for educational and training institutions and enforcing these standards using a regularly scheduled institutional self-study and an outside review. Accreditation is used by most health professions to define and enforce educational expectations. At times, these expectations may be laid out in detail down to the level of square footage per student for laboratory space and the number of hours devoted to specific subjects. In other health professions, educational subject areas may be outlined and institutions left to judge how to best implement the curriculum.

Credentialing implies that the individual, rather than the institution, is evaluated. "Credentialing" is a generic term indicating a process of verifying that an individual has the desirable or required qualifications to practice a profession. Credentialing often takes the form of **certification**. Certification is generally a profession-led process in which applicants who have completed the required educational process take an examination. Successful completion of formal examinations leads to recognition in the form of certification.

Certification also has come to define specialties and even subspecialties within a profession. Successful completion of a specialty or subspecialty examination may entitle a health professional to call him- or herself "board-certified." Certification is often a prerequisite for **licensure**, which is a state governmental function and usually requires more than certification. It may include residency requirements, a legal background check, continuing education requirements, etc. Licensure, when applicable, is usually required for practice of a health profession.

Thus, in order to understand what is meant by a particular health profession, it is important to understand the credentials that are expected or required. Let us take a look at the education required for public health, as well as for physicians and nurses.

WHAT ARE THE EDUCATIONAL OPTIONS WITHIN PUBLIC HEALTH?

Within public health, there is a growing array of health specialties. Some specialties require bachelor's degrees, such as environmental health specialists and health educators. However, many public health roles require graduate degrees that focus on disciplines including epidemiology, biostatistics, environmental sciences, health administration and policy, and social and behavioral sciences. **Box 9-1** discusses the development of what is being called the continuum of public health education.

BOX 9-1 Development of the Continuum of Public Health Education[2]

The history of public health education as a formal academic activity in the United States dates back approximately 100 years to the 1915 Welch-Rose Report. Funded by the Rockefeller Foundation, this report set the stage for development of separate schools of public health focused on graduate education designed for those with previous professional education, particularly as physicians, nurses, and engineers.

The focus on graduate-level education of those with previous professional education remained the norm for half a century after the publication of the Welch-Rose Report. This began to change in the 1970s and 1980s with the growth of schools of public health as well as programs in public health, often located in medical schools. By the 1980s, a substantial portion of the students entering graduate training in public health had a bachelor's degree but no prior professional training.

In addition, graduate training in public health increasingly became specialized, with master of public health (MPH) degrees often focusing not only on a generalist core but also on a specialty area, such as epidemiology, biostatistics, environmental health, health administration, health policy, health education, health communications, etc. This was accompanied by the growth of doctoral programs, including both PhDs and doctor of public health (DrPH) degrees.

Undergraduate public health education began as specialty areas, such as health education, environmental health, and health services administration, during the last half of the 1900s. For instance, health education developed its own

(continues)

BOX 9-1   Development of the Continuum of Public Health Education[2] (*continued*)

undergraduate degree programs, competencies, and certifying examination, the certified health education specialist (CHES).

A major change in public health education began in 2003 with the Institute of Medicine's recommendation that "all undergraduates should have access to education in public health."[3] This recommendation launched what came to be known as the Educated Citizen and Public Health movement, a collaborative effort of undergraduate education associations and public health education associations. The Educated Citizen and Public Health movement led to a series of recommendations, including the Critical Component Elements of an Undergraduate Major in Public Health. These recommendations are now being used by the Council on Education for Public Health (CEPH) as part of the accreditation process for undergraduate majors in public health, including those providing generalist education and specialty education, as well as those in institutions with and without graduate public health education.

As the 100th anniversary of the Welch-Rose Report neared, public health educators and practitioners joined with undergraduate educators and health profession leaders to form the Framing the Future Task Force: The Second Hundred Years of Education for Public Health. At the heart of the task force's deliberation was how to create a continuum of public health education. Key to the continuum was undergraduate public health education, including public health education as part of the curriculum of community colleges. The task force created the Community College and Public Health project, which is developing prototype curriculum models that encourage articulation of community college associate degrees and bachelor's degrees in both specialty areas as well as generalist degrees. In addition, community colleges are beginning to look at how to integrate public health into their own areas of strength and interest, including programs such as public health preparedness/disaster planning, health information systems, and health navigator/community health worker.

Thus, today, formal public health education includes degree programs at community colleges and four-year colleges as well as at the master's and doctoral level. The process of articulating these degrees and ensuring the development of career ladders is well underway. The continuum of public health education has been established as a goal and is rapidly becoming a reality.

In addition to the educational options that lead to becoming a public health professional, a large and growing number of options are available to combine public health education with other professions. Combined or joint degrees with medicine, nursing, and physician assistants are widely offered. Combinations with law, social work, international affairs, and a range of other fields are also being offered. Combined or joint degrees often allow students to reduce the total number of credit hours required to satisfy the requirement for the two degrees.

Public health professionals today include those who specialize in a wide range of disciplines and work in a variety of settings, from governmental public health to not-for-profit and for-profit institutions, as well as in educational and healthcare institutions. There are approximately 500,000 public health professionals in the United States, and it is estimated that in coming years, there will be a substantial shortage.[4]

Public health is one of the last health fields to formalize educational and professional requirements. Today, many public health professionals are trained exclusively in public health, and the process of formal credentialing is underway. The recognition of public health as a distinct professional field with its own educational process has been formalized through accreditation of public health schools and programs by the Council on Education for Public Health (CEPH). CEPH requires five areas of knowledge basic to public health: biostatistics, epidemiology, environmental health sciences, social and behavioral sciences, and health services management. Specific disciplines within public health, such as epidemiology and social and behavioral sciences, have provided recognition for specialized training through advanced degrees, such as the academically oriented doctor of philosophy (PhD) degree and the practice-oriented doctor of public health (DrPH) degree.

Specific technical areas have existed within public health for many years and have included competency examinations, especially in fields such as occupational and environmental health. Health educators in recent decades have formalized and standardized their education and increasingly taken on the structure of a profession, including examinations, certifications, and continuing education requirements.

Formal certification as a public health specialist has only been available since 2008, when the first certifying examination was given. The examination covers the five areas expected for a professional master's degree, such as a master's of public health (MPH). These are biostatistics, epidemiology, environmental health sciences, social and behavioral sciences, and health policy and management. In addition, new cross-cutting competencies have been defined and are being incorporated into the examination. These include communications and informatics, diversity and culture, leadership, professionalism, program planning, systems thinking, and public health biology.

The certifying examination tests core competencies, rather than more specialized competencies that students also frequently achieve as part of an MPH degree. Certification is a voluntary process, though it is expected that many employers will look for certification as an important credential in the future.[5] Licensure of public health professionals is not yet an issue. Thus, public health, along with health care, has increasingly formalized its educational requirements, formal credentialing, and competencies. This process is likely to continue.

WHAT IS THE EDUCATION AND TRAINING PROCESS FOR PHYSICIANS?

Physicians are a central part of what is called the practice of medicine. They can be categorized as allopathic or osteopathic physicians. Allopathic physicians graduate with an MD degree, while osteopathic physicians graduate from osteopathic medical schools and receive a DO degree. Graduates of both allopathic and osteopathic medical schools are eligible to apply for the same residency and fellowship programs for their postgraduate medical education. The number of osteopathic medical schools has grown rapidly in recent years and now totals approximately 30 nationwide. Allopathic medical schools number approximately 130 and have only recently begun to again grow in size and number.[a]

Within medicine, specialties and subspecialties continue to emerge. For instance, hospice and palliative medicine has recently been added to the list of specialties, and others, such as hospitalists, may be moving in that direction. **Table 9-1** outlines many of the current specialties and subspecialties within the field of medicine.[6] **Box 9-2** discusses the process

---

[a] Osteopathic and allopathic medical education curricula are quite similar today. The prerequisites for admission are similar, and both types of medical schools generally require the Medical College Admission Test (MCAT). However, osteopathic medical education retains its focus on manipulation of the muscular skeletal system and sees itself as providing a holistic approach to medicine, including a greater focus on prevention. A substantially higher percentage of DOs go into primary care as compared to MDs.

TABLE 9-1 Selected Specialties and Subspecialties of Medicine

Example of specialty area	Example of subspecialty area
Anesthesiology	Critical care medicine Hospice and palliative medicine Pain medicine
Emergency medicine	Hospice and palliative medicine Medical toxicology Pediatric emergency medicine Sports medicine Undersea and hyperbaric medicine
Family medicine	Adolescent medicine Geriatric medicine Hospice and palliative medicine Sleep medicine Sports medicine
Internal medicine	Adolescent medicine Cardiovascular disease Clinical cardiac electrophysiology Critical care medicine Endocrinology, diabetes, and metabolism Gastroenterology Geriatric medicine Hematology Hospice and palliative medicine Infectious disease Interventional cardiology Medical oncology Nephrology Pulmonary disease Rheumatology Sleep medicine Sports medicine Transplant hepatology
Obstetrics and gynecology	Critical care medicine Gynecologic oncology Hospice and palliative medicine Maternal and fetal medicine Reproductive endocrinology/infertility
Orthopaedic surgery	Orthopaedic sports medicine Surgery of the hand
Otolaryngology	Neurotology Pediatric otolaryngology Plastic surgery within the head and neck Sleep medicine

(continues)

TABLE 9-1 Selected Specialties and Subspecialties of Medicine (*continued*)

Example of specialty area	Example of subspecialty area
PATHOLOGY Anatomic pathology and clinical pathology Pathology—anatomic Pathology—clinical	Blood banking/transfusion medicine Chemical pathology Cytopathology Dermatopathology Forensic pathology Hematology Medical microbiology Molecular genetic pathology Neuropathology Pediatric pathology
Pediatrics	Adolescent medicine Child abuse pediatrics Developmental-behavioral pediatrics Hospice and palliative medicine Medical toxicology Neonatal-perinatal medicine Neurodevelopmental disabilities Pediatric cardiology Pediatric critical care medicine Pediatric emergency medicine Pediatric endocrinology Pediatric gastroenterology Pediatric hematology-oncology Pediatric infectious diseases Pediatric nephrology Pediatric pulmonology Pediatric rheumatology Pediatric transplant hepatology Sleep medicine Sports medicine
Physical medicine and rehabilitation	Hospice and palliative medicine Neuromuscular medicine Pain medicine Pediatric rehabilitation medicine Spinal cord injury medicine Sports medicine
Plastic surgery	Plastic surgery within the head and neck Surgery of the hand

TABLE 9-1 Selected Specialties and Subspecialties of Medicine (*continued*)

Example of specialty area	Example of subspecialty area
PREVENTIVE MEDICINE Aerospace medicine Occupational medicine Public health and general preventive medicine	Medical toxicology Undersea and hyperbaric medicine
Psychiatry Neurology Neurology with special qualifications in child neurology	Addiction psychiatry Child and adolescent psychiatry Clinical neurophysiology Forensic psychiatry Geriatric psychiatry Hospice and palliative medicine Neurodevelopmental disabilities Neuromuscular medicine Pain medicine Psychosomatic medicine Sleep medicine Vascular neurology
RADIOLOGY Diagnostic radiology Radiation oncology Radiologic physics	Diagnostic radiological physics Hospice and palliative medicine Medical nuclear physics Neuroradiology Nuclear radiology Pediatric radiology Therapeutic radiological physics Vascular and interventional radiology
Surgery Vascular surgery	Hospice and palliative medicine Pediatric surgery Surgery of the hand Surgical critical care
Urology	Pediatric urology

Data from American Board of Medical Specialties. Available at: http://www.abms.org/. Accessed July 24, 2013.

BOX 9-2 Medical Education

Medical education in 19th and early 20th century America was built upon the apprentice system. Future physicians, nearly all men, worked under and learned from practicing physicians. Medical schools were often moneymaking enterprises and primarily used lectures without patient contact or laboratory experiences. That changed with the introduction of the European model of science-based medical education, hospital-based clinical rotations, and a four-year education model. The 1910 Flexner Report formalized these standards, which soon became universal for medical education in the United States, in what came to be called the Flexner era of U.S. medicine. This era extended into the 1980s, and at some institutions, into the 2000s. It led to the growth and dominance of specialties and specialists within particular medical fields.

Hospital-based residency programs and fellowships leading to specialty and subspecialty training became the dominant form of clinical training. Emphasizing this trend, medical school education came to be called **undergraduate medical education**. Medical school was traditionally formally or informally divided into two years of basic science or preclinical training, followed by two years of hospital-based clinical rotations in specialty areas including surgery, internal medicine, obstetrics and gynecology, and psychiatry. This division of medical education is reflected in the examinations of the National Board of Medical Examiners, which traditionally included part 1 after the second year of medical school, part 2 prior to graduation, and part 3 after the first-year residency, which is often called the "internship." Additional specialty and subspecialty board examinations were linked to completion of training that occurs after medical school.

Change began to accelerate in medical education during the mid-1980s with the increasing movement of health care outside of hospitals, the increased medical school enrollment of women and minorities, a broader view of what should be included in medical education, and a better understanding of how learning takes place. Specific changes have occurred in the last two decades at all stages of medical education, and new proposals for change continue to be formally reviewed and implemented. These can be outlined as follows, starting with the premed college years and continuing through residency and fellowship training:

- Premedical training in the Flexner era was largely restricted to majors in the physical and biological sciences, plus specific social sciences such as psychology. Beginning in the early 1990s, medical schools encouraged a wider range of majors, while usually retaining biology, chemistry, and physics courses as prerequisites. Medical schools are increasingly receptive to a wide range of preparation for medical education, encouraging completion of courses in behavioral and social sciences, including public health and epidemiology.

- The comprehensive review of the Medical College Admission Test (MCAT) has resulted in changes to the MCAT. The changes include a new section emphasizing the behavioral and social sciences to parallel the sections emphasizing the physical and biological sciences. A framework known as scientific inquiry and reasoning skills (SIRS) will incorporate basic research methods and statistics into each of the content examinations.

- Admission to medical school was dominated by white males throughout the Flexner era. In the last 20–30 years, the percentage of women applicants has increased steadily. Today, the majority of medical students at many institutions are females. Likewise, the increase in minority applicants has paralleled the changes occurring in other aspects of U.S. education and society.

- The first two years of medical school in the Flexner era were dominated by lectures and laboratories. Basic sciences were the focus, with little or no patient contact. An important change in the last two decades includes widespread use of problem-based learning (PBL). PBL is characterized by small-group, student-initiated learning centered on "cases," or patient-oriented problems. New curricula in medical education, including evidence-based medicine, interviewing skills, and ethics, have become a standard part of coursework. A new simulated patient interview and physical examination are now part of the certifying examination process.

- Changes in the third and fourth years of medical school began in the 1960s, the era of student activism. Since then, the fourth year of medical school has been dominated by electives. Fourth-year students may choose formal courses, elective clinical experiences, or a wide array of other options. These usually include options for laboratory or clinical research;

(continues)

BOX 9-2 Medical Education (*continued*)

international experiences; and clinical rotations at other institutions, often called "audition" rotations, designed to increase a graduate's potential for selection as a resident.

- The growing trend of patient treatment outside of the traditional hospital setting has increased the range of types and locations of clinical experiences available. Most medical schools now require primary care experiences, along with traditional specialty rotations.

- Residency training has paralleled the changes in medical school, with greater outpatient and less inpatient, or hospital-based, education. Fellowship training beyond residency is now a routine part of the process of specialization. The general move toward more and more specialization has led to longer postgraduate training. The rigors of residency training remain, but limits have now been placed on it by the Residency Review Committees (RRCs), which govern

graduate medical education. An average of 80 hours per week is now the maximum standard for residents.

Further changes in medical education and residency programs can be expected in the near future. The increasing recognition that health care is a group, and not an individual, enterprise is leading to a focus on interprofessional education and practice. An appreciation that evidence is central to improving quality and controlling costs should continue to encourage the critical reading of clinical research as part of evidence-based medicine in medical school and in journal clubs as part of postgraduate education. The use of computer-based information systems should increase the sharing and coordination of information, the ability to monitor and control health care, and the ways that physicians communicate with colleagues and patients. Technology is also likely to have continued unexpected impacts on the ways that medicine is taught, learned, and practiced.

of medical education and the changes that have occurred in recent years and continue to evolve.[7]

Now let us take a brief look at the largest of the health professions—nursing.[8]

WHAT IS THE EDUCATION AND TRAINING PROCESS FOR NURSING?

Nursing as a profession dates from the middle of the 1800s, when it began to be organized as a profession in England. Florence Nightingale is often associated with the founding of nursing as a profession. In the United States, the nursing profession grew out of the Civil War and the essential role played by women in this conflict, who performed what we would today call nursing functions. Nursing has long been organized as a distinct profession and is governed by its own set of laws, often referred to as the "nursing practice acts."

Today, there are a wide range of health professionals that fall under the legal definition of nursing. Licensed practical nurses (LPNs) provide a range of services often under the direction of registered nurses (RN). An LPN's educational requirements vary widely from state to state, ranging from one year of education after high school to a two-year associate's degree. Certified nursing assistants (CNAs) or nursing aides have usually completed a short-term certification program and are allowed to perform only the basic care of patients.

Registered nurses are considered central to the nursing profession and they are usually responsible for hospital-based services. Each state defines its own requirements for RN licensure. Traditionally, many nurses graduated with a diploma that was offered through hospital-based programs. The move toward integrating nursing into the formal degree system has resulted in nurses with associate's degrees, bachelor of science in nursing (BSN) degrees, as well as graduate degrees. Being a registered nurse requires a state license that, depending on the state, may or may not require a BSN degree.

Advanced nursing degrees have been offered as a master's of science in nursing, or as an academic research-based degree, the PhD. Recently, a clinical doctorate, the doctor in nursing practice (DNP) is becoming central to graduate nursing education. The DNP is increasingly becoming the standard graduate degree for nursing, often replacing master's degrees.

Until recent years, there was little formal specialization within nursing, at least compared to physicians and other health professions. Nurse midwives and nurse anesthetists, however, are two traditional specializations within nursing. Graduate-level education and training of nurses has expanded rapidly in recent years. Nursing has added a series of advanced practice degrees, including nurse practitioners, as well as specialists such as pediatric, geriatric, and intensive care nurses. The DNP degree is becoming standard for a range of specialty areas within nursing. Recent changes in nursing have opened up the option to pursue a bachelor's degree in a range of fields followed by a shorter degree program leading to a BSN or a nurse practitioner degree.

WHAT ROLES DO PHYSICIANS, NURSES, AND OTHER CLINICAL HEALTH PROFESSIONS PLAY IN PUBLIC HEALTH?

As we have seen, the aim of the initial schools of public health was to train physicians, nurses, and other professionals who sought to play lead roles in local and state health departments. Thus, for many years, public health education was often combined with other professions. **Box 9-3** discusses the roles that clinicians still play in public health.

Remember that we have only touched on three basic types of health professionals: physicians, nurses, and public health professionals. There are several hundred other types of professions in the healthcare realm. As you think about a career in health, you should take a look at a range of health professions, using the concepts of education, training, and certification that we have discussed.

To understand the connections between the large number of diverse health professions, we need to look at how clinical care is organized into primary, secondary, and tertiary care.

WHAT IS MEANT BY "PRIMARY, SECONDARY, AND TERTIARY CARE"?

Primary, secondary, and tertiary care are traditional ways to categorize services delivered within the healthcare system.[9] **Primary care** traditionally refers to the first contact providers

---

BOX 9-3 Roles of Clinicians in Public Health

Public health is often distinguished from the clinical health profession by its focus on populations rather than individuals, public service rather than individual service, and disease prevention and health promotion rather than disease diagnosis and treatment, and its broad perspective on the determinants of disease. However, at the professional level, individuals have commonly combined the two approaches or moved from one to the other.

Clinicians have always played key roles in public health. From the early years of formal public health training nearly a century ago, until the 1960s and 1970s, the master of public health (MPH) degree was aimed primarily at physicians and nurses who were expected to take up leadership roles in health departments. Today, public health professionals come from much more diverse backgrounds, many entering master's programs directly after receiving a bachelor's degree. The role of clinicians in public health is also far more varied. For instance, today's pharmacists—now educated as doctors of pharmacy or PharmDs—play an increasingly important public health role in providing education about drugs for patients and practitioners and controlling prescription drug abuse. Prevention of dental and gum disease and early detection of oral cancers have significantly improved due to the careful attention of dentists and dental assistants. The dental profession has been a long-standing advocate of fluoridation of public water systems and other population health interventions.

Primary care specialists, including allopathic and osteopathic physicians, nurse practitioners, and physician assistants, are on the front lines of clinical prevention. Their involvement in screening, behavioral counseling, immunization, and the use of preventive medication is key to the success of these efforts. Primary care clinicians, as well as specialty care clinicians, also have important roles to play in being alert to new diseases or changes in well-known diseases; reporting adverse effects of drugs, vaccines, and medical devices; and coordinating case-finding efforts with public health agencies.

Within medicine, the field of preventive medicine has a long history. Formal specializations exist in public health and general preventive medicine, occupational medicine, as well as aerospace medicine.

Finally, all clinicians have the right and often the responsibility to advocate for improvements in patient care and of the health system as a whole. A few clinical specialties, such as pediatrics, regard advocacy as a core responsibility of the profession. Their work has had major impacts on child health policies, ranging from the use of child car restraints, to advocacy for pediatric HIV/AIDS care, to universal coverage of childhood vaccinations, as well as the provision of comprehensive insurance coverage for children.

The roles of clinicians in public health are likely to become ever more varied in coming years as public health and healthcare systems and institutions become more closely coordinated.

of care who are prepared to handle the great majority of common problems for which patients seek care. **Secondary care** often refers to specialty care provided by clinicians who focus on one or a small number of organ systems or on a specific type of service, such as obstetrics and gynecology or anesthesiology. **Tertiary care**, or subspecialty care, is usually defined in terms of the type of institution in which it is delivered, often academic or specialized health centers. Tertiary care may also be defined in terms of the type of problem that is addressed, such as trauma centers, burn centers, or neonatal intensive care units.

Primary care is widely seen as the foundation of a healthcare system, and a strong primary care system is viewed as a prerequisite for maximizing the potential benefits of health care. Traditionally, primary care was considered the domain of physicians. Today, a range of health professionals are involved in primary, as well as secondary and tertiary, care. In fact, the term "**medical home**" is becoming widely used, suggesting that primary care is increasingly viewed as a team effort.

Today, only about one third of physicians in the United States practice primary care. Increasingly, primary care is being delivered by physician assistants (PAs) and nurse practitioners (NPs), who in most states have authority to diagnose disease and prescribe medication either under the supervision of a physician (in the case of PAs) or under a nursing practice act (as in the case of NPs). A team approach to primary care is becoming standard practice. The Affordable Care Act (ACA) has encouraged the use of nurse practitioners as part of primary care by providing greater ability for them to bill directly for services without going through a physician.

It is important to understand the ideals of primary care, as well as today's realities.[7] Primary care is key to the healthcare system because it is where most care is delivered and it is often the entry point for subsequent specialty care. In addition, primary care is critical to the delivery of clinical preventive services and to the connections between health care and public health. Ideal primary care has been described using 6 Cs: contact, comprehensive, coordinated, continuity, caring, and community.

- "Contact" implies first contact with patients as they present for health care.
- "Comprehensive" refers to the ability of primary care practitioners or primary care teams to completely or at least initially address most health issues.
- "Coordinated" relates to the concept that primary care teams should have the responsibility to ensure that the parts of the healthcare system work together for the good of patients.

- "Continuity" is the role that primary care teams see themselves playing to hold together the components of the system.
- "Caring" implies a personalized relationship with each patient.
- "Community" implies that primary care provides the link with the broader community, including with public health institutions and services.

Despite the fact that many primary care practitioners continue to see this model of primary care as a highly desirable way to deliver clinical care, the realities of today's healthcare system deviate substantially from this model. **Table 9-2** outlines the 6 Cs and indicates ways that the current healthcare system differs from this primary care ideal.[9, b]

Thus, there is a large gulf between the ideals of primary care and their execution in practice. Part of the reason for this and other realities of health care can be better understood by looking at how health professionals are rewarded and compensated.

HOW ARE CLINICAL HEALTH PROFESSIONALS REWARDED AND COMPENSATED FOR THEIR SERVICES?

Physicians—and, increasingly, other health professionals—are compensated through a variety of mechanisms. Compensation levels depend on the site where care is delivered, the nature of the patient's insurance, and the type of institution in which the professional works or is employed.

Complicating the issues of coordination of services and continuity of care is the fact that patients can and are often encouraged to change insurance coverage on a yearly basis. Thus, clinicians now live in a complex, changing, and often confusing world in which issues of compensation can get in the way of quality care. Despite the best of intentions, many clinicians find themselves having to address compensation as another "C." **Table 9-3** outlines a number of methods of financial compensation to providers of health services and examines some of their advantages and disadvantages.

In addition to the mechanism of payment for services, another key factor that affects health professionals is the number of people in the profession. Let us look at how the right number makes a difference.

---

[b] A new approach, often called **concierge practice**, is attempting to provide primary care based upon many of these principles. Concierge practices often limit the number of patients they serve, provide more time for appointments, and guarantee same or next-day access to appointments. However, to provide these services, concierge practices often charge several thousand dollars per patient as a yearly charge, which is not covered by insurance. Thus, concierge practices have been limited to those who can afford to pay for these services.

TABLE 9-2 Ideals and Realities of Primary Care—the 6 Cs

	Primary care ideals	Realities
Contact	The point of first contact with the healthcare system—the entry point	Patients enter the healthcare system through many disconnected points, including ER, specialists, urgent care centers, nontraditional practitioners, etc.
Comprehensive	Primary care intends to be able to diagnose and treat the great majority of problems	Rapid increase in possible treatments and high-volume practices increase proportion of patient problems that are referred to specialists
Coordinated	Primary care intends to be the focal point for diagnosis and treatment, with coordination through referral to specialists for consultation and feedback	Primary care physicians increasingly being replaced by "hospitalists," who are full time in the hospital, provide care for inpatients, and direct patient access to specialists
Continuity	Patient followed over many years—continuous care provision	Patients increasingly required or encouraged to change physicians/providers for insurance purposes
Caring	Individualized care based on individual relationships	Primary care increasingly becoming an administrative entity without long-term individual relationships
Community	Primary care designed to connect the individual patient with community resources and community requirements (required examinations, reportable diseases, vaccinations, driver's licenses, etc.)	Healthcare professionals and public health have a long history of distant and—at times—contentious relationships

Data from Institute of Medicine. Defining Primary Care: An Interim Report. Washington DC: National Academies Press; 1994.

TABLE 9-3 Method of Financial Compensation to Providers of Health Services

Compensation method	Meaning	Examples	Advantages	Disadvantages
Fee-for-service	Clinician paid for each covered service	Physicians often paid for medical visits and procedure, but may not be paid for counseling for prevention	Reward linked directly to work performed Encourages efficiency of delivery of services	May encourage delivery of unnecessary, as well as necessary, services
Capitation	Clinicians are paid a set amount per time period for each patient for whom they are responsible, regardless of level of use of services	Primary care physicians in health plans may be paid a set amount per patient per month and are expected to provide all primary care services	Discourages unnecessary care, may encourage preventive care, allows for predictable budgeting	May discourage necessary care, may encourage referral to specialists unless specialty care is financially discouraged
Episode of care	Institution or clinician is paid a set amount for providing comprehensive services, such as hospital treatment based on the patient's diagnosis	Medicare pays for hospital care based on diagnosis related groups (DRGs), allowing a defined number of days per condition	Encourages rapid and efficient delivery of care	May encourage discharge prior to ability to provide self-care

(continues)

TABLE 9-3 Method of Financial Compensation to Providers of Health Services (*continued*)

Compensation method	Meaning	Examples	Advantages	Disadvantages
Salary	Set amount per time period	Governmental facilities generally pay clinicians on a seniority-based salary	May allow focus on quality	May discourage efficiency
Pay for performance "P4P"	Compensation adjusted based on measures of the quality of care delivered	Additional compensation for adherence to evidence-based guidelines. New P4P being instituted as part of Medicare reimbursement	Links income with quality, providing strong incentive for quality	Difficult to measure quality, outcomes may be related to factors outside clinician's control

HOW CAN WE ENSURE THE SYSTEM HAS THE RIGHT NUMBER OF HEALTHCARE PROFESSIONALS?

Financial compensation is the fundamental market mechanism for regulating the supply of most professionals. This mechanism has not generally worked well in the health professions. The demand for positions in medical schools, for instance, far exceeds the supply. Thus, much of the control over the number of professionals who are trained has been made by the profession itself through policies that control the number and size of accredited degree-granting institutions.

This control has had limited success. For instance, in the 1980s, dentists determined that there was an oversupply of dentists. A number of dental schools were closed and new dental schools were limited. Today, there is an undersupply of dentists. Balancing the supply and demand for health professionals is a complex undertaking, as illustrated by the current shortage of nurses.[10] The nursing shortage is discussed in **Box 9-4**.

We have now taken a look at the complex world of health care and public health professions, including the creation of health professions through education, training, and credentialing. We have also looked at issues of compensation

BOX 9-4 The Nursing Shortage and What Is Being Done About It

Nursing is the largest of the health professions, with almost 3 million registered nurses. The number of U.S.-trained registered nurses (RNs), however, has not kept up with demand. The shortage of nurses, especially those who work in the increasingly technical hospital environment, continues to grow. The projected size of the shortage is controversial, but estimates of a shortage of 200,000 or more RNs in the coming years are commonly quoted. Everyone agrees that nursing is one of the most (if not the most) rapidly growing professions in terms of available job positions. The shortage is made worse by the fact that the average age of nurses is increasing, because until very recently, there was a decline in the number of newly trained nurses. Why is there such a large and growing shortage? A number of factors contribute to this problem, reflecting changes in nursing and the U.S. society. There is

both a greater demand for nursing services and a supply that is not growing fast enough. Among the factors are:

- *Technology*—The increased availability and use of technology has increased the need for skilled nurses. Most of those who qualify for these technologically oriented jobs are recent graduates, and the number of recent graduates is very small compared to the demand.
- *More patients*—The aging baby boomer generation is expected to have a major impact on the need for nursing services. The large number of baby boomers born between 1946 and 1964 will need and expect increased nursing services.
- *Reduced supply*—Nursing has been viewed as a woman's profession, which has historically limited its

BOX 9-4 The Nursing Shortage and What Is Being Done About It (*continued*)

attractiveness to men. In addition, many women leave the profession or practice part time, which may be accelerated by the increasingly stressful nature of the work.

- *Restrictions on entry*—Until recently, nursing education was self-contained—to become a nurse, you needed to complete an undergraduate nursing degree, and the only way to pursue a graduate nursing degree was to already have a bachelor's degree in nursing.
- *Shortage of nursing faculty*—A shortage of nursing faculty and teaching facilities has also contributed to the shortage of nurses and the ability to rapidly expand the size of colleges of nursing.

A national effort is now underway to increase the number of nurses in training. The approaches being used include:

- *Better compensation*—higher salaries and more flexible work schedules
- *Increased educational opportunities*—scholarships to encourage admissions to nursing schools and more flexibility in entering nursing after bachelor's degree training in other fields
- *Increasing the applicant pool*—encouraging male and underrepresented minority group enrollment
- *Raising status of nursing*—greater independence and recognition

Enrollment in colleges of nursing is now increasing. However, it is not likely that the supply of U.S.-trained nurses will meet the rapidly increasing demand in the foreseeable future.

and how we can try to ensure the right numbers of health professionals. Now, let us turn our attention to examining the institutions in which health care is delivered.

KEY WORDS

- **Accreditation**
- **Credentialing**
- **Certification**
- **Licensure**
- **Undergraduate medical education**
- **Primary care**
- **Secondary care**
- **Tertiary care**
- **Medical home**
- **Concierge practice**

Discussion Questions

Take a look at the questions posed in the following scenarios, which were presented at the beginning of this chapter. See now whether you can answer them.

1. Upon your arrival at the hospital, the nurse specialist examines you and consults with the radiologists, the gastroenterologist, and the general surgeon. Your medication is reviewed by the pharmacist and your meals by the clinical nutritionist. Throughout the hospitalization, you are followed by a hospitalist. Once you get back home, the home care team comes to see you regularly for the first two weeks, and the certified physician assistant and the doctor of nursing practice (DNP) see you in the office. You realize that health care is no longer just about doctors and nurses. You ask yourself: What roles do all of these health professionals play in the healthcare system?

2. Jenna decides that after college, she wants to become a doctor and practice medicine. "I thought there was only one kind of doctor who could diagnose disease and prescribe medicine," she mentions at a career counseling meeting. "Not so, anymore," says her advisor. "There are allopathic and osteopathic physicians. In addition, there are nurse practitioners who are authorized to diagnose and prescribe medications, and there are physician assistants who do the same under a physician's supervision. The universe of 'doctors' now includes doctors of nursing practice, as well

as other doctoral degree professionals, such as pharmacists, occupational therapists, and physical therapists." *Understanding careers in health care can be as difficult for students as it is for patients*, Jenna thinks to herself. Now she understands why her advisor asked: "What do you mean by 'practice'? What do you mean by 'doctor'?"

3. Sarah was about to begin medical school and was expecting two years of "preclinical" classroom lectures focusing on the basic sciences, followed by the study of clinical diseases. Then, as she had heard from her physician father, she expected two years of clinical hospital "rotations" and electives investigating specialties. She is surprised to find that medical school has changed. There are small-group, problem-based learning sessions where she needs to be able to locate and read the research literature. There is contact with patients and their problems right from the beginning. There is increasingly a four-year approach instead of a preclinical and clinical approach to medical education. She wonders: Are these changes for the better? What else needs to be done to improve medical education?

4. You are interested in clinical care, as well as public health. *I need to make a choice*, you think to yourself. "Not necessarily," your advisor says. "There are many ways to combine clinical care with public health." After a little investigation, you find out that undergraduate public health education is increasingly seen as preparation for clinical education, and clinical prevention and population health are increasingly becoming part of clinical care. In addition, many careers, from health administration, to health policy, to health education, to clinical research, combine the individual orientation of clinical care with the population perspective of public health. So what is the best pathway to a public health career for you?

REFERENCES

1. Shi L, Singh D. *Essentials of the U.S. Health Care System*. Sudbury, MA: Jones and Bartlett Publishers; 2005.

2. Association of Schools and Programs of Public Health. Framing the future. the second hundred years of education for public health. http://www.asph.org/document.cfm?page=1184. Accessed November 11, 2013.

3. Gebbie K, Rosenstock L., Hernandez LM. *Who Will Keep the Public Healthy? Educating Public Health Professionals for the 21st Century*. Washington DC: National Academy Press; 2003:144.

4. Association of Schools and Programs of Public Health. ASPH Policy Brief. Confronting the Public Health Workforce Crisis. Executive Summary. http://www.asph.org/UserFiles/WorkforceShortage2010Final.pdf. Accessed November 11, 2013.

5. National Board of Public Health Examiners. Get certified. http://www.nbphe.org/getcertified.cfm. July 24, 2013.

6. American Board of Medical Specialties. Specialties and subspecialties. http://www.abms.org. Accessed July 24, 2013.

7. Ludmerer KM. *Time to Heal: American Medical Education from the Turn of the Century to the Era of Managed Care*. New York: Oxford University Press; 2005.

8. American Board of Nursing Specialties. Accredited certification programs. http://www.nursingcertification.org. Accessed July 24, 2013.

9. Institute of Medicine. *Defining Primary Care: An Interim Report*. Washington, DC: National Academy Press; 1994.

10. American Association of Colleges of Nursing. Nursing shortage. http://www.aacn.nche.edu/Media/FactSheets/NursingShortage.htm. Accessed July 24, 2013.

CHAPTER **10**

Healthcare Institutions

By the end of this chapter, the student will be able to:

- identify a range of inpatient healthcare facilities that exist in the United States.
- identify a range of outpatient healthcare facilities that exist in the United States.
- describe approaches being used to define and measure the quality of health care.
- describe types of coordination of care and methods available to facilitate coordination of care.
- identify ways that healthcare systems and Medicare demonstration projects are attempting to improve the quality of care.
- identify roles that may be played by electronic medical records in improving the delivery of health care.
- identify components of medical malpractice and disclosure of medical errors.

George did not have health insurance and went to the emergency room whenever he needed care. They always treated him there, but then tried to get him connected to a primary care facility. He was not eligible for care at the Veterans Administration facilities, so they sent him to the local community health center, which they called the "safety net" provider. George did go there and they tried to treat his problems and get him his medicine. When he got sick, however, George went back to the emergency department. Even George agreed that it was not

the best way to get care, but he wondered: What is needed to make the system work better?

Laura had breast cancer and it had spread. Her medical records were on file at the hospital, at four doctor's offices, in two emergency rooms, and at an outpatient imaging facility. No one seemed to know how to put the system together. Whenever her old records were essential, they asked her to go get a copy of them and bring them to her next appointment. That worked for a while, but when she ended up in the emergency room, her records just were not available. There must be a better way, Laura thought to herself. Has the healthcare system not discovered the Internet yet?

Fred ended his walk one day at the emergency room. He seemed confused about how to get home. "It looks like we are dealing with Alzheimer's," his doctor told Fred's wife, Sonya, at their next appointment. Taking care of Fred at home was not easy. Home health aides and occasional weekend relief called "respite care" eased the burden for a while. The new assisted-living facilities looked attractive, but Fred's family just could not afford one. When Fred fell and broke his hip, he required hospitalization for surgery. The hospital discharge planner arranged for a skilled nursing home for rehabilitation services paid for by Medicare. After a few weeks there, the only alternative was long-term or custodial care in a nursing home paid for by Medicaid. The care at the nursing home was not what the family had expected. The staff did clean Fred up before the announced family visits, but once when the family arrived unannounced, they were shocked to see Fred lying half-naked in his wheelchair. The end came almost two years from the day they moved him to the nursing home. Looking back, the family asked: Can the healthcare system do better at addressing the needs of Alzheimer's patients?

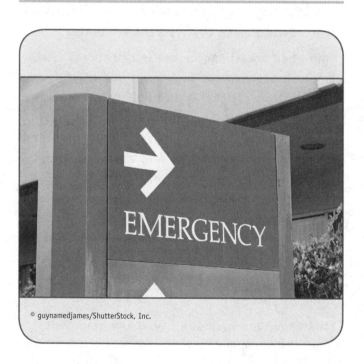

© guynamedjames/ShutterStock, Inc.

These are the types of situations faced by many patients as they try to navigate through the institutions that provide health care in the United States. Let us take a look at these different institutions.

WHAT INSTITUTIONS MAKE UP THE HEALTHCARE SYSTEM?

The number and types of healthcare institutions are almost as diverse and complicated as the number and types of healthcare professionals. In recent years, the complexity has grown as a range of facilities have developed to serve new needs and new financial reimbursement approaches.[1,2] Nonetheless, it is possible to understand the scope of healthcare institutions by categorizing them as **inpatient facilities** and **outpatient facilities**, with inpatient facilities implying that patients remain in the facility for at least 24 hours.

Inpatient facilities include hospitals, skilled nursing and rehabilitation facilities, nursing homes, and institutional hospices. Outpatient facilities include those providing clinical services by one or more clinicians and those providing diagnostic testing or treatment. We will provide an overview of inpatient and outpatient facilities and then ask: Do these facilities together provide a coordinated system of care? Let us begin by looking at inpatient facilities.

WHAT TYPES OF INPATIENT FACILITIES EXIST IN THE UNITED STATES?

We can classify inpatient facilities as: 1) hospitals generally designed for short-term stays by patients, and 2) long-term care facilities. Let us first take a look at hospitals.

The history of hospitals in the United States goes back to the colonial period. However, prior to the middle of the 1800s, hospitals were generally institutions for those without other sources of care, which included the poor, the military, and those with communicable diseases. Hospitals generally provided little more than shelter and food and separated the sick—especially those with communicable diseases—from the healthy.[1]

Today, the U.S. hospital is usually a modern high-tech enterprise that lies at the center of the healthcare system educationally, structurally, and psychologically. You can often identify the hospital from far away because it is frequently the largest and most modern facility in town. The psychological hold that the hospital has on U.S. health care is symbolized by the term "house" and the concept of "house staff," or residents who practically live full time in the hospital during their training.[3,a]

Hospitals share some common features, including:

- Hospitals are licensed by the state and usually accredited by a national organization, such as The Joint Commission (formally called the Joint Commission on the Accreditation of Healthcare Organizations [JCAHO]).

---

[a] The book *The House of God*, written in the 1960s, captured the mentality of the house staff of the era and has been unofficial required reading by subsequent generations of residents. It portrays house staff as having their own culture and portrays patients, as well as community physicians, in often disparaging ways.

- Hospitals have an organized physician staff and provide 24-hour-a-day nursing services.
- The hospital is governed by a governing board separate from the medical and nursing staff that has overall responsibility for the operation of the hospital consistent with state and federal laws.

The several types of hospitals in the United States differ in their purposes and organizational structures. Hospitals can be categorized as general hospitals and specialty hospitals. General hospitals attempt to serve a wide spectrum of patients and problems, though they may concentrate on serving only children or only those who qualify for services, such as a Veterans Administration (VA) hospital. In the past, specialty hospitals sought to serve the needs of patients who could not be accommodated in general hospitals, such as those with tuberculosis or severe mental illness. Today, these conditions are usually addressed in general hospitals. Today's specialty hospitals are more a result of the specialization of medical services. Institutions focused on cancer, heart disease, psychiatric illness, ophthalmology, and orthopaedics, for instance, are rapidly developing.

Hospitals are often categorized today by their funding source and financial arrangements. They can be divided into nonprofit and for-profit, or investor-owned, hospitals. Nearly 90% of the approximately 5,000 hospitals in the United States are nonprofits. These include the broad category of private nonprofit hospitals, hospitals run by state or federal government, and hospitals run by institutions, such as universities.[b]

Approximately half of these 5,000 hospitals are private nonprofit hospitals, many of which have affiliations with religious denominations, but accept patients of all faiths. State and local governments run nearly 20% of hospitals, many of which are described—along with private nonprofit hospitals—as community hospitals. Federal medical institutions include the Veterans Administration hospitals and the military hospital system. For-profit, or investor-owned, hospitals make up over 10% of all hospitals, many of which are owned by several large corporations specializing in providing healthcare services.

Hospitals today are often more than an inpatient facility. The most rapidly growing component of most hospitals is the spectrum of outpatient services they provide. In addition to emergency departments, hospitals usually also provide outpatient surgical and medical services, including diagnostic and treatment services, and may provide facilities for routine office-type visits.

The hospital should no longer be viewed as one building. Hospital networks or systems are increasingly being created, some of which provide a range of services, including skilled nursing and rehabilitative services, as well as long-term care.

We have classified inpatient facilities as including hospitals and long-term care facilities. Today, there are a range of long-term care facilities, some of which are not primarily operated as healthcare facilities.[1, 2] These facilities may include skilled nursing facilities, nursing homes, assisted living and dementia care, and, at times, hospice care. To fully understand the provision of long-term care, you also need to appreciate the types of services that are increasingly being provided in an individual's home.

It is important to distinguish between skilled nursing and rehabilitative services in contrast to nursing home or custodial services. Skilled nursing and rehabilitative services, like hospital services, are generally short term and aimed at accomplishing specific objectives, such as recovery from a stroke or injury. Though these services may continue for many months, they are not designed to provide long-term care beyond the point at which improvement can no longer be expected.

Nursing homes, on the other hand, are designed for long-term or custodial care while also providing a limited amount of healthcare services. Individuals in nursing homes usually require care because of their inability to perform the activities of daily living, such as dressing, feeding, and bathing themselves. Nursing homes may provide routine medical care and some acute care, but this type of facility is not primarily designed to improve the medical status of its residents.[c]

Nursing homes are generally operated according to a specific set of nursing home regulations determined by and enforced by the states. Federal minimal standards are set as part of the requirements to receive payment through the Medicare and Medicaid systems. Most nursing homes, like most hospitals, are run as private nonprofit institutions. However, for-profit, or investor-owned, nursing homes provide approximately 15% of the beds nationally. There are

---

[b] Hospitals are also categorized as teaching and nonteaching hospitals. A teaching hospital is one that has one or more accredited residency programs. Today, many community hospitals, as well as federal and state hospitals, have residency programs. The designation **academic health center** implies a medical school, one or more other health professions schools, and an affiliated hospital.

---

[c] Some states, such as California, have developed an additional long-term care model that is not part of the "medical model." That is, limited or no nursing care is provided and the facility is not obligated to provide services if the individual's health status changes substantially.

over 16,000 nursing homes in the United States, with over 1.5 million residents. Most, but not all, residents are elderly. Over 80% need help with mobility, nearly 66% are considered incontinent, and nearly 50% require assistance with eating. Alzheimer's patients are the most rapidly growing population in the nursing home system of care.[1, 2]

Although not strictly inpatient healthcare facilities, assisted-living facilities and home health care increasingly provide long-term care for those who have less severe impairments. Assisted-living facilities are not organized as healthcare facilities, but may provide or coordinate health care as part of their services. New concepts, such as continuing care retirement communities, attempt to provide a range of options, including independent-living, assisted-living, and nursing home facilities.

Most elderly and disabled individuals are not residents in long-term care institutions; rather, they live on their own or with family members. Thus, much attention in recent years has been paid to providing and financing home healthcare services, including home health aides, healthcare delivered at home, and respite care. Respite care provides short-term time away for primary caregivers such as family members.

The hospice movement today can be viewed as part of the long-term care system. It is care provided to those with a life expectancy of six months or fewer as determined by a physician. The goal of hospice care is to provide comfort, emotional support, and palliation—not to increase longevity. In some cases, hospice care may occur in a separate institution, but today, it is more often provided in the patient's place of residence.

WHAT TYPES OF OUTPATIENT FACILITIES EXIST IN THE UNITED STATES?

The variety of types of outpatient facilities is even more diverse and complicated than that of inpatient facilities. The basic distinction between clinical facilities and diagnostic testing or therapeutic facilities helps define the types of services provided.

Clinical services were traditionally viewed as being provided in "the doctor's office." None of these words—"the," "doctor's," "office"—does a good job of describing the current organization of clinical services. "The" implies one. Today, clinical services are rarely organized around one doctor or clinician. Group practice and multispecialty practices have become the rule. "Doctors" (or physicians) are by no means the only health professionals to organize and provide clinical services. Physical therapists, nurse practitioners, audiologists, optometrists, clinical psychologists, and a long list of other health professionals often provide their own office services. Rather than "doctor," the term provider is increasingly used to encompass this growing array of health professionals. Even the term "office" is no longer appropriate. In addition to the traditional office setting, many clinicians now provide services in shopping centers and work places, and even make house calls.

The average American makes over three visits for clinical services per year. An increasing number of these visits are provided outside of "the doctor's office" in the traditional sense. These sites now include a growing network of community health centers designed to provide what is called the "safety net" services for those who cannot or do not wish to seek other types of clinical services. **Box 10-1** provides an overview of community health centers.[4]

A key issue in the organization of health care is the delivery of quality services. Let us take a look at what we mean by "quality" and what mechanisms are being used to ensure the quality of healthcare services.

WHAT DO WE MEAN BY THE "QUALITY OF HEALTHCARE SERVICES?"

The quality of healthcare services may mean different things to different people. Administrators may focus on the structures, such as the availability of operating rooms or laboratory services. Clinicians may focus on the process, such as the technical competence of the practitioners. Patients may focus on different types of processes, like the personal relationships and their personal satisfaction. External reviewers may focus on the outcome—lives saved or disabilities prevented.

Quality can be assessed using what are called structure, process, and outcome measures. Structure focuses on the physical and organizational infrastructure in which care is delivered. Process concentrates on the procedures and formal processes that go into delivering care—for example, systems for ensuring credentialing of health professionals and procedures to ensure timely response to complaints. Outcome measures imply a focus on the result of care, from rates of infection to readmissions with complications.

Defining and measuring quality remains a controversial subject. However, the National Committee for Quality Assurance (NCQA) has developed a widely recognized framework to assist with this challenge.[5] **Table 10-1** outlines this framework.[d]

The complexity of inpatient and outpatient services in the United States has made the delivery of quality healthcare

---

[d] Note that NCQA's framework emphasizes structure and process measures with little emphasis on the actual outcomes of care.

BOX 10-1   Community Health Centers

Initially named neighborhood health centers, community health centers were established in 1965 as part of the Johnson administration's War on Poverty. The centers were designed based on a community empowerment philosophy that encouraged the flow of funds directly to nonprofit, community-level organizations, often bypassing state governments.

The Health Centers Consolidation Act of 1996 combined community health centers with healthcare services for migrants, the homeless population, and residents of public housing to create the consolidated health centers program under Section 330 of the Public Health Service Act. These centers are often called 330 grantees. To receive a 330 grant, a clinic must meet certain statutory requirements. It must:

- Be located in a federally designated medically underserved area (MUA) or serve a federally designated medically underserved population (MUP)
- Have nonprofit, public, or tax exempt status

- Provide comprehensive primary healthcare services, referrals, and other services needed to facilitate access to care, such as case management, translation, and transportation
- Have a governing board, the majority of whose members are patients of the health center
- Provide services to all in the service area regardless of ability to pay and offer a sliding fee schedule that adjusts according to family income

Community health centers have undergone rapid expansion in recent years and now serve approximately 20 million individuals annually at more than 4,000 sites in all 50 states and the District of Columbia. Most patients have low incomes and the majority qualify for Medicaid. According to a review, "health centers have proven to be an effective investment of federal funds, have garnered sustained goodwill and advocacy in the communities they serve, and, as a result, generally have enjoyed broad, bipartisan support."[4]

TABLE 10-1 Characteristics of Healthcare Quality—National Committee for Quality Assurance

Characteristic	Meaning	Examples	How is it measured?
Access and service	Access to needed care and good customer service	Enough primary care physicians and specialists Satisfaction of patients in terms of problems obtaining care	Patient satisfaction surveys, patient grievances and follow-up, interviews with staff
Qualified providers	Personnel licensed and trained and patients satisfied with services	System for checking credentials with sanctions Patient satisfaction with providers of care	Presence of system for checking credentials Patient satisfaction surveys
Staying healthy	Quality of services that help people maintain good health and avoid illness	Presence of guidelines for appropriate clinical preventive services Evidence that patients are receiving appropriate screening tests	Review of independently verified clinical records Review of responses from patients
Getting better	Quality of services that help people recover from illness	Presence of method for evaluating new procedures, drugs, and devices to ensure that patients have access to the most up-to-date care Providing specific services, such as smoking cessation	Review of independently verified clinical records Interviews with staff
Living with illness	Quality of services that help people manage chronic illness	Programs to assist patients to manage chronic conditions like asthma Provision of specific services, such as eye examinations for diabetics	Review of independently verified clinical records Interviews with staff

Data from NCQA Health Plan Report Care. Available at http://reportcard.ncqa.org/plan/external/Resources.aspx?Header=yes&Tab=Glossary#Accreditation. Accessed August 12, 2013.

services very challenging. The complexity of the system raises two closely connected questions:

- How can the pieces of the system be coordinated to provide integrated care?
- How can we improve and ensure the quality of health care?

The coordination and integration of healthcare delivery is often considered key to both the efficiency and the quality of health care. Let us begin by taking a look at how healthcare delivery can be coordinated among institutions.

HOW CAN HEALTH CARE BE COORDINATED AMONG THE MULTIPLE INSTITUTIONS THAT PROVIDE HEALTHCARE SERVICES?

The types of institutions that deliver health care in the United States have continued to proliferate in recent years. Each type differs in its governance, finance, accreditation, and organizational structure. It is not surprising that most patients, policy makers, and even clinicians do not have a good overview of the system. Connecting the institutions to achieve an organized system has become a major challenge.

Healthcare delivery systems aim to connect inpatient and outpatient services, as well as short-term and long-term clinical services, to provide a coordinated system of care. The desire for an integrated healthcare delivery system is not a new idea. For many years, the concept of "the patient's doctor" was seen as the mechanism to hold together the system. The doctor provided all care or coordinated the care with other clinicians. The doctor "followed" the patient into the inpatient facility and provided the patient's "follow-up" care after he or she left.

Like the concept of "the doctor's office," the concept of "the patient's doctor" is no longer a reflection of reality. Once again "the" rarely reflects the reality of multiple providers of care. Primary care physicians are now far less likely to follow the patient into the hospital or the nursing home and far less likely to be aware of the patient's multiple sources of and approaches to care.

Efforts to integrate the system are under way. We will look at two basic approaches that are being used: the development of integrated healthcare delivery systems and the use of integrated electronic medical records. These approaches are likely to be used together and form the basis for a future integrated system of healthcare delivery. In order to understand the uses and potential of these two approaches, we first need to think about the types of coordination of care that we want to see occur and the purposes they serve.

WHAT TYPES OF COORDINATION OF CARE ARE NEEDED AND WHAT PURPOSES DO THEY SERVE?

As we have discussed, the traditional approach to coordination of care revolved around the clinician–patient or doctor–patient relationship. Traditionally, the concepts of continuity of care and coordination of care have been almost synonymous. This approach assumed that the relationship between one doctor and one patient would provide the individualized knowledge, trust, and commitment that would ensure the coordination of care by ensuring the continuity of care. The concepts of primary care that we have discussed were built in large part upon this concept of one-to-one continuity.

Today, there is an increasing emphasis on ensuring coordination rather than one-to-one continuity. Coordination is sought between institutions and settings where care is delivered. The approach that leaves continuity of information and continuity of responsibility for care to individual clinicians alone has often failed to produce the desired results. As we will see, efforts are under way to formally link institutions, services, and information between the various healthcare delivery sites and institutions.

Institutional coordination often relies on financial coordination. If services are covered by insurance in one setting but not another, the system is not likely to function efficiently or effectively. When services are not covered at all, patients may receive excellent care in one setting only to lose the benefits of that care when necessary preparation or follow-up is not paid for and not accomplished in another setting.

Coordination is not just an issue within the healthcare delivery system; it is also an issue that straddles healthcare delivery and public health functions. Communicable disease control and environmental protections, such as controlling antibiotic resistance and lead exposure, cannot be successful without effective and efficient coordination between healthcare and public health professionals and institutions. **Table 10-2** outlines these types of coordination, their intended function, and the types of challenges that commonly occur with their implementation.

Let us take a look at the development of healthcare delivery systems as one approach to ensuring coordination of health care.

WHAT TYPES OF HEALTHCARE DELIVERY SYSTEMS ARE BEING DEVELOPED AND HOW CAN THEY HELP ENSURE COORDINATION OF HEALTH CARE?

We will use the term "healthcare delivery system" to imply a linkage of institutions and healthcare professionals

TABLE 10-2 Type of Coordination of Care, Intended Functions, and Challenges with Implementation

Type of coordination	Intended function	Challenges with implementation
Clinician–patient relationship	Continuity as a mechanism for ensuring coordination Development of one-to-one relationships built on knowledge and trust over extended periods of time	Multiple clinicians involved in care Team rather than individual concept of primary care Frequent changes in insurance coverage require change in health professionals
Institutional coordination	Coordination of individual's information between institutions needed to inform individual clinical and administrative decision making	Different structures and governance often lead to lack of coordination between inpatient facilities and between inpatient and outpatient facilities
Financial coordination	Implies that a patient has comprehensive coverage for services provided by the full range of institutions Aims to maximize the efficiency of the care received and minimize the administrative effort required to manage the payment system	Lack of comprehensive insurance coverage often means that essential services cannot be delivered or cannot be delivered at the most efficient or effective institutional site
Coordination between health care and public health	Coordination of services between clinical care and public health requires communication to ensure follow-up and to protect the health of others	Lack of coordination of services between public health services and clinical care is often based on lack of communications

that together take on the responsibility of delivering coordinated care.[e]

In a nation such as the United States, in which health care is provided by a range of providers and institutions, holding together one delivery system is not easy. A wide range of efforts are under way to connect the pieces. Let us take a look at some successful examples.

Care coordination challenges have been quite successfully met in the emergency response system. Today, there is a network of institutions, including government agencies and private emergency medical services providers that cooperate with hospital emergency departments to facilitate and expedite the care of the seriously ill and injured. The emergency response system helps to quickly respond to emergencies, provide onsite assistance and information, and identify the healthcare institution that is best prepared to handle

the emergency based on location, staffing, and capabilities. This system, while not perfect, demonstrates that coordination of care—at least urgent care—is possible.

Coordination of routine health care has proven to be a more difficult challenge. **Healthcare systems** are beginning to be developed, often based on common ownership or governance. These integrated systems are designed to provide a wide range of services, from outpatient clinical care, diagnostic testing, and treatment services, to inpatient, home health, skilled nursing, nursing home, and even hospice care.

Two of the longest standing and most developed healthcare systems are the Kaiser Permanente and Veterans Administration systems.[6, 7] These are discussed in **Box 10-2**. Many more healthcare systems are being formed by caregivers, such as multispecialty group practices, and by institutions, such as university medical centers. The coming years are likely to produce a number of successful models that will become examples that others will try to replicate.

In addition to the development of comprehensive healthcare delivery systems, experimentation is under way to improve the functioning of existing systems such as

---

[e] We will distinguish healthcare delivery systems, healthcare systems, and **health systems**. Healthcare delivery systems include the delivery of healthcare services to a defined population. A healthcare system also includes the financial arrangements needed to pay for the care. A health system, the broadest of the three terms, includes the public health system, as well as the health care system.

BOX 10-2 Healthcare Delivery Systems: Kaiser Permanente and the Veterans Administration

The Kaiser Permanente and the Veterans Administration healthcare systems are two of the largest organized healthcare systems in the United States. They have very different histories and philosophies, and they serve quite different populations. Nonetheless, they have both moved in the direction of developing an integrated set of healthcare delivery institutions linked together by an electronic health record and fostering evidence-based interventions. They share a common advantage in that they are financed by single sources, the Kaiser Permanente health plan and the federal government, respectively.

Kaiser helped introduce the concept of the health maintenance organization by offering a comprehensive package of preventive and curative services at a fixed monthly fee. The Kaiser Permanente health system has its roots in World War II, when employers offered health benefits when they were prohibited from raising wages. In the subsequent decades, Kaiser Permanente grew from its California base, enrolling over nine million individuals. It was created as a staff model prepaid health plan, enrolling patients who would receive all of their services directly from clinicians and institutions that were part of the plan. This allowed Kaiser Permanente to develop an integrated approach to healthcare delivery.

Kaiser, the management component, owns or contracts with hospitals, skilled nursing facilities, home healthcare systems, and a range of other institutions that provide care under their management. Permanente, the physician component, aims to provide an integrated set of inpatient and outpatient services. Kaiser Permanente competes actively in the market for healthcare services and often limits the amount and types of care that can be provided. Nonetheless, it has been able to develop an integrated healthcare delivery system, promote evidence-based interventions, and introduce an integrated electronic health record system.

The Veterans Administration healthcare system began as an outgrowth of World War I, though its roots go back to the Revolutionary War. After World War II, the Veterans Administration hospital system rapidly increased in size and developed strong relationships with medical schools and other health professional training schools for education and research. Today, the VA healthcare system is part of the cabinet-level Department of Veterans Affairs and serves over eight million patients each year.

For many years, the VA system was accused of poor quality care and lack of coordination of care because it emphasized inpatient services and patients often went back and forth between the VA and other healthcare delivery sites. In the mid-1990s, the VA health system underwent a major "systems reengineering," designed to improve quality. The changes included the development of an integrated electronic health record and an emphasis on evidence-based interventions for preventive, acute, and chronic care.

In recent years, the VA health system has been organized into a series of networks, including inpatient and outpatient facilities. Many of the networks aim to provide comprehensive outpatient and inpatient services, including skilled nursing and nursing home services, as well as outpatient and hospital services. Survey data collected a decade after the systems reengineering initiative began suggests that the VA health system provides an increasing quality of integrated care based upon evidence-based interventions.

The VA and Kaiser Permanente systems represent two of the largest healthcare systems in the United States. Both aim to serve a large number of patients and provide coordinated care utilizing evidence-based interventions and integrated healthcare records. The success of these two quite different healthcare systems suggests that an integrated system of care, patient information, and financing is possible and can be widely applied to improve the quality of health care.

Medicare. The Affordable Care Act has a large number of provisions that encourage demonstration projects for Medicare patients. These provisions are designed to improve performance and often focus on incentives for efficiency and coordination of care. **Box 10-3** discusses a number of the Medicare programs that are now under way.[8]

HOW CAN ELECTRONIC MEDICAL RECORDS BE USED TO FACILITATE COORDINATION OF CARE AND IMPROVE QUALITY?

There is widespread agreement that an electronic health record system could improve coordination of care, as well as achieve a number of other quality objectives. The Institute

---

BOX 10-3 The Affordable Care Act and Medicare

The ACA's impact on health services focuses primarily on funding experiments or demonstration programs designed to improve the delivery of health services. The ACA and other federal legislation encourage and authorize funding for the federal Centers for Medicare and Medicaid Services (CMS) to implement a series of new programs. Key programs are described by the CMS as follows:

Accountable Care Organizations (ACOs): ACOs will allow providers who voluntarily agree to work together to coordinate care for patients and providers who meet certain quality standards to share in any savings they achieve for the Medicare program. ACOs that elect to become accountable for shared losses have the opportunity to share in greater savings. ACOs will coordinate and integrate Medicare services, with success being gauged by roughly 30 quality measures organized in 4 domains. These domains include patient experience, care coordination and patient safety, preventive health, and at-risk populations. The higher the quality of care providers deliver, the more shared savings their Accountable Care Organization may earn, provided they also lower growth in healthcare expenditures.

Partnership for Patients: This partnership is a test care model to reduce hospital-acquired conditions and improve transitions in care. This public–private partnership supports the efforts of physicians, nurses, and other clinicians to make care safer and better coordinate patients' transitions from hospitals to other settings.

Bundled Payments for Care Improvement: The Bundled Payments for Care Improvement initiative seeks to improve patient care by fostering improved coordination through payments for multiple related services rather than for single services.

Comprehensive Primary Care Initiative: In addition to regular fee-for-service payments, CMS will pay primary care practices a monthly fee for clinicians to help patients with serious or chronic diseases follow personalized care plans; give patients 24-hour access to care and health information; deliver preventive care; engage patients and their families in their own care; and work together with other doctors, including specialists, to provide better coordinated care.

Federally Qualified Health Center (FQHC) Advanced Primary Care Practice Demonstration: This demonstration evaluates the impact of advanced primary care practice on improving care, focusing on prevention, and reducing healthcare costs among Medicare beneficiaries served by FQHCs (in other words, community health centers).

The results of these experiments and demonstration programs will take several years to determine. It is likely that these results will contribute to ongoing reform of the U.S. healthcare delivery system.

---

of Medicine (IOM) outlined the following potential roles for an electronic health information system. These roles aim in large part to provide the cornerstone for coordination of healthcare delivery.

- *Health information and data*—laboratory and pharmacy data, as well as records of a patient's history and findings on examination, including past medical records
- *Results management*—integration of findings from multiple providers at multiple sites
- *Order entry/management*—electronic ordering of tests and prescriptions to maximize accuracy and speed implementation
- *Decision support management*—computer reminders and prompts to encourage timely follow-up and adherence to evidence-based guidelines

- *Electronic communication and connectivity*—facilitation of communications between providers and between providers and patients
- *Patient support*—tools for patient education and patient involvement in decision making
- *Administrative processes*—facilitation of scheduling, billing, and other administrative services to increase efficiency and reduce costs
- *Reporting and population health*—improvements in the efficiency and completeness of required reporting and the speed and completeness of public health surveillance

The IOM also concluded that electronic record systems have the potential for helping achieve quality and efficiency objectives as outlined in **Box 10-4**.[9]

Efforts to implement a national system of electronic health records are under way. Nearly $20 billion was allocated

BOX 10-4 Use of Electronic Health Records to Improve Quality and Efficiency of Healthcare Delivery

The IOM report indicates that the electronic health record has the potential to improve the quality and efficiency of patient care in the following ways:

- *Improve patient safety*. Safety is the prevention of harm to patients. Each year in the United States, tens of thousands of people die as a result of preventable adverse events due to health care. Electronic records containing information on prescribed drugs and other treatments are expected to improve patient safety.
- *Support the delivery of effective patient care*. Effectiveness is providing services based on scientific knowledge to those who could benefit and at the same time refraining from providing services to those not likely to benefit. Only about one-half (55%) of Americans receive recommended medical care that is consistent with evidence-based guidelines. Reminder systems that require clinicians to accept or reject the recommendations of a clinical guideline are expected to increase the use of evidence-based guidelines.
- *Facilitate management of chronic conditions*. More than half of those with chronic conditions have three or more different providers and report that they often

receive conflicting information from those providers; moreover, many undergo duplicate tests and procedures, but still do not receive recommended care. Physicians also report difficulty in coordinating care for their patients with chronic conditions and believe that this lack of coordination produces poor outcomes. Electronic records can help inform clinicians of other care being given to their patients.

- *Improve efficiency*. Efficiency is the avoidance of waste—in particular, waste of equipment, supplies, ideas, and energy. Methods must be found to enhance the efficiency of healthcare professionals and reduce the administrative and labor costs associated with healthcare delivery and financing. Electronic records, if consistently and widely implemented in the healthcare arena, can be expected to reduce costs as they have in many other fields.

While there is widespread agreement that electronic medical records have the potential to improve health care, concerns have also been raised about privacy. In addition, the ease of ordering tests provided by many health information systems has raised concerns that these systems will result in additional ordering of costly and often unnecessary tests.

---

to this effort as part of the 2009–2010 stimulus plan. Recent efforts to include patients as direct users of their health information may spur more rapid acceptance of the electronic records. The need for security of data and control by patients over who has access and for what purposes is critical to the acceptance and use of an electronic system such as this. Assuming that security issues can be adequately addressed, you should expect to see widespread use of electronic records and an increased role for patients in accessing and managing their own medical records.[f]

Electronic health records are only one of the many ways that technology is changing the delivery and quality of healthcare services in the United States.

---

[f] Despite the national commitment to implement electronic health records, the usage by U.S. physicians in their offices is still far behind that of other developed countries. Financial incentives to utilize electronic medical records are producing rapid changes in physician behavior.

HOW IS TECHNOLOGY BEING USED TO IMPROVE THE QUALITY OF CARE?

The United States is among the leaders in adoption of new healthcare technologies, especially those that allow for technological approaches to disease diagnosis and treatment. In comparison with most other nations, the United States has more rapidly developed and accepted the use of medical technologies ranging from magnetic resonance imaging (MRI), to invasive cardiac procedures, to surgery for weight loss.

This country has generally relied on market mechanisms to develop, introduce, and disseminate or diffuse technology. This has resulted in extremely rapid innovation in areas with high levels of financial compensation and slower innovation in areas with less financial support. For instance, high-tech procedures ranging from heart surgery to hip replacements have been well compensated and have seen rapid innovation and diffusion. Well-compensated preventive procedures, such as mammography, have likewise seen widespread use. Other technologies, like telemedicine, are likely to have widespread applications only after financial reimbursement is provided.

Longer term innovations in technology have been fueled by the long-term U.S. investment in basic and applied research through the National Institutes of Health (NIH). The budget for the NIH was doubled during the 1990s, but has been relatively flat in recent years when adjusted for inflation. The innovations in care and in technology pioneered by the NIH have often led to new approaches and new health-related industries. In recent years, the NIH has begun to focus on translational research or efforts to bring the benefits of new knowledge and new technologies to individual patients and whole communities.

Increased knowledge of the human genome has laid the groundwork for new diagnostic and therapeutic approaches, as well as a better understanding of the causes of disease. Better understanding of brain function and better technology for measuring changes in the brain are leading to new strategies for dealing with diseases ranging from Alzheimer's to depression. Advances in technology continue to provide hope and new challenges to improving health care.

We have now looked at how the development of integrated healthcare delivery systems and electronic health records and other technologies are being used to try to improve the quality and efficiency of healthcare delivery. Now, let us take a look at mechanisms that are being developed to monitor and ensure quality of care.

WHAT MECHANISMS ARE BEING USED TO MONITOR AND ENSURE THE QUALITY OF HEALTH CARE IN THE UNITED STATES?

There are a variety of methods, including accreditation of academic institutions and individual credentialing to help ensure that health professionals are well educated and prepared for clinical practice. Increasing requirements for continuing education, recertification, and maintenance of licensure are being used to help ensure continued competence. Integrating financial compensation with quality of care through the use of pay-for-performance approaches is gaining momentum as an additional approach to ensuring quality.

In addition, there is a new emphasis on the use of evidence-based recommendations or clinical guidelines. Today, these recommendations are often available to clinicians in the form of protocols or step-by-step advice on approaches to the diagnosis and treatment of specific conditions. Computer systems increasingly prompt clinicians to take actions or confirm their actions with an aim to implement evidence-based

recommendations. The complexity of clinical practice and the limits of current research, however, mean that evidence-based recommendations are available for only a small percentage of the problems that clinicians face on a daily basis.

In addition to these approaches, a series of other mechanisms attempts to address issues of quality. They include:

- Hospital privileges and approval to perform specific procedures
- Accreditation of additional healthcare organizations, including clinical practices
- Malpractice liability, not only for physicians, but increasingly for other health professionals
- Disclosure of medical errors

Hospital privileges imply that hospitals may set criteria for allowing clinicians to practice in their facility. The criteria may include specialty and/or subspecialty boards. Approval to perform specific procedures implies the need to demonstrate competence either by training or experience or both.

Accreditation of hospitals and long-term care facilities has been a long-standing effort. It is often linked to reimbursement, and is thus essential to the survival of these institutions. Accreditation of clinical practices, especially large group practices, is a growing trend. The NCQA and The Joint Commission are encouraging this process and providing quality criteria that need to be met. While still a voluntary process, these new forms of accreditation are becoming a sign of quality that is useful when recruiting patients and dealing with insurance companies.

The U.S. healthcare delivery system has a unique body of law called **medical malpractice**. Medical malpractice is hailed by its supporters as the ultimate guarantor of quality. It is attacked by its detractors as leading to defensive medicine, increased costs, and shortages in vulnerable professions, such as obstetrics. Regardless of your view of malpractice, it has come to have a major impact on the relationship between clinicians and patients. **Box 10-5** examines the criteria for malpractice so you can understand what it means.[10]

Malpractice is an inherently adversarial process. Increasingly, patients, clinicians, and healthcare institutions are looking for alternatives. One recent approach is the disclosure of medical errors.

CAN DISCLOSING MEDICAL ERRORS CONTRIBUTE TO QUALITY OF CARE AND SERVE AS AN ALTERNATIVE TO MALPRACTICE?

In its report *To Error Is Human*, the IOM documented the extent to which medical errors produce harm to patients—they estimated over 40,000 deaths per year.[11] This makes

BOX 10-5 Medical Malpractice

Medical malpractice is a body of state law; therefore, it differs from state to state. It is part of the civil law, as opposed to criminal law, which means that a case may be decided by a jury based upon what is called the **preponderance of the evidence**. This implies that malpractice was more likely than not. Despite the differences that exist from state to state, malpractice law builds upon a tradition known as **negligence law**, which is intended to protect the individual from harm.

The occurrence of harm or a bad outcome resulting from health care is not the same as negligence or malpractice. Errors in judgment and unsuccessful efforts are only considered medical malpractice if the patient can establish all four of the following:

1. A duty was owed.
2. A duty was breached.
3. The breach caused an injury.
4. Damages occurred.

Let us look at each of these requirements.[a]

1. A duty was owed—This implies that a healthcare provider undertook the care or treatment of a patient. This duty may stem from services provided, ranging from a long-term relationship, a single visit, or a telephone call to a contractual relationship based upon an insurance agreement.
2. A duty was breached—This implies a failure of the healthcare provider to meet a relevant standard of care. The standard of care is defined in terms of the clinician's specialty. A healthcare provider is generally expected to possess the knowledge and skill and exercise the care and judgment expected of a reasonably competent clinician of the same specialty.

3. The breach caused an injury—The legal concept of causation is based on what is called proximal cause. In medical malpractice, responsibility for an injury lies with the last negligent act. **Proximal cause** asks whether the injury or other outcome would have occurred if the negligent act had not occurred. Causation can be divided among different "parties," including clinicians and institutions.
4. Damages occurred—Damages can be divided into direct, indirect, and punitive categories. Direct damages include lost earnings, as well as current and future medical expenses. Indirect damages may include pain and emotional distress. Punitive damages may be awarded when conduct is intentionally harmful or grossly negligent.[b]

Instructions to a jury in a medical malpractice case include efforts to convey the meaning of each of these components of malpractice law. However, juries have a great deal of latitude when interpreting their meaning. For example, the concept of proximal causation used in the law may not conform to the jurors' understanding of causation. For instance, assume a clinician refused to continue to provide prenatal care after the first 13 weeks. The jurors may decide based upon their own understanding of causation that the clinician's refusal was the cause of a subsequent birth defect.

Medical malpractice is a complex and changing field. Many factors affect whether or not a malpractice suit is brought. These include the extent of damages, the relationship between the patient and the healthcare provider, and the standards of practice of both medicine and law in the community.

---

[a] Physicians are not the only providers of health care who can be sued under malpractice laws. Other clinicians, such as pharmacists, may be sued, especially those who do not work directly under the authority of physicians. In addition, healthcare facilities as institutions may be sued and are often included as additional defendants in malpractice cases. In this section, we will refer to the defendant in a malpractice suit as a healthcare provider.

[b] Indirect damages may include what has been called a "loss of consortium," which includes services provided by a domestic partner, including companionship, homemaking, etc., and future reproductive capabilities of either sex. Gross negligence includes the intentional or wanton omission of care that would be proper to provide, or, alternatively, doing that which would be improper to do. Punitive damages are often justified as a method of deterring such conduct by other providers of care.

---

medical errors a slightly more common cause of death than either breast cancer or motor vehicle accidents. Errors may be due to deficiencies in the diagnostic or therapeutic process on the part of clinician(s). They may also be due to what are called **system errors**, problems resulting from deficiencies in the system for delivering health care.

Clinicians in the not-too-distant past often withheld key information from patients, including a diagnosis of cancer and the potential harms of recommended treatment. Today, disclosure of these types of information is an expected part of clinical practice. However, until recently, disclosure of medical errors had not been an expected part of clinical practice.

Beginning in 2001, The Joint Commission has required that patients be informed of all outcomes of care, including "unanticipated outcomes." Recent efforts to develop a system of disclosure have included a far more specific set of expectations, including conveying to the patient:

- Facts about the event
- Presence of error or systems failure
- Expression of regret
- A formal apology

In addition, institutions are expected to integrate the disclosure process with other aspects of patient safety and risk management activities; provide support for the process, including educating clinicians; and keep track of the use of disclosure at their institutions. Such formal efforts to disclose errors are becoming increasingly common in clinical care. It is still too early to determine the impact of these efforts on quality and their ability to reduce malpractice suits. However, there has already been a growing acceptance of disclosure as a way of addressing medical errors.[12]

We have examined the structure of the U.S. healthcare delivery system, including the types of services that are provided in the inpatient and the outpatient settings. We have seen the need for and difficulty in developing a coordinated system to provide continuity of care. We have also seen how the U.S. system is developing models of coordination linking institutions and providers in new ways. The use of technology is a major strategy used by the U.S. healthcare delivery system to hold itself together through electronic medical records and innovative approaches to diagnosis and treatment. The development of the healthcare delivery system is closely tied to the way that health care is financed and services are paid for. Therefore, let us turn our attention directly to the issue of paying for health care.

KEY WORDS

- **Inpatient facilities**
- **Outpatient facilities**
- **Academic health center**
- **Provider**
- **Structure, process, and outcome measures**
- **Healthcare delivery systems**
- **Healthcare systems**
- **Health systems**
- **Medical malpractice**
- **Preponderance of the evidence**
- **Negligence law**
- **Proximal cause**
- **System errors**

Discussion Questions

Take a look at the questions posed in the following scenarios, which were presented at the beginning of this chapter. See now whether you can answer them.

1. George did not have health insurance and went to the emergency room whenever he needed care. They always treated him there, but then tried to get him connected to a primary care facility. He was not eligible for care at the Veterans Administration facilities, so they sent him to the local community health center, which they called the "safety net" provider. George did go there and they tried to treat his problems and get him his medicine. When he got sick, however, George went back to the emergency department. Even George agreed that it was not the best way to get care, but he wondered: What is needed to make the system work better?

2. Laura had breast cancer and it had spread. Her medical records were on file at the hospital, at four doctor's offices, in two emergency rooms, and at an outpatient imaging facility. No one seemed to know how to put the system together. Whenever her old records were essential, they asked her to go get a copy of them and bring them to her next appointment. That worked for a while, but when she ended up in the emergency room, her records just were not available. *There must be a better way,* Laura thought to herself. *Has the healthcare system not discovered the Internet yet?*

3. Fred ended his walk one day at the emergency room. He seemed confused about how to get home. "It looks like we are dealing with Alzheimer's," his doctor told Fred's wife, Sonya, at their next appointment. Taking care of Fred at home was not easy. Home health aides and occasional weekend relief called "respite care" eased the burden for a while. The new assisted-living facilities looked attractive, but Fred's family just could not afford one. When Fred fell and broke his hip, he required hospitalization for surgery. The hospital discharge planner arranged for a skilled nursing home for rehabilitation services paid for by Medicare. After a few weeks there, the only alternative was long-term or custodial care in a nursing home paid for by Medicaid. The care at the nursing home was not what the family had expected. The staff did clean Fred up before the announced family visits, but once when the family arrived unannounced, they were shocked to see Fred lying half-naked in his wheelchair. The end came almost two years from the day they moved him to the nursing home. Looking back, the family asked: Can the healthcare system do better at addressing the needs of Alzheimer's patients?

REFERENCES

1. Shi L, Singh D. *Delivering Health Care in America: A Systems Approach*. 4th ed. Sudbury, MA: Jones and Bartlett Publishers; 2008.

2. Sultz HA, Young KM. *Health Care USA: Understanding Its Organization and Delivery*. 6th ed. Sudbury, MA: Jones and Bartlett Publishers; 2009.

3. Shem S. *The House of God: The Classic Novel of Life and Death in an American Hospital*. New York: Delta Trade Paperbacks; 2003.

4. Taylor J. *The Fundamentals of Community Health Centers, National Health Policy Forum*. Washington, DC: The George Washington University; 2004:23.

5. National Committee for Quality Assurance. Report cards. http://reportcard.ncqa.org/plan/external/Resources.aspx?Header=yes&Tab=Glossary#Accreditation. Accessed August 12, 2013.

6. Kaiser Permanente. Kaiser Permanente—more than 60 years of quality. http://xnet.kp.org/newscenter/aboutkp/historyofkp.html. Accessed July 24, 2013.

7. United States Department of Veterans Affairs. History of the Department of Veterans Affairs. http://www.va.gov/about_va/vahistory.asp. Accessed July 24, 2013

8. Centers for Medicare and Medicaid Services. The Affordable Care Act: helping providers help patients: a menu of options for improving care. http://www.cms.gov/Medicare/Medicare-Fee-for-Service-Payment/ACO/index.html?redirect=/aco. Accessed July 24, 2013.

9. Institute of Medicine Committee on Data Standards for Patient Safety. *Key Capabilities of an Electronic Health Record System: Letter Report*. Washington, DC: National Academies Press; 2004.

10. MedicalMalpractice.com. Elements to prove in medical negligence cases. http://www.medicalmalpractice.com/resources/medical-malpractice/medical-negligence-lawsuits/4-elements-prove-medical-negligence-. July 24, 2013.

11. Institute of Medicine. To Error Is Human: Building a Better Health Care System. Washington, DC: National Academies Press; 1999.

12. The Joint Commission. Medical errors disclosure—selected bibliography. http://www.jointcommission.org. Accessed July 24, 2013.

CHAPTER 11

Health Insurance and Healthcare Systems

LEARNING OBJECTIVES

By the end of this chapter, the student will be able to:

- identify the largest governmental insurance systems in the United States and explain the basic principles of their financing.
- describe the employment-based health insurance system in the United States and discuss how fee-for-service insurance and capitated insurance options have evolved in recent years.
- describe the features of the Affordable Care Act that represent key changes to the U.S. health insurance system.
- describe the basic structure and financing aspects of the healthcare systems in Canada and the United Kingdom and compare them to those of the United States.
- identify and describe six sources of excess costs in the U.S. healthcare system.
- identify strategies for reducing the costs of health care in the United States.

You take a job right out of college and need to select from among your company's comprehensive healthcare options. The choices appear to be quite complicated and none of them seems just right for you. You wonder: What are the key differences between comprehensive health insurance plans?

The Benjamin family has a teenaged son and a daughter who recently graduated from college and is looking for a job. Their son had a heart defect at birth requiring surgery. After starting his own business in 2009, John Benjamin had a great deal of difficulty getting insurance that he could afford because of his son's heart condition. Lynette Benjamin went back to work recently, primarily in order to take advantage of the health insurance offered by her employer. How is this family affected by the Affordable Care Act?

Jorge Rios's family is without health insurance. He works two jobs, neither of which provides health insurance. He earns a total income of slightly over the federal poverty level, which in his state means the family is not eligible for Medicaid. His state has recently accepted federal funds to expand its Medicaid program as part of the Affordable Care Act. Jorge was born in the United States, but his brother, who lives with the family, is undocumented. Jorge is now trying to pay off the bills for his brother's treatment when he was recently seen in the emergency department. How is this family affected by the Affordable Care Act?

The Johnson family's annual income is $300,000, so they thought they would never need to worry about money, until their son Bob was diagnosed with a brain tumor in 2008. They sought and he got the best available treatment. The hospital stays and the initial treatments went well and were covered by the comprehensive insurance provided by George Johnson's law firm. Things changed when one day the family received a notice saying that they were approaching the lifetime cap on treatment of brain tumors. How is this family affected by the Affordable Care Act?

Members of the Smith family live in the United States, Canada, and the United Kingdom. They have the same inherited disease. The recommended treatment is quite similar in the three countries and can be delivered as part of primary care. How might the delivery of care and the payment for care differ among the three countries?

You wonder how the United States ranks globally in terms of the performance of its healthcare system. You are surprised when you find out that its ranking is not number one, or even near the top. Why is that? you ask yourself.

The politicians seem to agree that health care is too expensive. However, some argue for greater regulation, while others argue for less. You ask yourself: What are the options for controlling costs and what are the consequences?

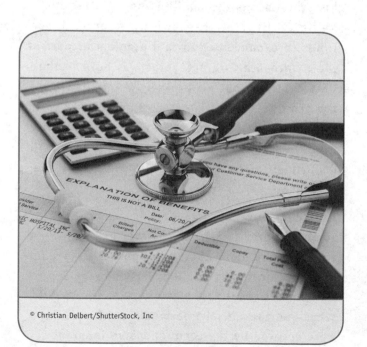

© Christian Delbert/ShutterStock, Inc

Understanding healthcare systems requires us to understand the workforce and institutions that make up the system. It also requires us to examine the central measures of success: the issues of quality, access, and cost of health care.

In this chapter, we will take a look at questions of access to and the costs of health care. Both of these issues are closely tied to the availability of health insurance to pay for health care. In the United States, there is no comprehensive right to health care. The ability to access most health care is dependent on having health insurance. Thus, to better understand the U.S. healthcare system, we will begin by taking a look at the finances. We need to know how much money is spent and how it is spent. This will require us to look at health insurance and the changes that are occurring as a result of the Patient Protection and Affordable Care Act (ACA).

Then, we will look at the overall features of the U.S. healthcare system and compare them to features of the systems in Canada and the United Kingdom. Equipped with these understandings, we will see how health systems can be scored or graded and how the United States compares with other nations. Finally, we will examine the issue of controlling costs while maintaining or improving health care quality—a major challenge facing the U.S. health system today. Let us start by looking at how much we currently spend on health care.

HOW MUCH MONEY DOES THE UNITED STATES SPEND ON HEALTH CARE?

The United States spends approximately $3 trillion per year on health care. That represents over 18% of the gross domestic product, or approximately $9,000 per person per year. Dollars spent have been growing faster than inflation for over 40 years. At the current rate of growth, the United States is estimated to spend 20% of its gross domestic product on health care by early in the next decade.[1]

Continuing that rate of growth takes money away from other activities, which makes it more difficult for the United States to compete globally or have discretionary resources to spend. Other developed countries, such as Canada, the United Kingdom, France, Germany, Japan, and Australia, spend about half as much per person and generally spend 10% or less of their gross domestic product on health care.

To understand how we spend so much of our money on health care, it is critical to know more about the U.S. health insurance system. Much of the money spent on health care, whether by individuals, businesses, or government, pays for insurance coverage. The majority of the remaining funds are spent to fill in the holes in insurance coverage through direct payments by patients called **out-of-pocket expenses**.

BOX 11-1   Important Insurance Terms

Cap—A limit on the total amount that the insurance will pay for a service per year, per benefit period, or per lifetime.

Copayment—An amount that the insured is responsible for paying even when the service is covered by the insurance. **Coinsurance**, in contrast, is the percentage of the charges that the insured is responsible for paying.

Covered service—A service for which health insurance will provide payment or coverage if the individual is eligible—in other words, any deductible has already been paid.

Customary, prevailing, and reasonable—These standards were used in the past by many insurance plans to determine the amount that would be paid to the provider of services. Under many employer-based plans, the provider may bill patients above and beyond this amount. This is known as balance billing.

Deductible—The amount that an individual or family is responsible for paying before being eligible for insurance coverage.

Eligible—An individual may need to meet certain criteria to be eligible for enrollment in a health insurance plan. These may include an income level for Medicaid, age and enrollment in the Social Security system for Medicare, or specific employment requirements for employer-based insurance. Health status is not generally a factor in eligibility.

Medical loss ratio—The ratio of benefit payments paid to premiums collected—indicating the proportion of the premiums spent on health services. Lower medical loss ratios imply that a larger amount of the premium is retained by the insurance company for administrative costs, marketing, and/or profit.

Out-of-pocket expenses—The cost of health care that is not covered by insurance and is the responsibility of the insured. These costs may be due to caps on insurance, deductibles, copayments, and/or balance billing.

Portability—The ability to continue employer-based health insurance after leaving a job—usually by paying the full cost of the insurance. A federal law, known as COBRA, generally ensures employees 18 months of portability but requires the employee to pay the entire cost of the health insurance.

Premium—The price paid by the purchaser for the insurance policy on a monthly or yearly basis.

Let us look at the basic types of insurance available in the United States. We start by examining government-financed insurance. We will then take a look at employment-based insurance. Finally, we will take a look at the changes that are occurring in health insurance in the United States. Before getting started, however, it is important to understand the language of health insurance. **Box 11-1** defines some important insurance terms.

WHAT TYPES OF GOVERNMENT-SUPPORTED HEALTH INSURANCE ARE AVAILABLE?

The two largest government programs of insurance are **Medicare** and **Medicaid**.[2, 3] Both programs began in the mid-1960s, but they have very different funding sources, coverage, and populations served.[a]

Medicare

Medicare began as a program for persons 65 and older. It was expanded to include disabled persons eligible for Social Security disability benefits and those with end-stage renal disease. Today, nearly 50 million Americans are eligible for Medicare, and the number is expected to increase to over 60 million by 2020.

When Medicare began, it was designed primarily to cover hospital services and doctors' services. It did not cover drugs, most preventive services, or nursing home care. Drugs are now partially covered by Part D of Medicare. Preventive services are covered only when specifically approved by Congress or when it can be shown that they actually save the Medicare system money. Skilled nursing or rehabilitative care, but not nursing home or custodial care, is covered by Medicare. Hearing aids and eyeglasses, perhaps the two most important medical devices for the elderly, are not covered by Medicare.

Medicare is a federal government program, which means that eligibility and benefits are consistent throughout the United States. Medicare is primarily funded by a payroll tax of 1.45% from employees and 1.45% from employers. There is no income limit on this tax, and high-income individuals pay a higher amount. Income from investments as

---

[a] The federal government also provides health care through the Veterans Administration, military health systems, and the Indian Health Service. The Veterans Administration is required to provide health care for military service–related conditions, but may—contingent upon resources—also provide care to veterans for nonservice-related conditions. The military healthcare system provides care directly or contracts for care through the TriCare system for all active duty military members and their families. American Indian and Alaskan Native members of federally recognized tribes are eligible for comprehensive health services, as well as public health services provided or funded through the Indian Health Service.

well as employment is now taxed. Self-employed individuals pay the employer as well as the employee share.

Medicare is a complicated program because there are four different parts: A, B, C, and D. The following describes the current basic costs and coverage of Medicare. The details are expected to change in coming years.

Part A covers hospital care, skilled nursing care, and home health care after a hospitalization, as well as hospice care. It is paid for primarily by the payroll tax, and no premium is required. An annual deductible is required before receiving payments.

Part B is a voluntary supplementary insurance that covers a wide range of diagnostic and therapeutic services provided by physicians, emergency departments, and other outpatient services. For most people, about 75% of the cost of Part B is funded by general tax revenues and about 25% by a monthly premium, which starts at approximately $100 per month. Those with higher incomes pay higher premiums, up to a maximum of approximately 80% of the cost of Part B. Those covered by Part B are still responsible for copayments of 20% for most services. There is also a deductible of approximately $150 per year. Health insurance policies called **Medigap** policies, which are offered by private insurance companies, are often obtained by individuals to cover all or most of the 20% copayment.

Part C is a special program designed to encourage Medicare beneficiaries to enroll in prepaid health plans.

Part D is a relatively new prescription drug coverage plan. It is a complicated plan that is open to those who are enrolled in Parts A and B of Medicare. It requires a monthly premium and an annual deductible. The exact terms depend on contracts through private plans that compete in part by offering lower costs or greater coverage. For example, coverage may include 75% of the costs of covered drugs once the deductible is satisfied, up to approximately $2,500 in drug costs. A gap, or "doughnut hole," in which no coverage is provided occurs above the $2,500 limit but is being gradually eliminated over the next few years. Once an enrolled individual reaches a "catastrophic level" of total annual drug costs of about $5,000, Medicare pays 95% of the additional cost of drugs.

Medicaid

Medicaid is a federal plus state program designed to pay for health services for specific categories of poor people and other designated categories of individuals. In the basic program, the federal government pays a variable amount of the cost ranging from 50 to 83%, depending on the per capita income of the state. These funds are designed to match the funds provided by a state based on the state's Medicaid formula. All states have chosen to be part of the basic program

and therefore must provide benefits for such groups as the disabled, children, and pregnant women based on the federal poverty level. The federal poverty level for a family of 4 is currently slightly under $25,000 per year. Thus, there have been a substantial number of poor and near-poor individuals, especially men, who have not been eligible for the basic Medicaid program. As we will discuss later in this chapter, eligibility for Medicaid is being expanded under the **Affordable Care Act** in states that choose to participate.

States at their discretion may include and receive federal matching funds for other categories of "medically needy" and may increase the eligible income level up to 185% of the federal poverty level. Most states cover custodial care in nursing homes for eligible individuals who have limited financial resources. As a result, Medicaid has become the largest source of insurance funds for nursing homes.[b]

In order to obtain federal matching funding through Medicaid, states that administer the program must provide basic services that include most inpatient and outpatient services, including preventive services. States may choose to offer other services, and the federal government will provide matching funds for a wide range of services including drugs, eyeglasses, and transportation services. Thus, for those who are eligible for Medicaid, the coverage is usually quite comprehensive. However, the reimbursement rates to clinicians are often comparatively low, and clinicians may choose not to participate in the Medicaid program.

A program begun in the late 1990s called the **State Child Health Insurance Program (SCHIP)** provides additional funds that states may use to enhance the health care of children. This may include raising the income level for Medicaid eligibility, starting eligibility more rapidly, and ensuring longer periods of eligibility. In 2009, Congress expanded and made this program more flexible, utilizing funds from an increase in the tax on cigarettes.

Medicaid now covers approximately 50 million individuals, about half of whom are children. Funds spent on the elderly, who constitute less than 10% of Medicaid beneficiaries, exceed those spent on children. The rising costs and increasing number of individuals eligible for the Medicaid program have led many states to require that Medicaid enrollees become members of a Medicaid-managed care organization in an effort to reduce costs and improve continuity of care.

---

[b] Medicaid requires that eligible individuals have very limited financial resources. Those with financial resources are generally expected to utilize most of these resources before becoming eligible. This process is known as "spending down." Complicated rules govern this process, including efforts to transfer the funds as gifts to others, including family members.

WHAT TYPES OF EMPLOYMENT-BASED HEALTH INSURANCE ARE AVAILABLE?

Employment-based insurance is the largest single category of insurance coverage in the United States. Approximately 50% of all Americans have the option to purchase some form of this type of insurance.

Employment-based insurance is in large part an accident of history. During World War II, employers were prohibited from raising wages. Instead, they offered healthcare benefits. Employment-based insurance grew rapidly in the 1950s and 1960s based on a principle known as **community rating**. Community ratings implied that the cost of insurance was the same regardless of the health status of a particular group of employees. Community rating has since been replaced by what is called **experience rating** or **medical underwriting**. This concept means that employers and employees pay based on their groups' use of services in previous years.[c]

In the 1950s and 1960s and in many parts of the country well into the 1990s, employment-based insurance provided payments to clinicians and hospitals based almost entirely on **fee-for-service** payments, often using the customary, prevailing, and reasonable criteria. Fee-for-service, as its name implies, consists of charges paid for specific services provided, and as a payment system, it encourages the provision of as many services as possible. Thus, this system has been accused of increasing healthcare costs through overuse of services.

In 1973, the federal government began to encourage an alternative approach to employment-based insurance called health maintenance organizations (HMOs). HMOs charge patients a monthly fee designed to cover a comprehensive package of services. Clinicians or their organizations are paid based upon the number of individuals that enroll in their practice. Their compensation is based on what is called **capitation**, which is a fixed number of dollars per month to provide services to an enrolled member regardless of the number of services provided. Classic HMOs are traditionally "staff model" HMOs, like Kaiser Permanente, that directly or indirectly provide the entire package of services.

Capitation, as opposed to fee-for-service, has the potential for underuse of services in an effort to reduce costs. HMOs, in contrast to a fee-for-service system, generally cover preventive services and thus argue that they do a better job of keeping people healthy.[d]

Classic fee-for-service systems and classic staff model HMOs represent the two traditional models of employment-based health insurance in the United States. Beginning in the 1990s, both these systems began to change in ways that brought them closer together.

Fee-for-service systems often evolved into what are called **preferred provider organizations**, or **PPOs**. Staff model HMOs developed options for what are called **point of service plans (POSs)**. PPOs imply that the fee-for-service insurance system decides to work with only a limited number of clinicians, called preferred providers. These providers, who form the plan's network, agree to a set of conditions that usually includes reduced payments and other conditions. Patients may choose to use other clinicians in what is called out-of-network care, but if they do so, they typically will pay more out of pocket.

Point of service plans imply that patients in an HMO may choose to receive their care outside the system provided by the health plan. Like a PPO patient who goes out of network, patients who choose the POS option must expect to pay more out of pocket. PPOs and POSs are today the most common forms of employment-based insurance. They now come in a variety of forms and together can be called mixed models. An employer may offer its employees a number of complicated mixed model choices, as well as ones that are closer to the classic fee-for-service plus HMO staff model, or classic HMOs. To better understand the types of options faced by employees, take a look at **Box 11-2**.

The basic elements of Medicare, Medicaid, and employment-based health insurance have been in place for several decades. A big change occurred in March 2010, when President Obama signed the Patient Protection and Affordable Care Act, often referred to as the Affordable Care Act (ACA) or Obamacare. The ACA legislation, which remains controversial, is in the process of being implemented. The law is a massive piece of legislation that will touch nearly every aspect of the U.S. healthcare and public health systems. However, it is important to recognize that the ACA is first and foremost what President Obama characterized as health insurance reform.

[c] It has been argued that community rating is a form of health insurance that is closer to the social justice approach to health care because individuals and groups with better health subsidize those with poorer health and greater expenses. This implies that experience rating has moved the system toward a market justice approach. Note that mental health services are now treated the same as services directed at physical health under all types of health insurance plans.

[d] It has been argued that the reason HMOs provide preventive services is related to the increased interest and use of these services by healthy individuals. Enrolling predominately healthy individuals has been called **skimming**. By enrolling these individuals, HMOs can reduce their overall costs because healthy individuals are far less likely to require large amounts of health care.

BOX 11-2 Prototype Health Insurance Options

Let us imagine that you go to work for a large employer that offers a full range of comprehensive health insurance options. The options fall into three basic categories: fee-for-service classic, mixed-model, and HMO classic. Your employer offers the following chart (**Table 11-1**) comparing the benefits and costs of each of these three options. Employers often subsidize the cost of insurance for the employee but not for the rest of the employee's family.

Now, let us put ourselves in the position of those who may need to choose among these options and think about which option they might choose.

- A healthy, single, 22-year-old male right out of college with an income of $30,000.
- A healthy, 30-year-old, recently married professional who intends to start a family in the next year. Their family income is $60,000.

- A 40-year-old married employee with a family of four with a family income of $80,000. Both husband and wife require ongoing treatments to prevent illness, including regular preventive care and expensive medications.
- A 35-year-old single parent of two young children and an income of $30,000. The mother and children need preventive care and the mother needs regular mental health care.
- A 55-year-old single professional with an income of $250,000 and no current major medical problems.

Today these types of choices face most employees of large organizations. No one plan is likely to be the best plan for everyone. In reality, there are often far more choices, and the best choice for each employee can be very difficult to determine. The classic models are rapidly disappearing, and a wide range of mixed models are now the usual options facing employees.

TABLE 11-1 Prototype Health Insurance Options

	Classic fee-for-service	Mixed model	Classic HMO
Monthly cost to employee	$200 for employee $1,200 for family of 4 $1,000 yearly deductible per person	$100 for employee $600 for family of 4 $500 yearly deductible per person	$50 for employee $300 for family of 4 No yearly deductible
Choice of physician and other clinicians	No restrictions—full coverage Physicians paid "prevailing fee"	No restrictions, 20% copayment for out of network Physician paid lower discounted fee for service	Staff physicians only Full coverage Physicians paid through capitation
Access to specialists, including OB-GYN	Access without referral—full coverage	Access with referral—full coverage Access without referral—20% copayment	Access with referral only
Drugs	Full coverage as ordered	$20 copayment for generic or approved/formulary drugs	$10 copayment for generic or approved/formulary drugs
Hospital	Full coverage as authorized by physician	80% coverage if preauthorized by plan	100% coverage if preauthorized by plan
Skilled nursing	Full coverage if ordered by physicians	80% coverage if found necessary by plan	100% coverage if found necessary by plan
Hospice	100% coverage based on physician authorization	80% coverage based on plan authorization	100% coverage based on plan authorization
Preventive services	Not covered	100% coverage in network 20% copayment out of network	100% coverage in network
Emergency department and out-of-area services	100% coverage	Requires prior authorization except in emergencies as defined by "reasonable person"	Requires prior authorization except in emergencies as defined by "reasonable person"

The ACA aims to provide increased access to healthcare services by reducing the number of uninsured, who numbered approximately 50 million people, or 15% of the population before passage of the ACA. It also aims to greatly reduce underinsurance, which affected approximately an additional 25 million people, most of whom received health insurance through their employment with small businesses. Underinsurance, with its inadequate coverage for severe illness, often led to bankruptcy when major illness occurred. Let us look at key health insurance approaches included in the ACA legislation.

WHAT ARE THE KEY HEALTH INSURANCE CHANGES INCORPORATED INTO THE ACA LEGISLATION?[4]

The following outlines the key health insurance changes that are incorporated into the ACA legislation.

Ensure more comprehensive and secure health insurance coverage: All insurance companies are restricted from denying coverage to those with preexisting conditions. Renewal of insurance is now guaranteed, in that insurance companies are prohibited from rescinding coverage except in the case of fraud. Caps on lifetime coverage and annual coverage are eliminated, and maximum annual out-of-pocket limits are generally required. Dependent children up to 26 years of age may remain on their parents' health insurance coverage.

Expand Medicaid: The ACA expands the Medicaid program for citizens and legal immigrants to include all those who make up to 133% of the federal poverty level. The federal government is paying for nearly all of the cost of this expansion. However, as a result of the 2012 Supreme Court ruling, states may choose not to participate.

Individual mandate: Individuals are required to purchase health insurance or face an additional tax. Most U.S. citizens and legal residents will be required to purchase health insurance or pay the additional tax. This provision, which is central to healthcare reform, was ruled constitutional as a tax by the 2012 U.S. Supreme Court ruling. The tax will gradually increase and take into account income. In 2016, the penalties will be the greater of $695 or 2.5% of taxable income per person.

Employer mandate: Employers with 50 or more employees are generally required to offer affordable health insurance or pay a penalty. The employer mandate was needed to encourage employers to continue offering or start offering health insurance. Without such a mandate, employers may have found it profitable not to offer health insurance and let their employees purchase their own health insurance with federal subsidies, shifting more of the costs of healthcare reform to the taxpayers.

Exchanges: The **health insurance exchanges**, or exchanges, are Web-based competitive marketplaces for the purchase of health insurance. They are intended initially for those who must purchase individual policies or for those employed by small businesses with fewer than 50 employees that do not offer health insurance with minimum expected coverage. The legislation encourages gradual expansion of the exchanges.

Exchanges are required to offer 4 types of insurance packages with average coverage as follows: bronze, covering ~60% of costs; silver, covering ~70% of costs; gold, covering ~80% of costs; and platinum, covering ~90% of costs. For adults who are under 30 years of age and eligible to receive health insurance as an individual through an exchange, a catastrophic plan with a high deductible and lower cost will be available. Catastrophic polices must include coverage of preventive services and limited primary care coverage but will not include the package of essential benefits. Subsidies are available for purchase of insurance through the exchanges for individuals and families. For instance, a subsidy is available for a family of 4 whose income is up to 4 times the federal poverty level, which currently is slightly over $90,000.

Competition is expected to help make the cost of policies purchased through the exchanges more affordable. Insurers may adjust the cost of policies for age, family size, geographic area, and tobacco use, but the ACA limits the extent to which this can occur.

Essential benefit packages included in insurance sold through the exchanges: The ACA mandates a package of essential benefits that must be included in insurance policies sold through exchanges except for the limited option to purchase catastrophic policies for those under 30. The essential benefit package includes at least ambulatory patient services, emergency services, hospitalization, maternity and newborn care, mental health, prescription drugs, rehabilitative services, habilitative services to address existing disabilities, laboratory services, wellness services, chronic-disease management, and pediatric services. Approved preventive services must be offered without **cost sharing**, or shifting costs to individuals. These include approved vaccines, recommended screening and preventive care for women, and preventive interventions given grades of A or B by the U.S. Preventive Services Task Force, indicating the net benefit is moderate to substantial.

Encourage cost sharing but limit its impact: Cost sharing is used as an incentive to discourage overuse of services under the ACA. Cost sharing, including deductibles and copayments, generally continues under the ACA. Limits are placed on cost sharing by the annual limit on out-of-pocket expenses. In addition, these costs will be subsidized for those with lower incomes. To encourage use of approved preventive interventions, cost sharing will not generally apply to approved preventive services. High coverage policies without cost sharing, known as "Cadillac" policies, will be discouraged by a tax to take effect in 2018.

Key provisions of the ACA, including new rules governing insurance coverage and the individual mandate, went into effect in January 2014. Implementation of the employer mandate was delayed until January 2015. Full implementation will not occur until at least 2018. However, it is already possible to speculate on what the U.S. health insurance system might look like when the ACA phase-in is completed.

WHAT MIGHT THE UNITED STATES HEALTH INSURANCE SYSTEM LOOK LIKE WHEN THE ACA PHASE-IN IS COMPLETED?

Greater protections for individuals and families: A range of provisions in the legislation provide protections for individuals and families who purchase health insurance. The legislation prohibits excluding or charging more for those with preexisting conditions. In addition, the ACA eliminates lifetime and annual caps and prohibits rescinding coverage except for fraud. These provisions should make coverage more predictable and secure with fewer personal bankruptcies due to serious illness. The availability of insurance through the exchanges should allow employees to more easily change jobs without fear of losing health insurance or needing to pay the full cost of the insurance.

Fewer uninsured: The individual mandate incorporated into the healthcare legislation as well as the penalties for businesses that do not offer adequate insurance are likely to increase the extent of coverage and reduce the problem of underinsurance. The ability of young adults to remain on their parents' policy until age 26 is also likely to increase coverage. It has been estimated that over 30 million additional individuals will be covered, but approximately 20 million, primarily undocumented aliens, will remain uninsured even when the ACA legislation is fully implemented.

Those without health insurance receive less preventive care, are diagnosed at more advanced stages of disease, receive less treatment once diagnosed, and have a higher mortality rate. They are much less likely to have a usual source of health care and are more likely to use the emergency department for routine care.[5]

More standardized coverage: The new exchanges provide standardized insurance packages with defined essential benefit packages, limits on cost sharing, and a choice of cost and payment levels. These packages are likely to be increasingly utilized by employment-based insurance as well. It should be easier for individuals and for families to compare insurance policies and know what they are purchasing.

More competition in offering insurance: The ACA ensures continuation of nongovernmental health insurance offered by for-profit as well as not-for-profit companies. The legislation encourages increased competition, including requiring the availability of multistate options in the exchanges. The ACA also creates a new type of private nonprofit health insurer, called a Consumer Operated and Oriented Plan, or "CO-OP." CO-OPs are directed by their customers and offer individuals and small businesses insurance options through the exchanges. CO-OPs are encouraged by the ACA through subsidies of start-up costs for a limited number of CO-OPs. The impact of the increased competition is not yet clear, but greater choice and lower costs are clearly the goals.

Expansion of the exchanges: Several provisions of the ACA, including efforts to encourage multistate plans and healthcare choice compacts intended to permit selling of insurance between states and to incorporate larger employee groups in the exchanges in later years, suggest that the legislation may lay the groundwork for a regional or national approach to purchasing health insurance. Keep an eye on the success in how the exchanges are working because they are central to the success of the ACA.

Higher taxes on high-income individuals: Medicare taxes increased in 2013 for high-income individuals, who are defined as those having an income from wages of $200,000 for those filing as individuals and $250,000 for those filing jointly. A new tax on investment income of up to 3.8% was also added. The income thresholds for these taxes are not indexed to inflation so that a growing percentage of the population will be subject to these taxes in the future.

Continuing efforts to control costs: The ACA does very little to directly control costs. The changes it makes in the structure and financing of the health insurance system should have some impact over the coming decade. The need to address the cost increases that are occurring in the employment-based insurance system as well as the government-supported systems will not go away. Expect continued debate and new efforts for many years to come.

We have described the basic components of the U.S. healthcare system, including the health professionals and institutions that provide health care, and addressed issues of quality and access. We are now ready to compare the U.S. healthcare system to that of other developed countries and examine the big issue of cost. First, let us look at a framework that we can use to describe and compare healthcare systems.

HOW CAN WE DESCRIBE HEALTHCARE SYSTEMS IN GENERAL AND THE UNITED STATES HEALTHCARE SYSTEM IN PARTICULAR?

One approach to describing healthcare systems is to define their characteristics using the following categories:

- Method of financing
- Method of insurance and reimbursement
- Methods for delivering services
- Comprehensiveness of insurance
- Cost and cost containment
- Degree of patient choice
- Administrative costs

Table 11-2 uses these categories to describe the complex U.S. healthcare system.

The U.S. system is often compared to those of Canada and the United Kingdom. Despite the fact that these countries have much in common, their healthcare systems have evolved in very different ways.

HOW CAN WE DESCRIBE THE HEALTHCARE SYSTEMS IN CANADA AND THE UNITED KINGDOM?

Let us use the same chart we used to describe the U.S. system to outline the features of the Canadian[6] and United Kingdom[7] healthcare systems. **Table 11-3** describes the Canadian healthcare system, and **Table 11-4** describes the healthcare system in the United Kingdom.

WHAT CONCLUSIONS CAN WE REACH FROM THESE DESCRIPTIONS OF THE HEALTHCARE SYSTEMS IN THE UNITED STATES, CANADA, AND THE UNITED KINGDOM?

These charts highlight key features of the three systems, while demonstrating substantial differences. When describing these

TABLE 11-2 Describing the U.S. Healthcare System

Category	Description
Financing	Cost approximately 18% of GDP and rising rapidly Complicated mix of federal, state, employer, and self-pay
Type(s) of insurance and reimbursement	Employment-based insurance plus government insurance through Medicare and Medicaid provide most insurance. New exchanges provide options for individuals and small business employees. Mix of fee-for-service, capitation, and salary with incentives are the most commonly used methods
Delivery of care	Mix of practice types with private practice dominant Physicians: 33% primary care; 66% specialists Primary care increasingly based upon nurse practitioners and physician assistants Hospitalists increasingly coordinate inpatient care Need for better continuity of care between institutions and between clinicians. New Accountable Care Organizations aiming to coordinate care for Medicare recipients.
Comprehensiveness of insurance	Until recently, 15% uninsured plus half again as many underinsured. Approximately 20 million expected to remain uninsured. Health insurance with cost sharing offered through employment-based insurance and through health insurance exchanges, as well as government programs including Medicaid and Medicare. Preventive services increasing, insurance obtained through exchanges requires coverage of approved preventive services and no copayments for approved preventive services; also generally requires coverage of essential benefits. Drug benefits provided through Medicare, Medicaid, exchange-purchased insurance, and most employment-based insurance.
Cost and cost containment	Emphasis on competition as means of controlling costs, plus cost sharing by patients
Patient choice	Considerable choice of primary care and often direct access to specialty care Greatly increased access for those with comprehensive insurance with high levels of provider reimbursement
Administrative costs	High: 25–30% of total costs, including administrative costs of health insurance, clinicians, and institutions, but this does not include administrative time spent by patients and their families

TABLE 11-3 Describing the Canadian Healthcare System

Category	Description
Financing	National policy to keep expenditures under 10% of GDP Combination of provincial and federal ~70% government through taxes ~30% private insurance payments by individuals
Type(s) of insurance and reimbursement	Government insurance for basic/essential services, individual policies with subsidies for the poor for most other services Negotiated fee-for-service reimbursement with single payer for basic services
Delivery of care	Mix of practice types with private practice dominant—emphasis on physicians in primary care Physicians ~50% primary care and ~50% specialists Primary care physicians generally admit to the hospital and are responsible for continuity of care Concerns about limited access to high-tech procedures
Comprehensiveness of insurance	Three-tiered: 1. Medically necessary basic services—universal coverage. Government funded and guaranteed to all without any cost sharing, including preventive services. No private insurance allowed for medically necessary services. 2. Private insurance and government-subsidized insurance for other medical services, including drugs, long-term care, home care with government payment for needy. Negotiated bulk purchasing of drugs on formulary keeps cost down. 3. Private insurance or self-pay for dental, vision, and many nonphysician services
Cost and cost containment	Capital purchases, such as of high-tech diagnostic equipment, are regulated and at times restricted Concern about waiting time for access Negotiated fees between providers and government with government as single payer having considerable negotiating power
Patient choice	Choice of primary care physician Referral often needed to see specialists
Administrative costs	Low—approximately 15% or less of total costs

characteristics, we can ask: On the spectrum of market justice versus social justice, where do the United States, Canada, and the United Kingdom lie?

It can be argued that the United States relies most heavily on market justice, while the United Kingdom places the greater emphasis on social justice. Canada lies somewhere in between. The ACA legislation has moved the United States in the direction of social justice while relying on market mechanisms to implement the changes.

In describing these systems, it can also be useful to identify areas in which the United States has unique approaches and unique results. The following distinguish the U.S. healthcare system not only from that of Canada and the United Kingdom, but also from the healthcare systems of most other developed countries:

- The United States spends considerably more per person and as a percentage of gross domestic product (GDP).

- The United States continues to have a higher percentage of uninsured individuals, even after the implementation of the ACA.
- The U.S. healthcare system is more complex for patients and providers of care and costs far more to administer.
- The U.S. healthcare system places more emphasis on specialized physicians and on nurse practitioners and physician assistants to provide primary care.
- The United States encourages rapid adoption of technology, especially for diagnosis and treatment.
- The United States places greater emphasis on giving patients a wider choice of clinicians.
- The United States has a more complex system for ensuring quality and a unique system of malpractice law.

Equipped with all this information, we will now see if it is possible to grade or score the performance of the U.S. healthcare system compared to those of other developed countries.

TABLE 11-4 Describing the United Kingdom's Healthcare System

Category	Description
Financing	Budget about 8% of GDP, has been rising Tax-supported comprehensive and universal coverage through National Health Service Private insurance system with overlapping coverage purchased as additional coverage by ~15% of the population with perception of easier access and higher quality
Type(s) of insurance and reimbursement	National Health Service is single payer with capitation, plus incentives for general practitioners, i.e., physicians responsible for a panel of patients Specialists generally salaried in National Health Service often earn substantial additional income through private insurance system
Delivery of care	Governmental system of healthcare delivery in National Health Service, including government-owned and administered hospitals Emphasis on physicians Primary care general practitioners ~66% Specialist physicians ~33% General practitioners generally do not admit to hospital
Comprehensiveness of insurance	National Health Service comprehensive with little cost sharing plus may cover transportation costs Incentives to provide preventive services and home care
Cost and cost containment	Overall limit on national spending ("global budgeting") Negotiated rates of capitation and salary with government as single payer with National Health Service having considerable negotiating power
Patient choice	National Health Service provides limited choice of general practitioners Waiting lines for services in National Health Service, especially specialists and high-tech procedures Referral to specialists generally needed Greater choice with private insurance
Administrative costs	Greater than Canada, less than United States

HOW CAN A HEALTHCARE SYSTEM BE SCORED?

The Commonwealth Fund's Commission on a High Performance Health System (the Commission)[e] has developed the National Scorecard on the U.S. Health System (National Scorecard).[8] The national scorecard uses a standardized set of measurements to try to objectively measure performance in 19 developed countries. **Box 11-3** outlines the criteria used to score these healthcare systems and the types of measurements that are used.

Let us take a look at how the United States scores in comparison with other developed countries based upon the national scorecard.

USING THE NATIONAL SCORECARD, HOW DOES THE UNITED STATES' HEALTHCARE SYSTEM PERFORM COMPARED TO THOSE OF OTHER DEVELOPED COUNTRIES?

The Commission scored the performance of 19 developed countries, including the United States, 14 European nations, Canada, Japan, New Zealand, and Australia. It set benchmarks high, but established realistic levels of performance for each area using the score of the top three countries as

e The Commonwealth Fund describes itself as "a private foundation working toward a high performance health system."[9] The national scorecard on U.S. Health Systems Performance was developed by a commission appointed by the Commonwealth Fund made up of individuals who, according to the Commonwealth Fund, are "distinguished experts and leaders representing every sector of health care, as well as the state and federal policy arena, the business sector, professional societies, and academia".[10]

BOX 11-3 Criteria and Measurements Used in the Commonwealth Fund's Commission on a High Performance Health System

The Commission's scorecard measures the following five areas of health system performance:

- *Healthy lives:* National health outcomes using such measures as life expectancy, infant mortality, HALEs at age 60, limitations in activities among adults under 65, and missed school days by children due to illness or injury
- *Quality:* Quality of preventive, curative, and rehabilitative health care using such measures as adults and children receiving recommended preventive services; control of chronic diseases; availability of services (including mental health) after hours and on an urgent basis; hospital quality of care, including the ratio of observed to expected mortality; and preventive measures in nursing homes
- *Access:* Availability of care using such measures as insurance coverage, including the percentage of uninsured and underinsured, as well as the impact of the cost of insurance
- *Efficiency:* Inappropriate, wasteful, or fragmented care using such measures as emergency department use for routine care, hospital admissions for preventable conditions, short-term readmission rates, and costs of administration
- *Equity:* Disparities in health services and health outcomes by racial/minority status and income using such measures as access to preventive and acute services, control of chronic diseases, insurance coverage, and measures of healthy lives

The scores from each of these areas are added together to produce overall scores.

TABLE 11-5 Performance of United States Compared to Best Performing Countries—2011

Area of performance	U.S. score (out of 100)
Healthy lives	70
Quality	75
Access	55
Efficiency	53
Equity	69
Overall score	64

Data from The Commonwealth Fund. Commission on a High Performance Health System. Available at http://www.commonwealthfund.org/Publications/Fund-Reports/2011/Oct/Why-Not-the-Best-2011.aspx. Accessed August 10, 2013.

Table 11-5 summarizes the performance of the United States on each of the criteria, as well as the overall score.

The score for access will hopefully improve on future surveys as the ACA changes in health insurance are fully implemented. Perhaps the greatest negative aspect of the U.S. healthcare system is the issue of high and escalating costs. This is reflected in the U.S. score for efficiency of 53 on the Commonwealth score. Let us complete our look at the U.S. healthcare system by examining the options for controlling costs.

HOW CAN THE COSTS OF HEALTH CARE BE CONTROLLED IN THE UNITED STATES?

To understand the options for controlling costs, it is important to first understand the reasons that costs are increasing. The United States is not alone in facing increased costs for health care. There are a number of forces at work in most developed countries that increase and most likely will continue to increase the costs of health care, including the following:

- *The aging of the population:* The success of public health and healthcare efforts over the last century has produced a population that is living longer. Longer life is strongly associated with the development of chronic diseases, many of which require expensive care over many years or decades.
- *Technological innovations have greatly expanded treatment options:* A wide range of interventions is now possible, some of which can have dramatic impacts on longevity and the quality of life. However, many others produce very modest improvements at high

the highest standard. Thus, high but realistic performance is given a score of 100.

The Commission has scored the performance of these 19 countries three times, most recently in 2011. The scores in the United States changed very little over the period of 2006 to 2011.

costs. It may be difficult to distinguish these different types of results.

- *The successes of medical care over the last half century have raised the expectations of patients*: Greater expectations for access to technology, preventive interventions, individualized care, rapid access to care, privacy, and protection of confidentiality are now all possible, but often are quite expensive.

Nearly all developed countries face these forces to a greater or lesser extent. Many countries in Europe, as well as Japan, face an even more rapidly aging population than the United States. How the healthcare systems respond to these challenges will determine in large part the overall costs of health care in each country.

The United States, however, also faces some issues to a far greater extent than other developed countries. The United States healthcare system has a far more complex, diverse, and changing structure. The sheer complexity of the system has led to a need for multiple levels of administration, which are not required in most other countries, where care is often paid by one source called a **single payer**. In addition, patients in the United States are often expected to fill out and process complex insurance applications and claim forms. Clinicians are often required to bill for each service provided, justify the services provided, and, in many cases, obtain approval for payments prior to treating patients. Today, a clinician's office usually has far more individuals involved in administering the system compared to those directly delivering care to patients.

The United States also has a far more complex and changing system of quality control. As we have seen, healthcare quality is monitored and maintained via a system that includes accreditation, certification, licensure, and malpractice, to name a few. The direct and indirect costs of this system may themselves contribute to the large and escalating cost of health care.

The Institute of Medicine recently examined the excess costs that are built into the U.S. systems of delivering and paying for health care.[9] **Box 11-4** describes its findings.

A variety of efforts has been and efforts are continuously being made to reduce costs in the United States. These include:

- *Cost control through reimbursement incentives*: The concept of capitation has been widely used as a mechanism for controlling or reducing costs. A special form of capitation, diagnosis-related groups (DRGs), has been successfully used to reduce the length of stay

---

BOX 11-4 Excess Costs of Health Care in the United States

The Institute of Medicine has identified the following six categories of excess costs of health care. For each category, the institute indicates the types of excess costs that occur. In addition, it has estimated the potential annual savings from each of the six categories of excess costs.

Unnecessary services and overuse—beyond evidence-established levels—$210 billion

- Discretionary use beyond benchmarks
- Unnecessary choice of higher-cost services

Inefficiently delivered services—$130 billion

- Mistakes—errors, preventable complications
- Care fragmentation
- Unnecessary use of higher-cost providers
- Operational inefficiencies at care delivery sites

Excess administrative costs—$190 billion

- Insurance paperwork costs
- Insurers' administrative inefficiencies
- Inefficiencies due to care documentation requirements

Prices that are too high—$105 billion

- Service prices beyond competitive benchmarks
- Product prices beyond competitive benchmarks

Missed prevention opportunities—$55 billion

- Primary prevention
- Secondary prevention
- Tertiary prevention

Fraud—$75 billion

- All sources—payers, clinicians, patients

Together, these excess costs come to over $750 billion per year, or approximately 25% of the dollars the United States spends on health care. Efforts to reduce these costs provide great opportunities for controlling healthcare costs without jeopardizing quality or access.

Data from Institute of Medicine. The Healthcare Imperative: Lowering Costs and Improving Outcomes-Workshop Series Summary. Available at: http://iom.edu/Reports/2011/The-Healthcare-Imperative-Lowering-Costs-and-Improving-Outcomes.aspx. Accessed June 27, 2013.

in hospitals. DRGs pay hospitals a set amount for a particular diagnosis, regardless of the length of hospital stay. However, reimbursement systems at times have moved the costs from one part of the system to another. Restrictions on payment for procedures may increase the number of procedures performed. Restriction on inpatient reimbursement may encourage an increase in outpatient or home care services.

- *Cost sharing*: This involves efforts to shift the costs of health care to individuals on the assumption that individuals will spend less when the costs are coming out of their pockets. Methods such as deductibles, copayments, and caps are all intended to reduce costs by shifting them to individual patients.

- *Regulation*: At times, efforts have been made to reduce costs by placing limits on how much care can be provided or how much compensation can be provided. Government-controlled health insurance, such as Medicare and Medicaid, is most easily targeted for

these types of regulation. The national issue of rates of compensation for clinicians and hospitals has become part of the political process.

- *Restrictions on malpractice*: It has been argued that the U.S. malpractice system encourages clinicians to practice "defensive medicine"—that is, to perform unnecessary tests to protect themselves against lawsuits. The extent of the problem and the impact of changes in malpractice are controversial, but efforts are being made to reduce the number of lawsuits that reach the court system and to restrict the amount of compensation that can be awarded beyond actual damages.

A more general approach to reducing costs favored by many in the United States is to increase competition between providers of health services, including institutions and individual clinicians and groups of clinicians. To better understand the potential for competition to succeed and the changes that are occurring to encourage competition, take a look at **Box 11-5**.[10]

BOX 11-5 Using Competition to Control Costs

The healthcare system in the United States is perhaps the most market-oriented system of any major nation. To successfully control costs through market mechanisms, a number of characteristics of a well-functioning market need to be in place. It has been argued that, until recently, the U.S. healthcare system has not reflected most of these characteristics. Advocates of a market approach often share these concerns, but argue that it is possible to modify the U.S. healthcare system so that it functions as a better market system.

Let us take a brief look at key features of a well-functioning market, examine the extent to which the U.S. healthcare system fulfills these conditions, and examine changes that are being made or considered to move the United States toward a more efficient market-based system.

- *Informed purchaser:* An informed purchaser is a key requirement for a well-functioning healthcare market. In the U.S. healthcare system, the employer often serves an intermediary role in selecting the health plans from which their employees may choose. Until recent years, employers paid little attention to the details of the health plans that they offered. However, that habit is changing rapidly. Cost information is now widely available to both employees and employers, and quality

measures are also becoming available. Employers often rely on accreditation standards, such as those of the National Committee for Quality Assurance, which now accredits a range of types of health plans and group practices. In addition, data on outcomes for surgical and medical procedures is increasingly available at the level of the hospital and group practice. In terms of purchasing health insurance, the exchanges are required to provide an increasing amount of information. In addition, health insurance navigators must be provided to assist consumers in choosing between insurance offerings provided through the exchanges.

- *Purchasing power:* The second requirement of a well-functioning market is the ability of those who need the product to have the purchasing power to obtain it. The subsidies that are available for health insurance purchased through the exchanges are designed to provide purchasing power to a wide range of previously uninsured and underinsured consumers.

- *Multiple competing providers:* Well-functioning markets give purchasers a choice of service providers. Consumers' choices then generally favor providers who offer the services at reduced costs and/or increased

(continues)

BOX 11-5   Using Competition to Control Costs (*continued*)

quality. The availability of choices for employed individuals has increased in recent years, especially for those whose employers pay a substantial portion of the premiums. Employees of large firms and organizations typically have a range of choices and can choose their health plan based on criteria including cost, quality, and/or convenience. For health insurance purchased through exchanges, two or more insurance providers are required, as well as choices between bronze, silver, gold, and platinum plans.

- *Negotiation:* Negotiation is the key to putting information, purchasing power, and competition together.

These negotiations increasingly take place through the employer. However, labor unions are becoming more involved in issues related to health benefits as well because health insurance constitutes an increasing percentage of their current, as well as future, benefits. The individual employee often has little negotiating power and needs to rely on his or her employee representatives and/or employers.

If the U.S. healthcare system continues to move in the direction of becoming a competitive healthcare market, it will need to ensure that these conditions are fulfilled as much as possible.

Understanding healthcare systems is a challenge for patients, as well as those who work in the system. Understanding the roles of healthcare professionals, institutions, and the issues of quality, access, and cost help us understand the system as a whole.

A well-functioning healthcare system is essential to the public's health. An efficient system that works in concert with organized public health efforts and leaves adequate financial resources to invest in programs directed at the health of the entire population is a key goal. The population health approach thus needs to pay considerable attention to the workings of the public and private healthcare system, as well as the workings of the public health system.

KEY WORDS

- Out-of-pocket expenses
- Cap
- Copayment
- Coinsurance
- Covered service
- Customary, prevailing, and reasonable
- Deductible
- Eligible
- Medical loss ratio
- Portability
- Premium
- Medicare
- Medicaid
- Medigap
- Affordable Care Act
- State Child Health Insurance Program (SCHIP)
- Community rating
- Experience rating or medical underwriting
- Fee-for-service
- Capitation
- Preferred provider organization (PPO)
- Point of service plan (POS)
- Skimming
- Health insurance exchanges
- Cost sharing
- Single payer

Discussion Questions

Take a look at the questions posed in the following scenarios, which were presented at the beginning of this chapter. See now whether you can answer them.

1. You take a job right out of college and need to select from among your company's comprehensive healthcare options. The choices appear to be quite complicated and none of them seems just right for you. You wonder: What are the key differences between comprehensive health insurance plans?

2. The Benjamin family has a teenaged son and a daughter who recently graduated from college and is looking for a job. Their son had a heart defect at birth requiring surgery. After starting his own business in 2009, John Benjamin had a great deal of difficulty getting insurance that he could afford because of his son's heart condition. Lynette Benjamin went back to work recently, primarily in order to take advantage of the health insurance offered by her employer. How is this family affected by the Affordable Care Act?

3. Jorge Rios's family is without health insurance. He works two jobs, neither of which provides health insurance. He earns a total income of slightly over the federal poverty level, which in his state means the family is not eligible for Medicaid. His state has recently accepted federal funds to expand its Medicaid program

as part of the Affordable Care Act. Jorge was born in the United States, but his brother, who lives with the family, is undocumented. Jorge is now trying to pay off the bills for his brother's treatment when he was recently seen in the emergency department. How is this family affected by the Affordable Care Act?

4. The Johnson family's annual income is $300,000, so they thought they would never need to worry about money, until their son Bob was diagnosed with a brain tumor in 2008. They sought and he got the best available treatment. The hospital stays and the initial treatments went well and were covered by the comprehensive insurance provided by George Johnson's law firm. Things changed when one day the family received a notice saying that they were approaching the lifetime cap on treatment of brain tumors. How is this family affected by the Affordable Care Act?

5. Members of the Smith family live in the United States, Canada, and the United Kingdom. They have the same inherited disease. The recommended treatment is quite similar in the three countries and can be delivered as part of primary care. How might the delivery of care and the payment for care differ among the three countries?

6. You wonder how the United States ranks globally in terms of the performance of its healthcare system. You are surprised when you find out that its ranking is not number one, or even near the top. *Why is that?* you ask yourself.

7. The politicians seem to agree that health care is too expensive. However, some argue for greater regulation, while others argue for less. You ask yourself: What are the options for controlling costs and what are the consequences?

REFERENCES

1. The Henry J. Kaiser Family Foundation. Health care costs: A primer. http://kaiserfamilyfoundation.files.wordpress.com/2013/01/7670-03.pdf. Accessed October 8, 2013.

2. Shi L, Singh D. *Delivering Health Care in America: A Systems Approach.* 4th ed. Sudbury, MA: Jones and Bartlett Publishers; 2008.

3. Sultz HA, Young KM. *Health Care USA: Understanding Its Organization and Delivery.* 6th ed. Sudbury, MA: Jones and Bartlett Publishers; 2009.

4. The Henry J. Kaiser Foundation. Health reform. http://kff.org/health-reform. Accessed June 27, 2013.

5. Institute of Medicine. *Hidden Costs, Value Lost: Uninsurance in America.* Washington, DC: National Academies Press; 2003.

6. Health Canada. Health care system. http://www.hc-sc.gc.ca/hcs-sss/index-eng.php. Accessed June 27, 2013.

7. National Health Service History. Chapter from *From Cradle to Grave: 50 Years of the NHS.* http://www.nhshistory.net/envoi1.html. Accessed June 27, 2013.

8. The Commonwealth Fund. Why not the best? Results from the national scorecard on U.S. health system performance, 2011. http://www.commonwealthfund.org/Publications/Fund-Reports/2011/Oct/Why-Not-the-Best-2011.aspx Accessed October 6, 2013.

9. The Commonwealth Fund. A private foundation working toward a high performance health system. http://www.commonwealthfund.org. Accessed October 6, 2013.

10. The Commonwealth Fund. Commission on a high performance health system. http://www.commonwealthfund.org/~/media/Files/Annual%20Report/2012/2012_AR_Commission%201219.pdf. Accessed October 6, 2013.

11. Institute of Medicine. The healthcare imperative: lowering costs and improving outcomes—workshop series summary. http://iom.edu/Reports/2011/The-Healthcare-Imperative-Lowering-Costs-and-Improving-Outcomes.aspx. Accessed June 27, 2013.

12. CATO Institute. Health care needs a dose of competition. http://www.cato.org/pub_display.php?pub_id=5070. Accessed June 27, 2013.

SECTION IV

Cases and Discussion Questions

WHEN NURSING MEETS MEDICINE

Maureen felt she had no other choice but to let the hospital administrator know when a physician had repeatedly prescribed the wrong dose of medication. How many times could she double-check with Dr. George Ludwig just to be sure that she had understood his orders? *Orders, they still call them*, she thought to herself. *That is certainly what they want them to be.*

The days of obeying orders were over for Maureen. She had been through nursing school, and after five years working in the hospital, she went back to get her doctor of nursing practice degree to become a nurse specialist so she could work in an intensive care unit. Now she was doing the weekend 12-hour nursing shift to make ends meet and finish her doctoral degree. Nurses were in short supply, so she could now for the first time speak her mind without fear of losing her job. Nursing, she realized, was by its very name designed to nurture and take care of patients, but that did not apply to physicians. Their arrogance was so deep, she did not think they saw it.

Hospital policy required nurses to follow the orders after first checking with the head nurse and then double-checking with the physician who wrote the order. Complaints could be filed with the hospital quality assurance committee, but the process took months and the nurse who initiated the process could be reprimanded if the committee found his or her complaints to be unfounded or trivial. Trivial, this was not, but when she confronted the hospital administrator, he confided, "Do not put me in the middle of this." The pharmacist finally agreed to call the doctor and check on whether he preferred the "standard dose" of medication or the "unusual dose" he had first ordered. Dr. Ludwig agreed that the standard dose was "worth a try," so Maureen went ahead and followed the doctor's new orders.

Not too many months later, Maureen found herself confronted with new decisions in her first job as a nurse specialist in the intensive care unit. She now worked under "standing orders," which allowed her to make many decisions on her own. For the first time, she felt like she was calling the shots and making the decisions that made a difference for patients.

On one shift, late in the middle of the night, she was running from bed to bed covering the intensive care unit when she realized that she had given a patient the wrong medication. Fortunately, it was not a life-threatening mistake. She sighed with relief. Checking the chart carefully, however, she winced when her eyes fell upon the name of the attending physician, Dr. George Ludwig.

Discussion Questions

1. How is Maureen's situation affected by the structure of the nursing profession?

2. How is Maureen's situation affected by the changes in roles of women that have occurred in the United States in the last 40 years?

3. How is Maureen's situation affected by the changes that have occurred in the delivery of health care over the last 10–20 years?

4. What changes do you think are needed in the healthcare system to prevent the types of mistakes illustrated in this case?

JACK AND CONTINUITY OF CARE

Jack was told that he had high blood pressure and high cholesterol when he was in the army. Because the conditions did not bother him, Jack paid little attention to them. His job did not provide health insurance, so he decided to take his chances rather than spend his last dollar paying for insurance through an exchange. Anyway, he was strong and athletic. Over the years, Jack gained weight, exercised less, and developed a "touch of diabetes."

When the diabetes produced symptoms, he went to the emergency room, where they did a good job of diagnosing his problem and sent him off with a prescription and a few pills to get started. The pills seemed to help, but Jack could not afford to fill the prescription or follow up with his "family doctor" because he did not have one. Jack did not understand all the terms the doctors and nurses used to describe his condition, but he knew it was serious and could get worse.

It was not long before he was sick again, so this time, he sought care at a community health center. He did not qualify for Medicaid, but the treatment was affordable. For a couple of months, he followed up and was feeling better, but on the next scheduled visit, they told him, "You need to be in the hospital—you are getting worse." They got him to the hospital, where he was admitted to the university service and assigned to a young resident who had just graduated from a well-known medical school. The resident reviewed his condition, developed a treatment plan, and explained to Jack what needed to be done. He ordered a TB skin test and collected sputum to check for TB because of Jack's chronic cough. Unfortunately, before the treatment could be implemented, the resident rotated to another service and Jack's new resident did not seem to pay much attention to him.

Jack decided to leave the hospital against medical advice and left no forwarding address. His TB skin test was never read. When his positive sputum culture for TB came back, the laboratory alerted the local health department. Not knowing where Jack lived, the health department was not able to follow up.

Before he left, the hospital made sure that Jack had signed all the forms to receive Medicaid payments for the hospitalization. However, Jack did not complete the forms because he did not plan to get any more medical care. That changed one day when the pain was more than he could stand. He decided to try another emergency room. This time, the place was very crowded and he had to wait hours to be seen. Once he was examined, the physicians and nurses tried to get information from him on his condition and treatment, but Jack could not provide much useful information.

He was prescribed pain medicine and sent home. He was told to follow up with a doctor in the next few days. By then, it was too late. One morning as he was getting up, Jack's left leg was weak and numb and he had lost his speech. He struggled to call 911. Despite the fact that he could not speak, the operator was able to send an ambulance by tracing his telephone location. The EMTs rushed to Jack's home and got him to the nearest hospital. Once again, the emergency room clinicians evaluated him, but this time, it was too late to be of much help. Jack was admitted for a stroke.

He stayed in the hospital for a week and made some improvement, but he needed help with the activities of daily living and could only speak a few words. The hospital was able to place him in a rehabilitation center because Jack, now 65, qualified for skilled nursing care under Medicare. He was transferred to the facility and received intensive rehabilitation services for the next month, until he no longer improved. At that point, Jack was no longer eligible for skilled nursing care. He was transferred to a Medicaid nursing home closer to his only relatives. The new facility had a large number of patients needing "custodial care." It provided all the services required by law, but Jack soon realized that he was just another stroke patient.

Discussion Questions

1. How does this case illustrate the lack of institutional continuity?

2. How does this case illustrate the lack of continuity between the healthcare and public health systems?

3. How does this case illustrate the lack of financial continuity?

4. What role does the lack of information play in this case? How can information technology serve to reduce or eliminate these lapses in continuity?

5. Which lapses in continuity require other types of interventions?

DONNA'S DOCTOR—TO ERROR IS HUMAN

Donna's heart was racing again and there just did not seem to be a reason for it. She was not upset and had not been exercising. She was only 48, and no one seemed to take her seriously when she told everyone that something was wrong with her heart. She knew it was more than her recent divorce and raising a couple of teenagers. Not even the diagnosis of menopause satisfied her.

She decided to change primary care doctors, having heard that Dr. Stein actually listened. He did listen and examined her carefully, but did not find anything. He ordered a 24-hour test to monitor her heart. Donna did her usual activity and the portable device recorded a basic electrocardiogram. She had one brief episode of racing heart. She recorded the time and length of the episode just as requested, and sure enough, she was having a brief episode of what the doctor called "atrial fibrillation" at the recorded time.

A week later, Donna got the results—episodes of atrial fibrillation. The upper chambers of her heart, called the atria, were beating very rapidly. Her lower chambers, called the ventricles, which pump the blood out of the heart, were doing just fine, so she was not in immediate danger.

"The real danger is blood clots and potentially a stroke," Dr. Stein told her, "and we should thin, or anticoagulate, your blood."

The thought of a stroke was enough to convince Donna to go ahead.

Anticoagulation can be done economically using a drug called Warfarin, often known by the brand name Coumadin, she was told, but it has to be done carefully. It can cause bleeding if it is not checked often. Taking Coumadin, Donna felt protected. She went back for the tests to adjust the dose. She felt better and now had lots of energy, but she still had some of those episodes of rapid heart rate.

When the hot flashes began, she knew that menopause had in fact arrived, but she felt better than ever and found herself skipping her blood tests because she wanted to be sure that she had time for her exercise routine. She did not realize that anything was wrong until she fell off her bike one day, hitting her head. Fortunately, she was wearing a helmet, so the injury did not seem too bad. However, she did feel dizzy afterward. And then a few hours later, her son told her that her speech was slurred.

"Have you been drinking, Mom?" he asked.

The look of disdain on his mother's face was enough to worry her son, who now insisted on taking her to the emergency room.

Dr. Stein met Donna and her son in the emergency room. He arranged an emergency MRI scan, which showed evidence of a small bleed, and the blood test showed her anticoagulation level was too high. The doctors rapidly reversed the level, and over the next few days, Donna's mental state returned to normal.

What a relief, she thought, *but there has to be a better answer than going back to anticoagulation.* Her doctors in the hospital asked for a consultation. First, the medical student, then the resident, and finally the professor came to look her over, examined her carefully, and then talked about her just outside her door, where she could hear bits and pieces of their conversation. "Dr. Stein sure missed the diagnosis"…"If she had only been compliant, none of this would have happened"…"An obvious case of hyperthyroidism"…"No need for Coumadin."

"The blood tests confirm overactivity of your thyroid, which is a condition called hyperthyroidism," the resident told her. "This caused your atrial fibrillation and your increased energy. You need treatment, but we do not do that here—we will give you a referral."

Donna could hardly absorb everything and did not get a chance to even ask questions.

She went back to Dr. Stein, who told her how badly he felt about missing the hyperthyroidism—he too had learned a lesson and he apologized for what had happened. He told her that there was very good treatment for hyperthyroidism and he would be pleased to take care of her after consultation with a specialist. Donna knew that doctors make mistakes, but she did not know that they admitted them. She knew that Dr. Stein was a good doctor and that he would pay extra attention to her. Donna hoped that things would go well and was confident that she was in good hands with Dr. Stein.

Discussion Questions

1. Did Dr. Stein's care fulfill the duty, breach, causation, and damages criteria for medical malpractice?

2. What additional aspects of Dr. Stein's care affected whether a malpractice case resulted?

3. What role do you think the disclosure of error played in preventing a malpractice suit?

4. What attitudes toward decision making in health care on the part of Donna influenced the approach she took to her health care?

HEALTH CARE IN THE UNITED STATES—FOR BETTER OR WORSE?

The final hours came as no surprise to his wife and family, who made daily visits to the hospital where Sam had been treated on and off for the final year of his life. His doctor had spared no expense to give him the most effective treatments available.

But wouldn't it have been nice if he could have died at home? they thought to themselves as they gathered at the funeral. *At least he held out until after the baby was born.*

Sam's diagnosis of colon cancer did not shock him. His father had died of colon cancer, and he had been thinking for some time that it was time to be checked. Surgery went well and he and his doctor were optimistic about the future. The surprise came about 18 months later, when during a follow-up examination, he was told that there might be a recurrence.

Chemotherapy seemed to do more harm than good. There did not seem to be a good answer. Sam's physician sought out the newest treatment, but it did not seem to help. The final shock to his system came after he received a dose of the wrong medicine administered by a nurse who was new to the unit. She was hired in response to the recent accreditation review, which criticized the hospital for understaffing.

Though his death was no surprise, the bills from the hospital and physician were an unexpected burden in the months and years that followed. The health insurance that was offered through Sam's employer did not pay for screening for the colon cancer that killed him. In addition, its loopholes, caps, and copayments left the family with bills that would require years to repay. It was not just the uncovered expenses that they had to pay out of pocket; it was the mountains of paperwork that arrived in the mail.

Nonetheless, the family understood. The doctors had done everything possible, treated Sam and them with respect, and responded quickly to their calls and continuous questions. Maybe things were not ideal, they concluded, but at least they did everything they could.

Discussion Questions

1. What strengths of the U.S. healthcare system are illustrated in this case?

2. What limitations of the U.S. healthcare system are illustrated in this case?

3. How would the Affordable Care Act affect the services provided in this case?

4. What steps would you recommend to improve the delivery of preventive and curative services to better serve patients like Sam?

5. How might Sam's health care have been different in other developed countries, such as Canada and the United Kingdom? In what ways might it have been better and in what ways might it have been worse?

EXCESS COSTS—HOW MUCH CAN BE SAVED?

Doris, an 80-year-old white female, had been previously healthy. Her mother had a history of hip fracture. Doris was told to take extra calcium to prevent osteoporosis, but she was never tested or prescribed any treatment.

One Saturday morning, Doris fell in her home and landed on her hip. She lay in pain for about an hour before she was able to reach the telephone and call for help. The ambulance took her to the nearest hospital rather than the hospital she had requested. The doctors at the hospital had none of her medical records and did not realize that she was allergic to penicillin, which they prescribed because of the deep skin abrasions she suffered in the fall. Within minutes after receiving a shot of penicillin, she experienced anaphylaxis, a severe allergic reaction, and required an emergency team to be called to provide immediate resuscitation.

Doris was admitted to the intensive care unit on a Friday night. She underwent X rays and was seen by five teams of doctors over the weekend. The doctors determined that she had a hip fracture and needed surgery as soon as possible. No surgeons were available to see her until Monday morning, at which time surgery was scheduled for Wednesday morning.

While Doris was in the hospital, the physicians decided to do a work-up for gallbladder disease because gallbladder disease is very common in her age group. The scans did show gallstones, and she was initially advised to have surgery for her gallstones. A consult recommended that rather than surgery, she seek health care if she ever had pain in the area of the gallbladder.

The physicians who took care of Doris in the hospital decided to treat her aggressively for osteoporosis using the newest and most expensive medication. The medication was covered by Medicare because Doris was in the hospital. The medication could be given by an injection and lasted for a year.

After discharge, Doris was supposed to receive physical therapy to be sure that she was ambulatory and did not develop blood clots in her legs. Unfortunately, the wrong telephone number and address were provided to the physical

therapy team, and it took a week before the physical therapists were able to locate Doris to begin physical therapy.

Doris began the therapy, but on the second day in the middle of the treatment, she became short of breath. The physical therapist recognized the signs of a pulmonary embolism, or a blood clot traveling to the lungs. She immediately called the ambulance, which took Doris to the same hospital where she stayed before.

The hospital staff recognized that Doris had been discharged less than one month earlier and were concerned that Medicare might not pay the bills for her readmission. They decided to transfer her to the hospital that she had originally requested. She was successfully treated for pulmonary emboli and was followed up as an outpatient on a weekly basis for several months.

Doris received over 40 mailings related to the billing for her hospitalization, many of which said, "This is not a bill." She did receive 10 separate bills, including ones from the two hospitals, three laboratories, the physical therapy group, and four different doctor groups. The bills for her care totaled $215,000, $212,000 of which was covered by Medicare or her Medigap policy. The bills included a $50,000 bill for the orthopedic surgery, which was fully covered, and a $1,000 bill for transportation to the second hospital, which was not covered by Medicare.

When Doris inspected the 10-page bill from the hospital, she noticed a bill to Medicare for equipment for three blood transfusions. "No one told me about that," she said to herself, so she called the hospital to confirm whether she in fact had had blood transfusions. The billing clerk checked with the hospital administration, let Doris know that this was a mistake, and apologized. A week later, Doris read in the newspaper that a large number of Medicare patients were being charged for equipment for blood transfusions they never received.

Discussion Questions

1. Identify ways that each of the IOM categories of excess costs played a role in this case.

2. Identify ways that excess costs could be reduced in this case.

3. Discuss ways in which a reduction in the costs of health care in the United States could affect the quality of health care favorably.

4. Discuss ways in which a reduction in costs of health care in the United States could affect the quality of health care unfavorably.

SECTION V

Public Health Institutions and Systems

Now that we have taken a look at the U.S. healthcare institutions and healthcare system, we need to turn our attention to the public health system. Treating healthcare and public health systems as separate systems is artificial because they have many points of overlap and collaboration. However, historically, public health institutions and systems have developed from different philosophies, have different goals, and have organizational structures and lines of accountability different from those of the healthcare system.

We will begin by outlining the current goals and roles of public health agencies. Then we will look at the current system of local/state, federal, and global public health institutions and examine how they are organized. We will explore why public health agencies need to coordinate with each other to achieve the goals of public health.

We will then return to our definition of population health—the totality of all evidence-based public and private efforts to preserve and promote health and prevent disease, disability, and death. This broad 21st century definition requires public health agencies and professionals to collaborate with a range of government agencies and healthcare professionals and institutions.

After getting an overview of what public health agencies do, we will focus in on one especially important and rapidly changing area of public health: foods and drugs. In Chapter 13, we will look at food and drugs as public health issues. Concerns about food and drugs have played an important role in forming today's approaches to population health and continue to play important roles in our thinking about the future.

Finally, we will take a look in Chapter 14 at a relatively new and increasingly important part of population health known as systems thinking. Systems thinking helps us put together the pieces and think about how they can and need to work together to address today and tomorrow's complex health challenges.

Let us now turn our attention in Chapter 12 to the current public health institutions and public health systems.

CHAPTER **12**

Public Health Institutions and Systems

LEARNING OBJECTIVES

By the end of this chapter, the student will be able to:

- identify goals of governmental public health.
- identify the 10 essential services of public health.
- describe basic features of local, state, and federal public health agencies in the United States.
- identify global public health organizations and agencies and describe their basic roles.
- identify roles in public health for federal agencies not identified as health agencies.
- illustrate the need for collaboration by governmental public health agencies with other governmental and nongovernmental organizations.
- describe approaches to connecting public health and the healthcare system.

A young man in your dormitory is diagnosed with tuberculosis. The health department works with the student health service to test everyone in the dorm, as well as in his classes, with a TB skin test. Those who are positive for the first time are advised to take a course of a medicine called INH. You ask: Is this standard operating procedure?

You go to a public health meeting and learn that many of the speakers are not from public health agencies, but from the Departments of Labor, Commerce, Housing, and Education. You

ask: What do these departments have to do with health?

You hear that a new childhood vaccine was developed by the NIH, approved by the FDA, endorsed for federal payment by the CDC, and recommended for use by the American Academy of Pediatrics. You ask: Do all these agencies and organizations always work so well together?

A major flood in Asia leads to disease and starvation. Some say it is due to global warming, others to bad luck. Coordinated efforts by global health agencies, assisted by nongovernmental organizations (NGOs) and individual donors, help get the country back on its feet. You ask: What types of cooperation are needed to make all of this happen?

A local community health center identifies childhood obesity as a problem in the community. They collect data demonstrating that the problem begins as early as elementary school. They develop a plan that includes clinical interventions at the health center and also at the elementary school. They ask the health department to help them organize an educational campaign and assist in evaluating the results. Working together, they are able to reduce the obesity rate among elementary school children by 50%. This seems like a new way to practice public health, you conclude. What type of approach is this?

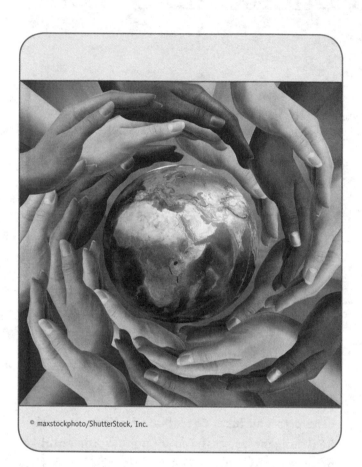

© maxstockphoto/ShutterStock, Inc.

These cases all reflect the responsibilities of public health agencies at the local, federal, and global levels. They illustrate public health working the way it is supposed to work. Of course, this is not always the case. Let us start by taking a look at the goals and roles of public health agencies.

WHAT ARE THE GOALS AND ROLES OF GOVERNMENTAL PUBLIC HEALTH AGENCIES?

Public health is often equated with the work of governmental agencies. The role of government is only a portion of what we mean by "public health," but it is an important component. It is so important, in fact, that we often define the roles of other components in terms of how they relate to the work of governmental public health agencies. That is, we may refer to them as nongovernmental public health.

In 1994, the United States Public Health Service put forth the Public Health in America statement, which provided the framework that continues to define the goals and services of governmental public health agencies.[1] These goals should already be familiar to you. They are:

- To prevent epidemics and the spread of disease
- To protect against environmental hazards
- To prevent injuries
- To promote and encourage healthy behaviors
- To respond to disasters and assist communities in recovery
- To ensure the quality and accessibility of health services

These are ambitious and complicated goals to achieve. To be able to successfully achieve them, it is important to further define the roles that governmental public health agencies themselves play, and by implication, the roles that other governmental agencies and nongovernmental organizations need to play to achieve these goals.

The Public Health in America statement built upon the Institute of Medicine's (IOM) 1988 report called *The Future of Public Health*.[2] The IOM defined three **core public health functions** that governmental public health agencies need to perform. The concept of "core function" implies that the job cannot be delegated to other agencies or to nongovernmental organizations. It also implies that the governmental public health agencies will work together to accomplish these functions because as a group, they are responsible for public health as a whole—no one agency at the local, state, or federal level is specifically or exclusively responsible for accomplishing the essential public health services.[a]

The core functions defined by the IOM are: (1) assessment, (2) policy development , and (3) assurance.[2]

- **Assessment** includes obtaining data that defines the health of the overall population and specific groups within the population, including defining the nature of new and persisting health problems.
- **Policy development** includes developing evidence-based recommendations and other analyses of options, such as health policy analysis, to guide implementation, including efforts to educate and mobilize community partnerships.
- **Assurance** includes governmental public health's oversight responsibility for ensuring that key components

---

[a] This does not imply that components of the work cannot be contracted to nongovernmental organizations. This activity is increasingly occurring. The concept of core function, however, implies that public health agencies remain responsible for these functions even when the day-to-day work is conducted through contracts with an outside organization.

of an effective health system, including health care and public health, are in place even though the implementation will often be performed by others.

The three core functions, while useful in providing a delineation of responsibilities and an intellectual framework for the work of governmental public health agencies, were not tangible enough to provide a clear understanding or definition of the work of public health agencies. Thus, in addition to the goals of public health, the Public Health in America statement defined a series of **10 essential public health services** that build upon the IOM's core functions, guide day-to-day

responsibilities, and provide a mechanism for evaluating whether the core functions are fulfilled. These 10 services have come to define the responsibilities of the combined local, state, and federal governmental public health system.

WHAT ARE THE 10 ESSENTIAL PUBLIC HEALTH SERVICES?

Table 12-1 outlines the 10 essential public health services and organizes them according to which IOM core function they aim to fulfill.[1] A description of each service is presented in column two and examples of these essential services are

TABLE 12-1 10 Essential Public Health Services

Essential service	Meaning of essential service	Examples
Core function: assessment		
1. Monitor health status to identify and solve community health problems	This service includes accurate diagnosis of the community's health status; identification of threats to health and assessment of health service needs; timely collection, analysis, and publication of information on access, utilization, costs, and outcomes of personal health services; attention to the vital statistics and health status of specific groups that are at a higher risk than the total population; and collaboration to manage integrated information systems with private providers and health benefit plans.	Vital statistics Health surveys Surveillance, including reportable diseases
2. Diagnose and investigate health problems and health hazards in the community	This service includes epidemiologic identification of emerging health threats; public health laboratory capability using modern technology to conduct rapid screening and high-volume testing; active communicable disease epidemiology programs; and technical capacity for epidemiologic investigation of disease outbreaks and patterns of chronic disease and injury.	Epidemic investigations CDC–Epidemic Intelligence Service State public health laboratories
Core function: policy development		
3. Inform, educate, and empower people about health issues	This service includes social marketing and media communications; providing accessible health information resources at community levels; active collaboration with personal health care providers to reinforce health promotion messages and programs; and joint health education programs with schools, churches, and worksites.	Health education campaigns, such as comprehensive state tobacco programs
4. Mobilize community partnerships and action to identify and solve health problems	This service includes convening and facilitating community groups and associations, including those not typically considered to be health-related, in undertaking defined preventive, screening, rehabilitation, and support programs; and skilled coalition-building to draw upon the full range of potential human and material resources in the cause of community health.	Lead control programs: testing and follow-up of children, reduction of lead exposure, educational follow-up, and addressing underlying causes
5. Develop policies and plans that support individual and community health efforts	This service requires leadership development at all levels of public health; systematic community and state-level planning for health improvement in all jurisdictions, tracking of measurable health objectives as a part of continuous quality improvement strategies; joint evaluation with the medical/healthcare system to define consistent policy regarding prevention and treatment services; and development of codes, regulations, and legislation to guide public health practice.	Newborn screening and follow-up programs for PKU and other genetic and congenital diseases

(continues)

TABLE 12-1 10 Essential Public Health Services (*continued*)

Essential service	Meaning of essential service	Examples
Core function: assurance		
6. Enforce laws and regulations that protect health and ensure safety	This service involves full enforcement of sanitary codes, especially in the food industry; full protection of drinking water supplies; enforcement of clean air standards; timely follow-up of hazards, preventable injuries, and exposure-related diseases identified in occupational and community settings; monitoring quality of medical services (e.g., laboratory, nursing home, and home health care); and timely review of new drug, biological, and medical device applications.	Local: Fluoridation and chlorination of water State: Regulation of nursing homes Federal: FDA drug approval and food safety
7. Link people to needed personal health services and ensure the provision of health care when otherwise unavailable	This service (often referred to as "outreach" or "enabling" services) includes ensuring effective entry for socially disadvantaged people into a coordinated system of clinical care; culturally and linguistically appropriate materials and staff to ensure linkage to services for special population groups; ongoing "care management"; and transportation.	Community health centers
8. Ensure the provision of a competent public and personal health-care workforce	This service includes education and training for personnel to meet the needs of public and personal health services; efficient processes for licensure of professionals and certification of facilities with regular verification and inspection follow-up; adoption of continuous quality improvement and lifelong learning within all licensure and certification programs; active partnerships with professional training programs to ensure community-relevant learning experiences for all students; and continuing education in management and leadership development programs for those charged with administrative/executive roles.	Licensure of physicians, nurses, and other health professionals
9. Evaluate effectiveness, accessibility, and quality of personal and population-based health services	This service calls for ongoing evaluation of health programs, based on analysis of health status and service utilization data, to assess program effectiveness and to provide information necessary for allocating resources and reshaping programs.	Development of evidence-based recommendations
All three IOM core functions		
10. Research for new insights and innovative solutions to health problems	This service includes continuous linkage with appropriate institutions of higher learning and research and an internal capacity to mount timely epidemiologic and economic analyses and conduct needed health services research.	NIH, CDC, AHRQ, other federal agencies

Data from Public Health in America. Essential Public Health Services. Available at http://www.health.gov/phfunctions/public.htm. Accessed July 25, 2013.

listed in column three. We have now looked at the core public health functions and the 10 essential services of public health agencies. **Figure 12-1** puts these together to allow you to see the connections.

Public health services are delivered through a complex web of local and federal agencies, as well as via increasing involvement of global organizations. Let us take a look at the work of public health agencies at each of these levels.

Figure 12-2 provides a framework to guide our review of the delivery of public health services. It diagrams the central role of governmental public health agencies and the complicated connections required to accomplish their

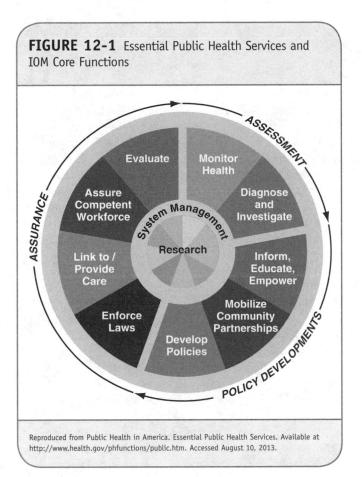

FIGURE 12-1 Essential Public Health Services and IOM Core Functions

Reproduced from Public Health in America. Essential Public Health Services. Available at http://www.health.gov/phfunctions/public.htm. Accessed August 10, 2013.

FIGURE 12-2 Framework for Viewing Governmental Public Health Agencies and Their Complicated Connections

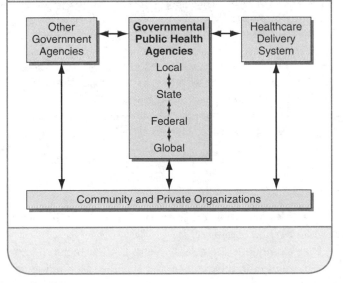

responsibilities. We will begin by taking a look at the structure and function of governmental public health agencies at the local/state, federal, and global levels. Then we will examine the key connections with other governmental agencies, community organizations, and private organizations, and finally the connections with the healthcare delivery system as a whole.

WHAT ARE THE ROLES OF LOCAL AND STATE PUBLIC HEALTH AGENCIES?

The U.S. Constitution does not mention public health. Thus, public health is first and foremost a state responsibility. States may retain their authority, voluntarily request or accept help from the federal government, or delegate their responsibility and/or authority to local agencies at the city, county, or other local levels.[b]

Box 12-1 describes a brief history of public health agencies in the United States. It is a complex history and has resulted in more structures than there are states—more because large cities often have their own public health systems.[3] In addition, the District of Columbia and several U.S. territories have their own systems and often have the authority to make public health system decisions as if they were states.

To understand the role of local health departments, it is useful to think of two models.[4] In the first model, which we will call the **home rule** or local autonomy model, authority is delegated from the state to the local health department. The local health department, or the local government, has a great deal of autonomy in setting its own structure and function and often raising its own funding.

In the second model, which we will call the branch office model, the local health department can be viewed as a branch office of the state agency with little or no independent authority or funding. There are several thousand local health departments across the country. The majority of these lie somewhere in between these two extreme models; however, these models provide a framework for understanding the many varieties of department structures. Thus, when we speak of local public health, we may be speaking of a state agency with branch offices or a relatively independent local agency. Regardless of which model a state uses, many public health responsibilities of local public health

[b] This delegation may occur at the discretion of the state government or it may be included in the state's constitution, providing what is called home rule authority to local jurisdictions. In general, jurisdictions with home rule authority exercise substantially more autonomy.

BOX 12-1   Brief History of Public Health Agencies in the United States

An understanding of the history of U.S. public health institutions requires an understanding of the response of local, state, and federal governments to public health crises and the complex interactions between these levels of government.

The colonial period in the United States saw repeated epidemics of smallpox, cholera, and yellow fever focused in the port cities. These epidemics brought fear and disruption of commerce, along with accompanying disease and death. One epidemic in 1793 in Philadelphia, which was then the nation's capital, nearly shut down the federal government. These early public health crises brought about the first municipal boards of health, made up of respected citizens authorized to act in the community's interest to implement quarantine, evacuation, and other public health interventions of the day. The federal government's early role in combating epidemics led to the establishment in 1798 of what later became known as the U.S. Public Health Service.

Major changes in public health awaited the last half of the 1800s, with the great expansion of understanding of disease and the ability to control it through community actions. The Shattuck Commission in Massachusetts in 1850 outlined the roles of state health departments as responsible for sanitary inspections, communicable disease control, food sanitation, vital statistics, and services for infants and children. Over the next 50 years, the states gradually took the lead in developing public health institutions based upon delivery of these services.

Local health departments outside of the largest cities did not exist until the 1900s. The Rockefeller Foundation stimulated and helped fund early local health departments and campaigns in part to combat specific diseases, such as hookworm. There was no standard model for local health departments. Local health departments developed in at least 50 different ways in the 50 states and were chronically underfunded.

The federal government played a very small role in public health throughout the 1800s and well into the 20th century. An occasional public health crisis stimulated in part by media attention did bring about federal action. The founding of the Food and Drug Administration in 1906 resulted in large part from the journalistic activity known as "muckraking," which exposed the status of food and drug safety. The early years of the 1900s set the stage for expansion of the federal government's role in public health through the passage of the 16th Amendment to the Constitution, which authorized federal income tax as a major source of federal government funding.

The Great Depression, in general, and the Social Security Act of 1935, in particular, brought about a new era in which federal funding became a major source of financial resources for state and local public health departments and nongovernmental organizations. The founding of what was then called the Communicable Disease Center (CDC) in 1946 led to a national and eventually international leadership role for the CDC, which attempts to connect and hold together the complex local, state, and federal public health efforts and integrate them into global public health efforts.

The Johnson administration's War on Poverty, as well as the Medicare and Medicaid programs, brought about greatly expanded funding for healthcare services and led many health departments to provide direct healthcare services, especially for those without other sources of care. The late 1980s and 1990s saw a redefinition of the roles of governmental public health, including the Institute of Medicine's definition of core functions and the development of the 10 essential public health services. These documents have guided the development of a broad population focus for public health and a move away from the direct provision of healthcare services by health departments.

The terrorism of September 11, 2001, and the subsequent anthrax scare moved public health institutions to the center of efforts to protect the public's health through emergency response and disaster preparedness. The development of flexible efforts to respond to expected and unexpected hazards is now a central feature of public health institutions' roles and funding. The success of these efforts has led to new levels of coordination of local, state, federal, and global public health agencies utilizing state-of-the-art surveillance, laboratory technology, and communications systems.

departments are quite similar, and they usually have authority and responsibility for at least the following:[4]

- Immunizations for those not covered by the private system

- Communicable disease surveillance and initial investigation of outbreaks
- Communicable disease control, often including at a minimum tuberculosis and syphilis case finding and treatment

- Inspection and licensing of restaurants
- Environmental health surveillance
- Coordinating public health screening programs, including newborn and lead screenings
- Tobacco control programs
- Public health preparedness and response to disasters

Health departments in many parts of the United States have also served as the healthcare provider for those without other sources of health care. This has been called the **health-care safety net**. In recent years, many health departments have reduced or discontinued these services, often transferring them to the healthcare system or integrating their efforts into community health centers. The concept of core functions holds that while these activities can be performed by other organizations or agencies, the public health agencies still retain responsibility for ensuring access to and the quality of these services.

The work of local public health agencies cannot be viewed in isolation. The state health department usually retains important roles even in those states where the local departments have home rule authority. These responsibilities often include collecting vital statistics, running a public health laboratory, licensing health professionals, administering nutrition programs, and regulating health facilities, such as nursing homes. In addition, drinking water regulation, administration of the state Medicaid program, and the office of the medical examiner may also fall under the authority of the state health department.

The 2003 IOM report *The Future of the Public's Health in the 21st Century*, in conjunction with the Futures Initiative of the Centers for Disease Control and Prevention (CDC), initiated the establishment of a voluntary national accreditation program for state and local health departments to advance quality and performance in health departments. Through these efforts, the Public Health Accreditation Board (PHAB) was formed, and in early 2013, the first set of health departments achieved national accreditation. The accreditation standards and measures address each of the 10 essential public health services to evaluate health department processes and services and their outcomes.[5]

Today, the federal government has a great deal of involvement in national and global issues of public health and often works closely with local agencies. Let us take a look at the structure and role of the federal government in public health.

WHAT ARE THE ROLES OF FEDERAL PUBLIC HEALTH AGENCIES?

The federal government's role in public health does not explicitly appear in the U.S. Constitution. It has been justified largely by the Interstate Commerce clause, which provides federal government authority to regulate commerce between the states. Federal public health authority often rests on the voluntary acceptance by the states of funding provided by the federal government. This may come with requirements for state action in order to qualify for the funding.

The Department of Health and Human Services (HHS) is the central public health agency of the federal government. It includes operating agencies, each of which report directly to the cabinet-level secretary of HHS. **Table 12-2** outlines most of these agencies, their roles and authority, and their basic public health structure and activities.[6]

The National Institutes of Health (NIH) is far and away the largest agency within HHS, with a budget of over $30 billion—as much as all the other six agencies' budgets combined. However, most of its efforts are devoted to basic science research and the translation of research into clinical practice. Some of the federal agencies, such as the Health Resources and Services Administration (HRSA), Substance Abuse and

TABLE 12-2 Key Federal Health Agencies of the Department of Health and Human Services

Agency	Roles/authority	Examples of structures/activities
Centers for Disease Control and Prevention (CDC) and the Agency for Toxic Substances and Disease Registry (ATSDR)	The CDC is the lead agency for prevention, health data, epidemic investigation, and public health measures aimed at disease control and prevention. The CDC administers the ATSDR, which works with the Environmental Protection Agency to provide guidance on health hazards of toxic exposures.	The CDC and ATSDR work extensively with state and local health departments. The CDC's Epidemic Intelligence Service (EIS) functions domestically and internationally at the request of governments.

(continues)

TABLE 12-2 Key Federal Health Agencies of the Department of Health and Human Services (*continued*)

Agency	Roles/authority	Examples of structures/activities
National Institutes of Health (NIH)	Lead research agency; also funds training programs and communication of health information to the professional community and the public.	17 institutes in all—the largest being the National Cancer Institute. The National Library of Medicine is part of NIH Centers, which also include the John E. Fogarty International Center for Advanced Study in the Health Sciences. NIH is the world's largest biomedical research enterprise, with intramural research at NIH and extramural research grants throughout the world.
Food and Drug Administration (FDA)	Consumer protection agency with authority for safety of foods and safety and efficacy of drugs, vaccines, and other medical and public health interventions.	Divisions responsible for food safety, medical devices, drug efficacy, and safety pre- and postapproval.
Health Resources and Services Administration (HRSA)	Seeks to ensure equitable access to comprehensive quality health care.	Funds community health centers, HIV/AIDS services, scholarships for health professional students.
Agency for Healthcare Research and Quality (AHRQ)	Research agenda to improve the outcomes and quality of health care, including patient safety and access to services.	Supports U.S. Preventive Services Task Force, evidence-based medicine research, and Guidelines Clearinghouse.
Substance Abuse and Mental Health Services Administration (SAMHSA)	Works to improve quality and availability of prevention, treatment, and rehabilitation for substance abuse and mental illness.	Research, data collection, and funding of local services.
Indian Health Service (IHS)	Provides direct health care and public health services to federally recognized tribes.	Services provided to approximately 550 federally recognized tribes in 35 states. Only comprehensive federal agency responsibility for health care plus public health services.

Mental Health Services Administration (SAMHSA), and the Indian Health Service, provide or fund individually-oriented health services in addition to population-oriented preventive services. The Indian Health Service is unique because it is responsible for both public health and healthcare services for a defined population.

The Centers for Disease Control and Prevention (CDC) is perhaps the agency most closely identified with public health at the federal level. **Box 12-2** describes its first 50 years, from 1946 to 1996, in a reprint of its official history first published in the *Morbidity and Mortality Weekly Report* (*MMWR*), a weekly publication of the agency.[7] Today, the CDC is a global partner in conducting research and epidemiologic investigations in addition to working closely with states to monitor and prevent disease through health surveillance, taking an action-oriented approach to disease prevention, and maintaining health statistics through the National Center for Health Statistics, which has been a part of the CDC since 1987.

The CDC's role in connecting federal, state, and local governmental public health efforts is central to the success of the system. Approximately half of the CDC's over $10 billion total budget is channeled to state and local health departments. A key function of the CDC is to provide national leadership and to coordinate the efforts of local/state and federal public health agencies.

To understand the local/state and federal public health system, it is important to appreciate that less than 5% of all health-related expenditures in the United States goes to governmental public health agencies, and of that, less than half goes to population-based prevention as opposed to providing healthcare services as a safety net for individuals. In addition, the role of governmental public health is limited by social attitudes toward government. For instance, we have seen that there are constitutional limitations on the authority of public health and other government agencies to impose actions on individuals. These may limit public health

BOX 12-2   History of the CDC

The Communicable Disease Center was organized in Atlanta, Georgia, on July 1, 1946; its founder, Dr. Joseph W. Mountin, was a visionary public health leader who had high hopes for this small and comparatively insignificant branch of the Public Health Service (PHS). It occupied only one floor of the Volunteer Building on Peachtree Street and had fewer than 400 employees, most of whom were engineers and entomologists. Until the previous day, they had worked for Malaria Control in War Areas, the predecessor of CDC, which had successfully kept the southeastern states malaria-free during World War II and, for approximately 1 year, from murine typhus fever. The new institution would expand its interests to include all communicable diseases and would be the servant of the states, providing practical help whenever called.

Distinguished scientists soon filled CDC's laboratories, and many states and foreign countries sent their public health staffs to Atlanta for training.... Medical epidemiologists were scarce, and it was not until 1949 that Dr. Alexander Langmuir arrived to head the epidemiology branch. Within months, he launched the first-ever disease surveillance program, which confirmed his suspicion that malaria, on which CDC spent the largest portion of its budget, had long since disappeared. Subsequently, disease surveillance became the cornerstone on which CDC's mission of service to the states was built and, in time, changed the practice of public health.

The outbreak of the Korean War in 1950 was the impetus for creating CDC's Epidemic Intelligence Service (EIS). The threat of biological warfare loomed, and Dr. Langmuir, the most knowledgeable person in PHS about this arcane subject, saw an opportunity to train epidemiologists who would guard against ordinary threats to public health while watching out for alien germs. The first class of EIS officers arrived in Atlanta for training in 1951 and pledged to go wherever they were called for the next 2 years. These "disease detectives" quickly gained fame for "shoe-leather epidemiology" through which they ferreted out the cause of disease outbreaks.

The survival of CDC as an institution was not at all certain in the 1950s. In 1947, Emory University gave land on Clifton Road for a headquarters, but construction did not begin for more than a decade. PHS was so intent on research and the rapid growth of the National Institutes of Health that it showed little interest in what happened in Atlanta. Congress, despite the long delay in appropriating money for new buildings, was much more receptive to CDC's pleas for support than either PHS or the Bureau of the Budget.

Two major health crises in the mid-1950s established CDC's credibility and ensured its survival. In 1955, when poliomyelitis appeared in children who had received the recently approved Salk vaccine, the national inoculation program was stopped. The cases were traced to contaminated vaccine from a laboratory in California; the problem was corrected, and the inoculation program, at least for first and second graders, was resumed. The resistance of these 6- and 7-year-olds to polio, compared with that of older children, proved the effectiveness of the vaccine. Two years later, surveillance was used again to trace the course of a massive influenza epidemic. From the data gathered in 1957 and subsequent years, the national guidelines for influenza vaccine were developed.

CDC grew by acquisition.... When CDC joined the international malaria-eradication program and accepted responsibility for protecting the earth from moon germs and vice versa, CDC's mission stretched overseas and into space.

CDC played a key role in one of the greatest triumphs of public health, the eradication of smallpox. In 1962 it established a smallpox surveillance unit, and a year later tested a newly developed jet gun and vaccine in the Pacific island nation of Tonga.... CDC also achieved notable success at home tracking new and mysterious disease outbreaks. In the mid-1970s and early 1980s, it found the cause of Legionnaires disease and toxic-shock syndrome. A fatal disease, subsequently named acquired immunodeficiency syndrome (AIDS), was first mentioned in the June 5, 1981, issue of MMWR.

Although CDC succeeded more often than it failed, it did not escape criticism. For example, television and press reports about the Tuskegee study on long-term effects of untreated syphilis in black men created a storm of protest in 1972. This study had been initiated by PHS and other organizations in 1932 and was transferred to CDC in 1957. Although the effectiveness of penicillin as a therapy for syphilis had been established during the late 1940s, participants in this study remained untreated until the study was brought to public attention. CDC was also criticized because of the 1976 effort to vaccinate the U.S. population against swine flu, the infamous killer of 1918–1919. When some recipients of the vaccines developed Guillain-Barre syndrome, the campaign was stopped immediately; the epidemic never occurred.

As the scope of CDC's activities expanded far beyond communicable diseases, its name had to be changed. In 1970 it became the Center for Disease Control and in 1981, after extensive reorganization, Center became Centers. The words "and Prevention" were added in 1992, but, by law, the well-known three-letter acronym was retained. In health emergencies, CDC means an answer to SOS calls from anywhere in the world, such as the recent one from Zaire where Ebola fever raged.

Fifty years ago, CDC's agenda was non-controversial (hardly anyone objected to the pursuit of germs), and Atlanta was a backwater. In 1996, CDC's programs are often tied to economic, political, and social issues, and Atlanta is as near Washington as the tap of a keyboard.

Reproduced from Centers for Disease Control and Prevention, MMWR 1996;45: 526-528.

agencies' abilities to address issues ranging from tuberculosis and HIV control to responses to emergencies.

The social attitudes of Americans may also limit the authority and resources provided to public health agencies. Americans often favor individual or private efforts over governmental interventions when they believe that individuals and private organizations are capable of success. For instance, some Americans resist active efforts in schools to provide information and access to contraceptives, while others resist the type of case-finding efforts for HIV/AIDS that have been used successfully in investigating and controlling other communicable diseases.

Today, governmental public health is a global enterprise. Let us take a look at the roles of global health organizations and agencies.

WHAT ARE THE ROLES OF GLOBAL HEALTH ORGANIZATIONS AND AGENCIES?

Public health is increasingly becoming a global enterprise. Global governmental efforts have grown dramatically in recent years. The World Health Organization (WHO) was created in 1948. Its impact has become more prominent in the 2000s with the increasing importance of global health issues. The WHO is a part of the United Nations organizations, which also include the United Nations Children's Fund (UNICEF) and the Joint United Nations Programme on AIDS/HIV (UNAIDS).[8]

Today, the World Bank and other multilateral financial institutions are the largest funding source for global health efforts.[9] National governmental aid programs, including the United States Agency for International Development (USAID), also play an important role in public health. **Table 12-3** outlines the structure/governance, roles, and limitations of global public health agencies.

The complexity of local, state, federal, and global public health agencies raises the question of whether or not these agencies can and do work together. It should not surprise you that close collaboration, while the goal, is often difficult to achieve with so many organizations involved. Thus, it is important to ask: How can public health agencies work together?

TABLE 12-3 Global Public Health Organizations

Type of agency	Structure/governance	Role(s)	Limitations
World Health Organization	United Nations Organization Seven "regional" semi-independent components, e.g., Pan American Health Organization covers North and South America	Policy development, e.g., tobacco treaty, epidemic control policies Coordination of services, e.g., SARS control, vaccine development Data collection and standardization, e.g., measures of health care quality, measures of health status	Limited ability to enforce global recommendations, limited funding, and complex international administration
Other UN agencies with focused agenda	UNICEF UNAIDS	Focus on childhood vaccinations Focus on AIDS	Limited agendas and limited financing
International financing organizations	The World Bank Other multilateral regional banks, e.g., InterAmerican and Asian Development Banks	World Bank is largest international funder. Increasingly supports "human capital" projects and reform of healthcare delivery systems and population and nutrition efforts Provides funding and technical assistance, primarily as loans	Criticized for standardized approach with few local modifications
Bilateral governmental aid organizations	USAID Many other developed countries have their own organizations and contribute a higher percentage of their gross domestic product to those agencies than does the United States	Often focused on specific countries and specific types of programs, such as the United States' focus on HIV/AIDS, and maternal and child health	May be tied to domestic politics and global economic, political, or military agendas

HOW CAN PUBLIC HEALTH AGENCIES WORK TOGETHER?

Coordination among public health agencies has been a major challenge that is built into our local, state, and federal systems of governance. Increasingly, coordination also requires a global aspect as well. Efforts on all levels have a long way to go. There are signs of hope with progress in such fields as tobacco control, food safety, and the response to SARS. **Box 12-3** discusses the dramatic events of the 2003 SARS epidemic, providing an example of what can be done and what needs to be done to address future public health emergencies.[10]

Collaboration needs to be an everyday effort, and not just a requirement for emergencies or epidemics. Let us look at the relationships and needed collaboration among governmental public health and other governmental agencies, nongovernmental organizations, and the healthcare delivery system.

WHAT OTHER GOVERNMENT AGENCIES ARE INVOLVED IN HEALTH ISSUES?

To address health issues, it is important to recognize the important roles that government agencies not designated as health agencies play in public health. Such agencies exist at the local/state, federal, and global levels. To illustrate the involvement of these agencies in health issues, let us begin with the roles of nonhealth agencies at the federal level.

A number of federal agencies serve public health functions even though they are not defined as health agencies. The roles they play are important, especially when we take the population health perspective, which includes the totality of efforts to promote and protect health and prevent disease, disability, and death.

Environmental health issues are an important part of the role of the Environmental Protection Agency (EPA). Reducing injury and hazardous exposures in the workplace are key goals of the Occupational Safety and Health

---

BOX 12-3　SARS and the Public Health Response

The SARS (Severe Acute Respiratory Syndrome) epidemic of 2003 began with little notice, most likely somewhere in the heartland of China, and then spread to other areas of Asia. The world took notice after television screens filled with reports of public health researchers sent to Asia to investigate the illness subsequently contracting and dying from the disease. Not an easily transmissible disease except for between those in very close contact, such as investigators, family members, and healthcare providers, the disease spread slowly but steadily through areas of China. Among those infected, the case-fatality rate was very high, especially without the benefits of modern intensive care facilities.

The disease did not respond to antibiotics and was thought to be a viral disease by its epidemiological pattern of spread and transmission, but at first, no cause was known. The outside world soon felt the impact of the brewing epidemic when cases appeared in Hong Kong that could be traced to a traveler from mainland China. Fear spread when cases were recognized that could not be explained by close personal contact with a SARS victim.

The epidemic continued to spread, jumping thousands of miles to Toronto, Canada, where the second greatest concentration of disease appeared. Soon, the whole world was on high alert, if not quite on the verge of panic. At least 8,000 people worldwide became sick and almost 10% of them died. Fortunately, progress came quite quickly. Researchers coordinated by the World Health Organization (WHO) were able to put together the epidemiological information and laboratory data and establish a presumed cause, a new form of the coronavirus never before seen in humans, leading to the rapid introduction of testing.

The WHO and the CDC put forth recommendations for isolation, travel restrictions, and intensive monitoring that rapidly controlled the disease even in the absence of an effective treatment aimed at a cure. SARS disappeared as rapidly as it emerged, especially after systematic efforts to control spread were put in place in China. Not eliminated, but no longer a worldwide threat, SARS left a lasting global impact. The WHO established new approaches for reporting and responding to epidemics—these now have the widespread formal acceptance of most governments.

Once the world could step back and evaluate what happened, it was recognized that the potential burden of disease posed by the SARS epidemic had worldwide implications and raised the threat of interruption of travel and trade. Local, national, and global public health agencies collaborated quickly and effectively. Infection control recommendations made at the global level were rapidly translated into efforts to identify disease at the local level and manage individual patients in hospitals throughout the world. It is a model of communicable disease control that will be needed in the future.

Administration (OSHA), which is part of the Department of Labor.

Protecting health as part of preparation and response to disasters and terrorism is central to the role of the Department of Homeland Security. The Department of Agriculture shares with the FDA the role of protecting the nation's food supply. The Department of Housing and Urban Development influences the built environment and its impacts on health. The Department of Energy plays important roles in setting radiation safety standards for nuclear power plants and other sources of energy.

The multiple federal agencies involved in health-related matters often means that coordination and collaboration are required across agencies. This is certainly the case with food safety and disaster planning and response. It is true as well for efforts to address problems that cut across agencies, such as lead exposure or efforts to reduce the environmental causes of asthma.

The collaboration needed to address complex public health issues lends itself to a health in all policies approach, which acknowledges that the variety of influences impacting population health are outside the control of the health sector. Collaborative efforts are not restricted to governmental agencies. We will now explore the roles of nongovernmental organizations in public health.

WHAT ROLES DO NONGOVERNMENTAL ORGANIZATIONS PLAY IN PUBLIC HEALTH?

Nongovernmental organizations (NGOs) play increasingly important roles in public health in the United States and around the world. The United States has a long tradition of private groups organizing to advocate for public health causes, delivering public health services, and providing funding to support public health efforts. In recent years, these efforts have been expanding globally as well.

The American Red Cross and its network of international affiliates represent a major international effort to provide public health services. The organization plays a central role in obtaining volunteers for blood donations and ensuring the safety and effectiveness of the U.S. and world supply of blood products in collaboration with the U.S. Food and Drug Administration. The ability of the Red Cross to obtain donations, mobilize volunteers, and publicize the need for disaster assistance has allowed it to play a central role in providing lifesaving public health services.

Many private organizations provide public health education, support research, develop evidence-based recommendations, and provide other public health services. Many of these are organized around specific diseases or types of disease, such as the American Cancer Association, the American Heart Association, the American Lung Association, and the March of Dimes, which today focuses on birth defects. Other private organizations focus primarily on advocacy for individuals with specific diseases, but these organizations also may advocate for specific public health interventions. For instance, Mothers Against Drunk Driving (MADD) has had a major impact on the passage and enforcement of drunk driving laws. HIV/AIDS advocacy groups have influenced policies on confidentiality, funding, and public education.

Globally, NGOs increasingly play a key role in providing services and advocating for public health policies. CARE and Oxfam International are examples of the types of organizations involved in global health-related crises. Physician groups, including Physicians for Social Responsibility and Doctors without Borders, have been active in advocating for public health efforts, seeking funding for public health needs, and addressing the ethical implementation of public health programs.

New combinations of governmental and nongovernmental organizations are increasingly developing to fill in the gaps. At the global level, the Global Fund to Fight AIDS, Tuberculosis and Malaria, a public-private effort, provides funding for evidence-based interventions to address these diseases. It is funded not only by governments, but also by private foundations, such as the Bill and Melinda Gates Foundation.

Private foundations have long played major roles in funding public health efforts and also stimulating governmental funding. The Rockefeller Foundation's efforts were instrumental in developing local health departments and initiating schools of public health in the United States during the early years of the 1900s. The Kellogg Foundation, the Robert Wood Johnson Foundation, and most recently the Gates Foundation have all played key roles in advancing public health efforts in areas ranging from nutrition to tobacco control to advancing new public health technologies.

Foundation funding has been the catalyst in initiating new funding efforts and sustaining those that are not adequately funded by governments. They cannot be expected, however, to provide long-term support for basic public health services. Thus, additional strategies are required. One key strategy is to link public health efforts with the efforts of healthcare professionals and the healthcare system.

HOW CAN PUBLIC HEALTH AGENCIES PARTNER WITH HEALTH CARE TO IMPROVE THE RESPONSE TO HEALTH PROBLEMS?

We have already seen a number of traditional connections between public health and health care. Clinicians and public health professionals increasingly share a common

BOX 12-4 National Vaccine Plan

In 1994, a National Vaccine Plan was developed as part of a coordinated effort to accomplish the following goals:

1. Develop new and improved vaccines.
2. Ensure the optimal safety and effectiveness of vaccines and immunizations.
3. Better educate the public and members of the health profession on the benefits and risks of immunizations.

A recent Institute of Medicine (IOM) report evaluated progress since 1994 on achieving these goals and made recommendations for the development of a revised National Vaccine Plan.[11] The IOM highlighted a number of successes since 1994 in achieving each of the goals of the plan. These successes illustrate the potential for improved collaboration between public health systems and healthcare systems.

In terms of the development of new and improved vaccines since 1994, over 20 new vaccine products resulting from the collaborative efforts of the National Institutes of Health (NIH), academic, and industry researchers were approved by the Food and Drug Administration (FDA). Novel vaccines introduced include vaccines against pediatric pneumococcal disease, meningococcal disease, and the human papillomavirus (HPV)—a cause of cervical cancer.

In terms of safety, vaccines and vaccination approaches with improved safety have been developed since 1994, including those directed against rotavirus, pertussis (whooping cough), and polio. The FDA Center for Biologics Evaluation and Research (CBER), which regulates vaccines, now has an expanded array of regulatory tools to facilitate the review and approval of safe and efficacious vaccines. The FDA and the Centers for Disease Control and Prevention (CDC) have collaborated on surveillance for and evaluation of adverse events. Efforts have also been made to increase collaboration with the Centers for Medicare and Medicaid Services, the Department of Defense, and the Department of Veterans Affairs to improve surveillance and reporting of adverse events following immunization in the adult populations these agencies serve.

In terms of better education of health professionals and the public, progress has also been made. The American Academy of Pediatrics (AAP) collaborates with the CDC for its childhood immunization support. The American Medical Association (AMA) cosponsors the annual National Influenza Vaccine Summit, a group that represents 100 public and private organizations interested in preventing influenza.

Despite the growing collaboration and success in vaccine development and use, new issues have appeared in recent years. Vaccines are now correctly viewed by the health professionals and the public as having both benefits and harms. In recent years, the public has grown more concerned about the safety of vaccines, including the issue of the use of large numbers of vaccines in children. The limitations of vaccines to address problems, such as HIV/AIDS, have also been increasingly recognized. Hopefully, the continued efforts to develop and implement national vaccine plans will build upon these recent successes and address the new realities and opportunities.

commitment to evidence-based thinking, cost-effective delivery of services, and computerized and confidential data systems. They also increasingly share a commitment to provide quality services to the entire population and eliminate health disparities. The potential for successful collaboration between public health and health care is illustrated by the National Vaccine Plan, which is discussed in **Box 12-4**.[11]

In the mid-1990s, the Medicine-Public Health Initiative was implemented to investigate better ways to connect public health with medicine, in particular, and health care, in general. Connecting these two fields has not always had easy or successful results. Additional structures are needed to formalize effective and efficient bonds. Models do exist and new ideas are being put forth to connect clinical care and public health. **Box 12-5** discusses one such model, called **community-oriented primary care (COPC)**.[12]

Despite efforts in the healthcare system to reach out to the community and address public health issues (such as COPC), it remains the primary responsibility of governmental public health to organize and mobilize community-based efforts. Working with nongovernmental organizations and healthcare professionals and organizations is imperative to effectively and efficiently accomplish the goals of public health. But how exactly can public health agencies accomplish these goals?

HOW CAN PUBLIC HEALTH TAKE THE LEAD IN MOBILIZING COMMUNITY PARTNERSHIPS TO IDENTIFY AND SOLVE HEALTH PROBLEMS?

An essential service of public health is the mobilization of community partnerships and action to identify and solve health problems. These efforts by public health agencies are

BOX 12-5 Community-Oriented Primary Care (COPC)

Community-oriented primary care (COPC) is a structured effort to expand the delivery of health services from a focus on the individual to also include an additional focus on the needs of communities. Serving the needs of communities brings healthcare and public health efforts together. COPC can be seen as an effort on the part of healthcare delivery sites, such as community health centers, to reach out to their community and to governmental public health institutions.

Table 12-4 outlines the six steps in the COPC process and presents a question to ask when addressing each of these steps. Notice the parallels between COPC and the evidence-based approach. In both cases, the process is actually circular because evaluation efforts often lead to recycling to move the process ahead.

A series of principles underlies COPC, including:

- Healthcare needs are defined by examining the community as a whole, not just those who seek care.
- Needed healthcare services are provided to everyone within a defined population or community.
- Preventive, curative, and rehabilitative care are integrated within a coordinated delivery system.
- Members of the community directly participate in all stages of the COPC process.

The concept of COPC, if not the specific structure, has been widely accepted as an approach for connecting the organized delivery of primary health care with public health. It implies that public health issues can and should be addressed when possible at the level of the community with the involvement of healthcare providers and the community members themselves.

TABLE 12-4 The Six Sequential Steps of Community-Oriented Primary Care (COPC)

Steps in the COPC process	Questions to ask
1. Community definition	How is the community defined based upon geography, institutional affiliation, or other common characteristics, e.g., use of an Internet site?
2. Community characterization	What are the demographic and health characteristics of the community and what are its health issues?
3. Prioritization	What are the most important health issues facing the community and how should they be prioritized based upon objective data and perceived need?
4. Detailed assessment of the selected health problem	What are the most effective and efficient interventions for addressing the selected health problem based upon an evidence-based assessment?
5. Intervention	What strategies will be used to implement the intervention?
6. Evaluation	How can the success of the intervention be evaluated?

Data from District of Columbia Area Health Education Center. The Conceptual Framework for COPC. Available at http://dcahec.gwumc.edu/education/session4/index.html. Accessed August 10, 2013.

critical to putting the pieces of the health system together to protect and promote health and prevent disability and death.

Increasingly, community members themselves are becoming active participants in addressing health and disease in their communities. One approach to engage community members in the process is through **community-based participatory research (CBPR)**. Through CBPR, community members are involved in all phases of the research process, contributing their expertise while sharing ownership and responsibility over the research, and assisting to build trust, knowledge, and skill to facilitate the research and development and implementation of interventions.

Examples of successful collaboration include state tobacco control programs that have been led by public health agencies, but rely heavily on nongovernmental organizations, healthcare professionals, and other governmental agencies. These efforts have been able to substantially reduce statewide cigarette smoking rates.

BOX 12-6 Child Oral Health and Community-Oriented Public Health (COPH)

The problem of childhood dental disease illustrates the potential for community-oriented public health (COPH). A lack of regular dental care remains a major problem for children in developed, as well as developing, countries. The need for this type of care is often high on the agenda of parents, teachers, and even the children themselves.

Public health efforts to improve oral health go back to the late 1800s and early 1900s, when tooth brushing and toothpaste were new and improved technologies. The public health campaigns of the early 1900s were very instrumental in making tooth brushing a routine part of U.S. life. The history of public health interventions in childhood oral health is a story of great hope and partial success. The benefits of the fluoridation of drinking water were well grounded in evidence. The American Dental Association and the American Medical Association have supported this intervention for over half a century. Resistance from those who view it as an intrusion of governmental authority, however, has prevented universal use of fluoridation in the United States. After over a half century of effort, fluoridation has reached less than 66% of Americans through the water supply.

Today, new technologies from dental sealants to more cost-effective methods for treating cavities have again made oral health a public health priority. However, the number of dentists has not grown in recent years to keep up with the growing population. In addition, dental care for those without the resources to pay for it is often inadequate and inaccessible. Thus, a new approach is needed to bring dental care to those in need. Perhaps a new strategy using a COPH approach can make this happen.

Community-oriented public health can reach beyond the institutional and geographical constraints that COPC faces when based in a community health center or other institutions serving a geographically defined population or community. COPH as a governmentally led effort allows a greater range of options for intervention, including those that require changes in laws, incentives, and governmental procedures. These may include authorizing new types of clinicians, providing services in nontraditional settings such as schools, funding innovations to put new technologies into practice, and addressing the regulatory barriers to rapid and cost-effective delivery of services.

Efforts to organize coordinated programs for lead control have also been met with success. Collaborative efforts between public health and health care have identified and treated children with elevated lead levels. Cooperation with other agencies has provided for the removal of lead paint from homes and testing and control of lead in playgrounds, water, and, most recently, toys.

It is possible to view the coordinated mobilization of public and private efforts as community-oriented public health (COPH). We can see this as a parallel to COPC. In COPC, healthcare efforts are expanded to take on additional public health roles. In COPH, public health efforts are expanded to collaborate with healthcare delivery institutions, as well as other community and other governmental efforts. Child oral health, an example of COPH, is illustrated in **Box 12-6**.[13]

Developing community partnerships is a time-consuming and highly political process that requires great leadership and diplomatic skills. Central authority and command and control approaches are generally not effective in the complex organizational structures of the United States. New approaches and new strategies are needed to

bring together the organizations and individuals who can get the job done.

We have now looked at the organization of the public health system and the challenges it faces in accomplishing its core functions and providing its essential services. The role of public health will continue to evolve as current and emerging issues impact the health of the population.

KEY WORDS

- **Core public health functions**
- **Assessment**
- **Assurance**
- **Policy development**
- **10 essential public health services**
- **Home rule**
- **Healthcare safety net**
- **Nongovernmental organizations**
- **Community-oriented primary care (COPC)**
- **Community-based participatory research (CBPR)**
- **Community-oriented public health (COPH)**

Discussion Questions

Take a look at the questions posed in the following scenarios, which were presented at the beginning of this chapter. See now whether you can answer them.

1. A young man in your dormitory is diagnosed with tuberculosis. The health department works with the student health service to test everyone in the dorm, as well as in his classes, with a TB skin test. Those who are positive for the first time are advised to take a course of a medicine called INH. You ask: Is this standard operating procedure?

2. You go to a public health meeting and learn that many of the speakers are not from public health agencies, but from the Departments of Labor, Commerce, Housing, and Education. You ask: What do these departments have to do with health?

3. You hear that a new childhood vaccine was developed by the NIH, approved by the FDA, endorsed for federal payment by the CDC, and recommended for use by the American Academy of Pediatrics. You ask: Do all these agencies and organizations always work so well together?

4. A major flood in Asia leads to disease and starvation. Some say it is due to global warming, others to bad luck. Coordinated efforts by global health agencies, assisted by nongovernmental organizations (NGOs) and individual donors, help get the country back on its feet. You ask: What types of cooperation are needed to make all of this happen?

5. A local community health center identifies childhood obesity as a problem in the community. They collect data demonstrating that the problem begins as early as elementary school. They develop a plan that includes clinical interventions at the health center and also at the elementary school. They ask the health department to help them organize an educational campaign and assist in evaluating the results. Working together, they are able to reduce the obesity rate among elementary school children by 50%. This seems like a new way to practice public health, you conclude. What type of approach is this?

REFERENCES

1. Public Health in America. Essential public health services. http://www.health.gov/phfunctions/public.htm. Accessed July 25 2013.

2. Institute of Medicine. *The Future of Public Health*. Washington, DC: National Academies Press; 1988.

3. Turnock BJ. *Public Health: What It Is and How It Works*. 4th ed. Sudbury, MA: Jones and Bartlett Publishers; 2009.

4. Turnock BJ. *Essentials of Public Health*. Sudbury, MA: Jones and Bartlett Publishers; 2007.

5. Public Health Accreditation Board. Standards and measures. http://www.phaboard.org/accreditation-process/public-health-department-standards-and-measures. Accessed July 25, 2013.

6. United States Department of Health and Human Services. Organizational chart. http://www.hhs.gov/about/orgchart. Accessed July 25, 2013.

7. Centers for Disease Control and Prevention. History of CDC. *Morbidity and Mortality Weekly Report*. 1996;45:526–528.

8. World Health Organization. About WHO. http://www.who.int/about/en. Accessed July 25, 2013.

9. The World Bank. Health. http://www.worldbank.org/en/topic/health. Accessed July 25, 2013.

10. Duffin J, Sweetman A. *SARS in Context: Memory, History, Policy*. Montreal, Canada: McGill-Queen's University Press; 2006.

11. Institute of Medicine. Initial guidance for an update of the National Vaccine Plan: a letter report to the national vaccine program office. http://www.nap.edu/catalog/12257.html. Accessed July 25, 2013.

12. Gofin J, Gofin R. *Essentials of Global Community Health*. Sudbury MA: Jones and Bartlett Learning; 2011.

13. Pfizer Global Pharmaceuticals. *Milestones in Public Health: Accomplishments in Public Health over the Last 100 Years*. New York, NY: Pfizer Global Pharmaceuticals; 2006.

CHAPTER 13

Food and Drugs as Public Health Issues

© Elena Itsenko/ShutterStock, Inc.

LEARNING OBJECTIVES

By the end of this chapter, the student will be able to:

- describe six ways that food affects health and disease.
- identify the steps in a foodborne outbreak investigation.
- identify the roles played by the FDA, CDC, and U.S. Department of Agriculture in food safety.
- describe the phases of drug approval by the FDA.
- explain the safety limitations of traditional approaches to drug approval.
- describe the role of postmarket surveillance in drug safety.
- describe recent changes in the FDA laws for food and also for drugs.
- identify other categories of products besides foods and drugs regulated by the FDA.

"We are what we eat," you hear said again and again. "Sure," you say, "too little is bad, too much is bad, but what other ways can food affect our health?"

An outbreak of hepatitis A occurs among employees eating in your cafeteria. To your surprise, the local health department and the CDC quickly investigate the outbreak and trace its source to seafood grown and harvested in an Asian country and to the factory that handled the food in the United States far from your home. *How is food being traced*, you wonder, *to allow outbreaks to be so rapidly and efficiently investigated*?

Jessica wondered why she needed a pregnancy test each month to refill her prescription for acne medication. She was not even currently sexually active. The pharmacist told her that she needed to come in with proof of a recent pregnancy test because serious birth defects are so common with this medication. *What a pain and what an embarrassment*, she thought to herself. *Why is all this bureaucracy needed anyway*?

John's cancer was in remission but he was still taking chemotherapy and he often felt very sleepy. His doctor asked whether he wanted to try a new drug that was just approved by the FDA and showed evidence of reducing fatigue. John knew he was taking a chance but he readily agreed. The side effects were worse than expected and John's doctor told him some of them had never been reported before. "I guess I am part of the experiment," he told his doctor. "Yes, with new drugs, we are always on the lookout for surprises," his doctor said. John asked himself if it was worth it to be one of the first to try out a new drug.

Veronica saw it on TV and on the Web. It was a new dietary supplement that showed promise for reducing blood pressure, and that was just what Veronica needed. The fine print on the bottle said that it was not for the treatment or prevention of any disease. A low dose seemed to have some effect and a higher dose was even better. When Veronica started feeling a little dizzy, she went to the emergency room, where they found that she was losing blood in her stools. The dietary supplement was thought to be the cause of her bleeding and her reduced blood pressure. Veronica asked, "Do I need to treat dietary supplements as if they are drugs?"

Carlos's doctor told him he wanted to try him on a new treatment for his headaches because the standard treatment was not working. He told Carlos that the drug had been on the market for several years but was not officially recommended for headaches by the FDA. "I have been hearing that it works for headaches and I would like to try it out, if you agree," the doctor said. Carlos wondered, *Is that the way medicine is practiced*?

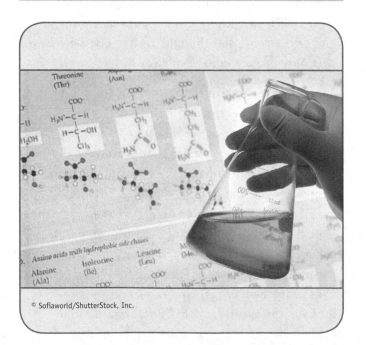

© Sofiaworld/ShutterStock, Inc.

Issues of food and drugs are central to public health. In this chapter, we will take a look at where we are in addressing the ongoing public health issues related to food and drugs. To understand where we are today, we need to take a look at the history of food and drugs and public health issues.

WHAT ARE IMPORTANT MILESTONES IN THE HISTORY OF FOOD AND DRUGS AS PUBLIC HEALTH ISSUES IN THE UNITED STATES?[1]

Until the early years of the 1900s, narcotics, cocaine, and other addictive substances were widely sold in the United States totally within the law. Drugs were falsely advertised to produce miraculous cures and labeling of ingredients was not required. There were few limitations on what could be advertised or what substances the miracle cures of the day could contain. Abuses in the food industry included use of poisonous preservatives and dyes in food. Unsanitary conditions in the meatpacking industry were vividly portrayed in Upton Sinclair's classic novel *The Jungle*.

The "muckrakers," aggressive journalists of the early 1900s, brought to public attention many dangers from food and drugs. In 1906, these efforts resulted in the passage of federal legislation establishing what later became the Food and Drug Administration (FDA) as part of the United States Department of Agriculture (USDA). The Federal Food and Drugs Act of 1906 is often considered a key accomplishment of what has been called the Progressive Era of U.S. politics.

Though this legislation creating the FDA provided the foundation for modern food and drug regulation, the original law only required that products include accurate labeling indicating their ingredients. The burden was on the FDA to demonstrate safety problems before a drug could be removed from the market. It was not until the late 1930s that the authority of the FDA was expanded. This expansion was justified by use of the interstate commerce clause because most drugs are part of commerce between two or more states.

In 1937, a Tennessee drug company producing a pediatric liquid form of sulfa, the first antibiotic, precipitated the changes in FDA law. The solvent in this untested product was a highly toxic chemical related to antifreeze. Over 100 people died from kidney disease, mostly children. The public outcry brought Congress to action with the passage of the 1938 Federal Food, Drug, and Cosmetic Act. These amendments required safety testing prior to making a new drug available to the market. The process of safety regulation soon resulted in an additional requirement that certain drugs be prescribed only by a physician, while others were available as nonprescription drugs, or over-the-counter drugs. In addition, Congress expanded the authority and created a separate entity now called the Food and Drug Administration. Congress gave the FDA authority to regulate cosmetics, authorized factory inspections, and gave the FDA increased authority to regulate both foods and drugs.

Over the years, the FDA's authority has been repeatedly increased in the wake of highly publicized tragedies. The production and distribution of a batch of polio vaccine that itself caused polio led to the regulation of vaccines in the 1950s. The Dalkon Shield, an intrauterine device (IUD) that produced thousands of cases of infection and subsequent infertility, brought about increased regulation of medical devices in the mid-1970s.

Perhaps the most famous U.S. drug disaster was the one that did not happen. In the early 1960s, FDA safety regulations resulted in a delay in approving a new, very effective sleeping pill called thalidomide. In Europe, the drug produced thousands of grossly deformed newborns with greatly shortened arms and legs, an event that did not occur in the United States. Ironically, the thalidomide case resulted in the Kefauver-Harris Drug Amendments, which focused on efficacy, not safety, and mandated efficacy testing before a drug could be approved and marketed. This landmark legislation laid the groundwork for today's process of drug approval and for the evolution of evidence-based medicine and public health.

The authority of the FDA, however, did not continue to expand. The 1980s and 1990s produced a social movement that sought smaller government and less authority over the lives of individuals. In addition, in the early 1990s, a U.S. Supreme Court decision allowed advertising of prescription drugs. The enormous expansion of prescription drug promotion encouraged a flood of direct advertisement to consumers and a rapid expansion of the quantity of prescription drugs marketed and prescribed. The greatly increased use of drugs in recent years has been associated with a large increase in drug side effects. As we will see, the FDA is now trying to address this 21st century issue based on new federal legislation.

On the food front, the 2000s have brought globalization of our food supply. The United States now obtains food products from well over 100 countries. Food increasingly originates in distant places, across the country, or from abroad and is processed in multiple locations. These foods are far more likely than locally grown and unprocessed foods to produce disease. The complexity of our food sources and food processing has magnified the potential for food-related disease, including outbreaks of disease. As we will see, several federal agencies are also now addressing this issue using tools provided by new federal food legislation as well as new technology.[2] Thus, the early years of the 2000s have brought new challenges and new approaches to both food and drug safety.

FOOD AND FOOD SAFETY

"We are what we eat" is a now familiar expression that suggests a wide range of ways that food can affect our health and lead to disease. Let us begin by taking a look at possible ways that food can affect our health.

What Ways Can Food Affect Health and Disease?

There are a large number of ways that food can affect our health and can produce disease. Among the most important are:

- Too little food
- Too much food
- Deficiencies of vitamins and minerals
- Contaminants
- Individual susceptibilities
- Foodborne communicable diseases

Let us take a look at each of these:

Too little food: Undernutrition consisting of inadequate intake of calories and protein was among the most common causes of disease in the 1900s and earlier centuries, and it still is a common cause of disease, especially in today's developing world. Today, undernutrition remains an issue in a number of areas of the world, including some poor and remote areas of the United States. The world's food supply today is adequate to prevent undernutrition. Undernutrition today represents a society's failure to ensure basic services.

Too much food: Obesity is rapidly approaching tobacco use as the number one cause of death and disability in the United States. Over 30% of the adult population is now considered obese, having a body mass index (BMI) of over 30. An even larger percentage of the adult population is considered overweight, having a BMI of over 25. The epidemic of obesity is rapidly expanding to include children. The rapid increase in type 2 diabetes and the potential for longer term complications have put obesity at or near the top of the U.S. public health agenda.

Deficiencies of vitamins and minerals: A growing list of vitamins and minerals, often called **micronutrients**, are now recognized as essential in small quantities to good health. These include vitamins A, B, C, D, E, and K, as well as the B-complex vitamins. The need for minerals—including iron, which is needed to prevent anemia, and iodine, which is needed to prevent thyroid enlargement or goiter—has been known for many years. A long list of minerals is being recognized as important to optimal health, including magnesium, selenium, copper, and zinc. A classic case of the importance of vitamins to public health is illustrated in **Box 13-1** which takes a look at the history of pellagra.

Supplementation of foods with vitamins and minerals has been an important public health intervention for many years. Supplementation of foods with vitamin D has been used for decades to prevent bone disease. Other vitamins and minerals are increasingly being added to food products. For instance, folic acid, or vitamin B9, has been recognized as a key to the closure of the fetus's spinal

BOX 13-1 Vitamin Deficiency Disease—Pellagra

The concept that food deficiencies could produce disease did not become fully accepted until the early 1900s. In 1905, Englishmen William Fletcher, researching the disease beriberi, found that eating unpolished, or brown, rice prevented beriberi and eating polished, or white, rice did not. Dr. Fletcher concluded that there were special nutrients contained in the husk of the rice. These nutrients were soon called "vitamins," after "vita," meaning "life" and "amine," which were compounds found in rice husks.[3]

Pellagra is the most deadly vitamin deficiency disease in the history of the United States. Between 1900 and 1940, approximately 3 million Americans developed pellagra, and over 100,000 died. In the rural southeastern United States in the early years of the 1900s, physicians frequently began reporting the previously rare disease. Pellagra produces some or all of the features that came to be called the "four Ds": diarrhea, dermatitis (skin outbreaks, especially after sun exposure), dementia, and death. Initially, it was thought that pellagra was a communicable disease.

In 1914, the United States Public Health Service sent a public health physician named Joseph Goldberger to directly observe patients with pellagra and their living environment. He noted the following:

- Pellagra was almost exclusively present in poor rural areas, suggesting a socioeconomic relationship.
- Pellagra did not occur among nurses, attendants, or employees in hospitals or orphanages that took care of individuals with the disease, challenging the conclusion that pellagra was a communicable disease.
- Pellagra was present in association with cheap and filling diets, suggesting a dietary cause.

Goldberger and his U.S. Public Health Service colleagues conducted extensive cohort and case-control studies of mill towns in rural South Carolina where pellagra was common. They found a clear socioeconomic gradient, with far more disease among those with lower socioeconomic status. They looked for evidence of communicability through crowding and also a link with poor sanitation but found no evidence for either. They did find a lower incidence among men, especially those who worked in the mills and were often served a hearty and varied lunch. Regular consumption of food products low in nutrients and high in calories were strongly associated with pellagra.

After the occurrence of this epidemiological field investigation, Goldberger continued using epidemiological methods acceptable at the time to investigate a nutritional cause of pellagra.

- He identified 172 children with pellagra and 168 children without pellagra in the same orphanage. Both groups were given a new, more varied diet. Within weeks, almost all children were cured of symptoms of pellagra. After a year, no new cases of pellagra had occurred.
- In a prison where pellagra had never been reported, he identified a dozen volunteers who were offered pardons for participation. They were given an experimental diet consistent with the diet Goldberger had initially observed. Evidence of pellagra occurred in 6 of the 11 inmates within 9 months. When the initial diet was resumed, all 6 inmates recovered.
- In an effort to refute the theory that pellagra was infectious, Goldberger injected himself, his wife, and 16 healthy volunteers with blood from patients with pellagra. He also collected extracts from the nose, urine, and feces and mixed them with food consumed by volunteers. Despite episodes of diarrhea and nausea, no evidence of pellagra was ever noted.

Goldberger's studies demonstrate the strengths and limitations of traditional public health and clinical approaches to studying the cause of disease. Goldberger was able to successfully challenge the communicable disease theory of pellagra and strongly suggested the existence of a nutritional deficiency. However, convincing proof of the vitamin deficiency theory of pellagra required laboratory research as well. The definitive proof that pellagra was a vitamin deficiency had to wait until the late 1930s, when Conrad Elvehjem and his colleagues showed that nicotinic acid or vitamin B3 cured pellagra-like illness in dogs. Nicotinic acid was rapidly tried in humans and had a dramatic effect on the prevention and treatment of pellagra, demonstrating effectiveness even in the absence of a control group.[4]

column and skull during the first month of pregnancy. Supplementation of food with folic acid is now being used as an important intervention to prevent what are called neural tube defects, especially spina bifida, which is failure of the spinal column to close.[a]

Contaminants: Contamination of food comes in many varieties, both naturally occurring as well as introduced by humans either intentionally or unintentionally. Aflatoxins are a naturally occurring contaminant that in chronic high exposure can contribute to hepatoma or primary liver cancer. Aflatoxins are fungi or mold that may grow on peanuts, tree nuts such as pecans, corn, wheat, and oilseeds such as cottonseed. The FDA restricts the quantity of aflatoxins that can be present in susceptible foods, but as a naturally occurring contaminant, it is not considered practical to totally remove aflatoxins from the food supply.[5] Residual pesticides used on fruits and vegetables and antibiotics used to increase the weight of animals represent important potential contaminants introduced as part of commercial agriculture.

Humans may intentionally introduce contaminants to food as a form of terrorism. Alternatively, contaminants such as glass or metal products or food products such as nut or seafood shells may be included in food products unintentionally as part of harvesting or processing.

Individual susceptibilities: An increasing range of individual susceptibilities to diseases related to food are being recognized. Many of these are genetic or what has been called inborn errors of metabolism. For instance, phenylketonuria, or PKU, is a genetic inability to metabolize the amino acid phenylalanine, leading to mental deterioration and death at an early age. Genetic testing and avoidance of phenylalanine have allowed many of those with PKU to live normal lives. Individual susceptibility may be a form of allergic reaction, producing symptoms ranging from a skin reaction to life-threatening anaphylaxis. Peanut allergy, for instance, is being recognized as a relatively common form of allergy that has the potential to cause anaphylaxis.

Foodborne communicable diseases: Last but by no means least is the potential for foods to serve as a vehicle for transmission of disease-producing organisms, or pathogens. Food can be a vehicle for transmission of disease pathogens, including bacteria such as *Salmonella*, *Campylobacter*, and toxin-producing *E. coli*. Virus-related foodborne illnesses include hepatitis A and noroviruses. Noroviruses are highly contagious viruses and are increasingly recognized as the leading cause of foodborne outbreaks, especially in crowded environments ranging from nursing homes, to dormitories, to cruise ships.

Let us take a closer look at foodborne outbreaks of disease whose control has long been a part of public health efforts. In fact, when we speak of food safety, we are often referring to control of communicable diseases transmitted by food.

How Important Is Foodborne Communicable Disease as a Cause of Morbidity and Mortality?

The CDC estimates that each year, roughly 1 in 6 Americans gets sick, over 100,000 are hospitalized, and over 3,000 die of foodborne diseases. As with many communicable diseases, the very young, the very old, and those who are immunologically compromised due to disease are the most vulnerable. Most foodborne disease is not related to outbreaks. Nonetheless, outbreak investigations are an important means to understand the sources of food contamination and the methods for its control.[6]

What Are the Steps in Foodborne Outbreak Investigation?

According to the CDC, the following steps should be followed in an outbreak investigation.[7]

1. *Detecting a possible outbreak*: Detecting an outbreak is the first step. An outbreak with hundreds of ill persons can be missed if the people are located over a wide geographic area. Public health officials may detect outbreaks through public health surveillance. By continuously gathering reports of illnesses, they know how many illnesses to expect in a given time period in a given area. If a larger number of people than expected appear to have the same illness in a given time period and area, it is called a **cluster**. When ill persons in a cluster are found to have something in common to explain why they have the same illness, the group of illnesses is called an **outbreak**.

2. *Defining and finding cases*: Often, the initial illnesses that are recognized are only a part of the total outbreak. Finding more persons who are ill with the same condition is important to help public health officials understand the size, timing, severity, and possible sources of the outbreak. To determine who has the same disease, public health officials utilize or at times

---

[a] In recent years, food supplementation has also included adding physiologically active substances such as caffeine to other foods. Power drinks that have caffeine supplements have been an important and potentially dangerous form of food supplementation.

develop what is called a **case definition** to spell out which persons will be defined as having the disease as part of the outbreak.[b]

3. *Generating hypotheses about likely sources*: When exposure to a food is suspected, the investigators need to narrow the list to the foods that the ill persons remember eating before they got sick. Health officials interview persons who are or were ill to find out where and what they ate in the days or weeks before they got sick.

4. *Testing the hypothesis*: Case-control studies are the most common type of study conducted so investigators can analyze information collected from ill persons and comparable well persons to see whether ill persons are more likely than people who did not get sick to have eaten a certain food or to report a particular exposure. Food testing can also provide useful information and help to support a hypothesis. For instance, finding bacteria with the same DNA fingerprint in an unopened package of food and in the stool samples of people in the outbreak can be convincing evidence of a source of illness.

5. *Finding the point of contamination and the source of the outbreak*: If a likely source is identified, investigators may try to determine how the food was contaminated. If the people who got sick ate food prepared in only one kitchen, it is likely the contamination occurred in that kitchen. If an outbreak is linked to a food prepared in a number of different kitchens, such as food from many stores of the same chain, or to a food that was bought from many stores and eaten without further preparation, it is likely that contamination happened somewhere in the food production chain before the final kitchen. In that case, investigators do what is called a **source traceback** to find out where contamination occurred.

6. *Controlling the outbreak*: Once a food is found to be the source of illness, control measures are often needed

immediately. If contaminated food stays on store shelves, in restaurant kitchens, or in home pantries, more people may get sick. Outbreak control measures may include cleaning and disinfecting food facilities, temporarily closing a restaurant or processing plant, recalling food items, and/or informing the public how to make the food safe or how to avoid it completely. Public health officials may decide on control measures based on strong epidemiological evidence on the disease's etiology. They do not need to wait for proof of contamination from the laboratory.

7. *Deciding that an outbreak is over*: An outbreak is considered over when the number of new illnesses reported drops back to the number normally expected in a particular geographic area. Even when new illnesses from the outbreak appear to have stopped, public health officials still continue active public health surveillance for a few weeks to be sure cases do not start to increase again. If that happens, they continue or restart their investigation because the source may not have been completely controlled, or a second contamination may have occurred.

Figure 13-1 displays the seven steps in a food outbreak investigation as defined by the CDC.

Most foodborne outbreak investigations are handled by local or state health departments. However, the CDC may be called in by state health departments to help with an outbreak investigation. The CDC's Epidemic Intelligence Service (EIS) can provide comprehensive outbreak investigation resources for a wide range of types of outbreaks, including but not limited to foodborne outbreaks.

Investigation of foodborne diseases remains an important public health effort, but prevention of foodborne disease is the goal. Let us see what is being done to prevent foodborne diseases.

What Is Being Done To Prevent Foodborne Diseases?

The FDA has a key regulatory role in food safety, including setting safety standards for food processing and distribution. The FDA shares this authority and responsibility with the USDA, which regulates meat, poultry, and eggs. The CDC has a lead role in collecting data on disease related to food along with its role in investigating possible foodborne outbreaks.

The successful implementation of food safety requires collaboration between the CDC, FDA, and USDA. This type of interagency collaboration is frequently needed in public health but often not easy to achieve. One example of

---

[b] A case definition is a set of criteria used to define which persons will be considered to have a disease as part of an outbreak. There may be more than one definition, such as definite, probable, or suspect. Alternatively, case definitions may be laboratory confirmed or not laboratory confirmed. Use of multiple definitions can be useful for epidemiologists who are investigating an outbreak or large-scale epidemic. Note that an epidemic like an outbreak represents a greater than usual occurrence of disease over a defined period of time. An epidemic implies a much greater number of cases, usually over a larger geographic area. For some diseases, such as influenza, the CDC defines the difference between an epidemic and an outbreak based on the percentage of the deaths that are due to influenza.

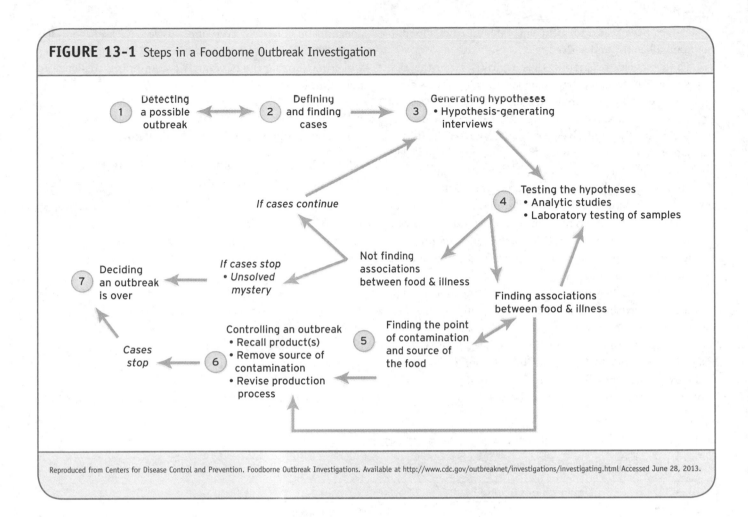

FIGURE 13-1 Steps in a Foodborne Outbreak Investigation

Reproduced from Centers for Disease Control and Prevention. Foodborne Outbreak Investigations. Available at http://www.cdc.gov/outbreaknet/investigations/investigating.html Accessed June 28, 2013.

successful collaborative efforts has been the FoodNet program. The FoodNet program aims to identify and investigate foodborne disease not only from outbreaks but also from routine exposures.

The Foodborne Diseases Active Surveillance Network, or FoodNet, has been tracking trends for infections commonly transmitted through food since 1996. FoodNet provides data for food safety policy and prevention efforts. It estimates the number of foodborne illnesses, monitors trends in incidence of specific foodborne illnesses over time, attributes illnesses to specific foods and settings, and disseminates this information.[8]

In 2010, the Food Safety Modernization Act was passed, giving the FDA and the USDA increased authority to ensure the safety of foods. Key to the law was the ability to track foods, including their origin, date of production, and other data that could be useful in locating the source of the food if a disease outbreak occurred and investigating the outbreak's cause. The law requires:[9]

- Farmers and food processors to maintain distribution records so that the FDA can more quickly trace an outbreak to its source
- Foreign food suppliers to meet the same safety standards as domestic suppliers
- Regular inspection of all food processing facilities, with more frequent inspections in higher risk facilities

In the United States, What Other Programs Aim to Prevent Food-Related Disease and Disability?

In addition to its regulatory role, the USDA administers a series of **food security** programs. Food security as defined by the World Health Organization requires that "all people at all times have access to sufficient, safe, nutritious food to maintain a healthy and active life."[10]

Food security programs cover nearly 15% of the U.S. population. The largest program, formerly called food stamps and now called the Supplemental Nutrition Assistance Program (SNAP), aims to provide access to healthy diets by making relatively expensive items such as fresh fruits and vegetables accessible to those with low incomes. The USDA also runs the WIC program, or the Special Supplemental Nutrition Program for Women, Infants, and Children. WIC serves over 4 million women and children under 5 by providing federal grants to states for supplemental foods, healthcare referrals, and nutrition education for low-income pregnant women, postpartum women, and infants and children up to age 5 at nutritional risk.[11]

A large number of local, national, and global agencies are involved in food-related issues. Many of these are described in **Table 13-1**.

Food safety and food benefits have been long-standing issues in public health. The 2000s have brought new threats and new approaches for dealing with these threats. This century has also brought new possibilities for providing safe and nutritious food to everyone. As we have seen, food has multiple impacts on health and disease. Reducing the harms while maximizing the benefits is a continuing challenge to public health at all levels.

DRUGS AND DRUG SAFETY

Now let us turn our attention to drugs and drug safety.

Why Is Drug Safety Considered an Important 21st Century Public Health Issue?

The Institute of Medicine (IOM) has concluded that nearly 100,000 Americans die each year as a result of adverse effects of drugs.[12] Thus, from the population perspective as well as for individual patient care, drug testing and monitoring for safety are important public health issues.

Drug safety as a public health issue has gained increasing recognition in recent years. Highly publicized adverse effects of medications, including Vioxx® and other new arthritis drugs, are believed to have contributed to heart disease in tens of thousands of patients. Medications for diabetes, weight loss, and a long list of other conditions have been taken off the market because of side effects. The aging of the

TABLE 13-1 Agencies and Their Role in Food Issues

Level	Organizations involved	Roles
Global	Food and Agriculture Organization of the United Nations (FAO)	The United Nations agency with overall responsibility for the food supply, with special emphasis on ensuring an adequate supply of food worldwide
	World Health Organization (WHO)	Not a regulatory agency, but establishes policy and makes recommendations regarding the safety of the world food supply through its Department of Food Safety and Zoonoses (FOS)
	Codex Alimentarius Commission (CAC)	Initiated as a joint program of FAO and WHO that develops food standards, guidelines, and codes of practice; these now form the basis for the rules of global trade under the jurisdiction of the World Trade Organization (WTO)
Federal	United States Food and Drug Administration (FDA)	Overall responsibility for food safety regulation in the United States
	United States Department of Agriculture (USDA)	Regulatory responsibilities for meat, poultry, and eggs in the United States
	United States Environmental Protection Agency (EPA)	Regulation of pesticide usage and the establishment of water quality standards
	Centers for Disease Control and Prevention (CDC)	Not a regulatory agency, but responsible for ongoing surveillance, as well as acute investigations in collaboration with state and local health departments
State/local	State and local health departments	Restaurant inspections, outbreak investigations
Consumer	Consumer protection agencies	Education in safe food purchasing, preparation, and storage

population and increasing reliance on medications widely promoted in the media have also raised concerns about more frequent and often unexpected side effects of drugs.

To understand the FDA's traditional approach to drug testing and monitoring, we need to look at the phases of testing as used by the FDA. The FDA has traditionally divided the testing and approval process for drugs into preclinical research, **phase 1, phase 2, phase 3, and phase 4**, which is also called postmarket surveillance.[13] Let us take a look at each of these phases.

What Do We Mean By "Preclinical Research" on Drugs?

Drug testing begins before any human beings have received the drug. Prior to studying a drug on humans, the FDA requires animal safety studies. Animal testing is usually administered to two different species at levels well above the equivalent dosage expected to be used in humans. Studies are done primarily to detect cancer, teratogenicity (fetal malformations), and effects on fertility. In addition, toxic effects on drug-sensitive organs such as the liver, kidneys, and bone marrow are also investigated.

Unfortunately, the effects on animals may either fail to detect subsequent effects in humans or demonstrate high-dose effects that are difficult to interpret. For instance, thalidomide, the sleeping pill that caused severe limb shortening in newborns, did not demonstrate these effects in animal testing.

Humans may absorb, metabolize (alter its chemistry), and excrete (remove from the body) drugs differently than animal species. High-dose effects on one animal species alert us to the possibility of similar effects in humans but by no means guarantee their occurrence. In addition, humans have an enormous range of reactions to drugs even when given by the same route with the dose adjusted for body weight. Thus, it should not be surprising that animal testing can easily miss the rare but serious side effects occasionally experienced by humans.

What Is Phase 1?

The initial administration of a drug to human beings is called phase 1. A phase 1 study focuses on the pharmacology of the drug—that is, its absorption, metabolism, and excretion. It aims to establish the dosage range and route of administration to be used in subsequent studies. It also looks at safety issues.

Phase 1 studies are capable of identifying common and serious side effects—even those that are not initially suspected. Thus, it is a critical component of the drug safety testing process. Phase 1 focuses on effects on organs that are known to be especially sensitive to the actions of drugs. These include the liver, kidney, bone marrow, and testicles. The liver may be especially prone to drug effects because it often concentrates drugs as it participates in their metabolism and excretion. The kidneys likewise may be exposed to high doses as part of the excretion process. The rapid rate of cell division in the bone marrow and testicles may make them especially vulnerable to the effects of drugs.

Phase 1 may also focus on effects that may be expected based on the known actions of a particular class of drugs or a particular drug, perhaps based on animal studies. A new antidepressant may be subjected to examination of the electrical conduction system of the heart because antidepressants are known to produce heart rhythm changes, or arrhythmias. A new diuretic that removes salt and water from the body would be thoroughly examined for a range of electrolyte and metabolic effects because this class of medication is known to have a range of effects on the chemistry of the blood.

The duration of the exposure to the drug as part of phase 1 may be quite short—usually days to weeks. The length of exposure may be governed by the length of time needed to determine issues of absorption, metabolism, and excretion. Thus, phase 1 testing cannot be expected to detect longer term or chronic effects.

A phase 1 study is usually quite small, perhaps including only a few dozen individuals. The type of patients who are asked to participate in phase 1 studies is quite variable. Depending on the intended use of the drug, the patients may be severely ill with little or no chance of benefiting from the drug. Alternatively, they may be healthy volunteers who do not have a need for the drug. As a rule, patients at highest risk, such as pregnant women and young children, will not be part of a phase 1 study, even if they are the intended eventual recipients of the drug. Phase 1 studies by their very nature are designed to be short term. They intend to detect effects that occur in the short term and are predictable or produce clinical symptoms. Thus, it is expected that additional attention to safety will be needed.[c]

One of the major limitations of phase 1 in particular and safety assessment in general is the wide range of special sensitivities to drug actions that occur among a small number of people. These sensitivities may occur for a variety of reasons.

---

[c] The process of phase 1 testing, like the overall process of safety assessment of drugs, is undergoing revision and hopefully improvement. For instance, advances in our understanding of the mechanism of drug action on a molecular basis may in the future allow us to do a better job of understanding what, where, and how a drug is acting, allowing researchers to focus on the impacts on the molecular as well as the clinical level.

These individuals may be unusual in the way they metabolize drugs, the way their other drugs interact with the new drug, or the way the presence of other diseases complicates the reactions to the new drug.

What Are Phase 2 and Phase 3?

Phase 2 and 3 studies are primarily designed to establish efficacy of a drug for a particular use or indication. That is, they aim to establish that on average, the drug improves outcomes under research conditions. Phase 2 consists of small, sometimes uncontrolled, trials designed to determine whether there is a suggestion of efficacy. Phase 2 trials are important because they serve as a precondition for moving ahead with the expense, time, and potential harm of conducting large randomized controlled trials, which are at the heart of phase 3.

Side effects identified in phase 1 trials are given special attention, but phase 2 trials are not primarily focused on safety. Randomized controlled trials are the gold standard for establishing efficacy for one particular indication. Their key role in establishing efficacy often means that they are designed around the specific requirements for determining efficacy for a particular disease on a particular type of patient. Randomized controlled trials, even those that are well designed for establishing efficacy, have limitations in establishing safety. The key limitations of randomized controlled trials for evaluating safety can be summarized as follows:

- Too small—The sample size for randomized controlled trials is determined by the requirements of establishing efficacy. Thus, the number of patients generally ranges from several hundred to several thousand. Identifying rare but serious side effects often requires tens or even hundreds of thousands of users.[d]
- Too short—The duration of randomized controlled trials is geared to the length of time necessary to establish efficacy for the particular indication that is being investigated. Thus, an antibiotic for acute infections may be tested for 10–14, days while a new drug for acute depression may be tested for 1–2 months. Long-term follow-up for safety is not an inherent part of randomized controlled trials.

- Too simple—The individuals eligible for inclusion in a randomized controlled trial are carefully defined by inclusion and exclusion criteria. These criteria make it easier to establish efficacy. Thus, patients with other complicating diseases or those on a variety of other drugs that make them especially susceptible to adverse effects of treatment are rarely included in randomized controlled trials.[e]

New drugs are approved on the basis of data collected in preclinical testing and phases 1, 2, and 3. These phases provide a great deal of assurance that the drug works or has efficacy to improve outcome for the average person in the groups that have been investigated. Phases 1, 2, and 3 do not, in and of themselves, establish that the drug has effectiveness—that is, that it works under the conditions of clinical practice. Furthermore, while safety is considered all throughout the approval process, the limitations of safety assessment leave open the possibility that new and more frequent side effects will be seen when the drug is widely used in clinical practice.[f]

What Are the Implications of FDA Approval of a Drug?

Understanding the process of assessing safety requires that we first understand what the FDA is indicating when it approves a drug. In general, FDA approval implies:

- The drug may be advertised and marketed for a particular indication, the one for which it was studied and approved.
- Once the drug is approved, it may be used by prescribing clinicians for any patient. That is, the prescribing

---

[d] An important statistical principle for establishing safety is known as the rule of three. The rule of three tells us that in order to be 95% confident that we will observe at least one case of a rare but serious side effect—for example, one with a true probability of once per 20,000 uses—we are required to observe 60,000 individuals. A sample size of this magnitude is generally only possible once the treatment is used in clinical practice.

[e] In addition to limitations due to the focus on efficacy, for many years, phase 2 and phase 3 testing routinely excluded those felt to be at the highest risk of complications—usually pregnant women and children. Recent changes have now made inclusion of children routine in phase 2 and 3 if the intention is to include children among those recommended to receive the drug if it is approved. Pregnant women are still generally omitted from phase 2 and 3 trials except in the unusual circumstance that a treatment is intended for women known to be pregnant.

[f] Accelerated approval is given to some new drugs for serious and life-threatening illnesses that lack satisfactory treatments. Accelerated approval may occur before measures of efficacy and safety that would usually be required for approval are available. Less traditional measures called **surrogate endpoints** are used. Surrogate endpoints may not be a direct measurement of how a patient feels, functions, or survives, but they are considered likely to predict a desirable outcome. For example, a surrogate endpoint could be short-term lowering of HIV load. The FDA requires ongoing studies of drugs approved under accelerated approval rules. If studies do not confirm the initial results, the FDA can withdraw the approval.

clinician has the authority to use the treatment for indications or at dosages not specifically approved by the FDA. Use of FDA-approved drugs for indications not approved by the FDA is called **off-label prescribing**.

Thus, once approved, a drug may be prescribed for other conditions, at alternative doses, and for longer durations than those recommended for the particular indication for which the drug was approved. Frequently, clinicians will find that a drug works well in patients with more or less severe disease than those studied in the randomized controlled trial and will use the drug for these patients. Alternatively, a drug may be studied only for those who have failed other treatments, but clinicians in practice may use the drug as an initial treatment. Occasionally, there will be suggestive evidence that the drug works for other conditions not previously approved, and clinicians will utilize the drug for these indications as well as the approved indications. A full evaluation of safety needs to take into account the actual uses of the drug in clinical practice. We can think of large-scale and long-term use in clinical practice as providing the gold standard for drug safety.

Many drugs are taken by individuals without a prescription. **Box 13-2** looks at how nonprescription drugs differ from prescription drugs.

BOX 13-2 Nonprescription Drugs[14]

Nonprescription drugs, often called over-the-counter drugs, are designed to be used without a clinician's prescription. Their sale is not limited to pharmacies. Nonprescription drugs are not necessarily designed to be used by one individual, as is the case with prescription drugs. While the FDA regulates the advertising of prescription drugs, the Federal Trade Commission (FTC) regulates the advertisement of nonprescription drugs.[a]

There are over 300,000 nonprescription drug products available in the United States. Many of them contain the same ingredients. The FDA reviews the active ingredients and the labeling of over 80 therapeutic classes of drugs, such as pain-killers and antacids, instead of reviewing individual drug products. For each category, a monograph is published, which the FDA describes as a "recipe book" covering acceptable ingredients, doses, formulations, and labeling. These monographs define the safety, effectiveness, and labeling of all nonprescription active ingredients. Companies can follow the recipe book and produce and market a nonprescription drug without the need for FDA preapproval.

New nonprescription drugs that utilize new active therapeutic agents need to satisfy the FDA requirement for a new drug or be converted from a prescription drug to a nonprescription drug. Conversion from a prescription to a nonprescription drug is becoming an increasingly common action. In general, conversion requires that the drug is able to be safely used without the supervision of a prescribing clinician. In addition, the drug labeling must be tested to ensure that it can be generally understood by the groups of individuals for whom it is intended.

Nonprescription drugs such as aspirin and acetaminophen can have strong impacts on their own and can interact with prescription and nonprescription drugs. Some nonprescription drugs can have life-threatening side effects at levels only modestly greater than those recommended on the label. Acetaminophen, for instance, can cause life-threatening liver disease with long-term use at levels only modestly above those recommended for short-term pain relief. Thus, the increased use of nonprescription drugs on their own and along with prescription drugs poses a potential public health hazard that needs continuing monitoring and ongoing education.

---

[a] The term "over the counter" will not be used here because it implies an interaction with an informed individual. Today, many nonprescription products can be purchased through vending machines, automated checkout counters, and the Internet without any human contact. In addition, a new option is being used by the FDA that may be called "behind the counter." Behind-the-counter drugs require identification of the purchaser and limitations on the quantity of drugs that can be purchased. Pseudoephedrine, often purchased as the brand name Sudafed®, is a nonprescription decongestant that was placed behind the counter after it was recognized that it could be used to make methamphetamine.

Data from United States Food and Drug Administration. Drug Applications for Over-the-Counter (OTC) Drugs. Available at http://www.fda.gov/drugs/developmentapprovalprocess/howdrugsaredevelopedandapproved/approvalapplications/over-the-counterdrugs/default.htm. Accessed June 28, 2013

How Are Adverse Effects of a Drug Monitored in Phase 4, after FDA Approval?[15]

For many years, the system for detection of adverse side effects of drugs was limited to what is known as the **spontaneous reporting system**. In this system, those who prescribe the drug, and increasingly, patients themselves, are encouraged to report side effects to the FDA. However, they are not required to do so.

When a drug or vaccine produces a rare and dramatic side effect following soon after treatment is begun, spontaneous reporting systems may be useful in detecting their occurrence. For instance, a small number of cases of a rare and acute life-threatening condition called intussusception of the colon was seen in children within a few weeks of receiving a new rotavirus vaccine for the prevention of gastroenteritis. The unusual nature of the side effect, its dramatic presentation, and its clear time relationship to the vaccination provide convincing evidence that the side effect was due to the vaccine.

This example can be viewed as the exception rather than the rule. Spontaneous reporting systems often do not work this well because they have a number of limitations, including the following:

- Even with serious side effects, only a small percentage may be reported, especially when the effect is not dramatic or closely linked in time to the treatment.
- Side effects that result from a variety of causes or are similar to the consequences of the disease being treated may be difficult to recognize and attribute to the treatment.
- Unsuspected side effects may escape detection or not be attributed to the treatment.

The spontaneous reporting system cannot be expected to rapidly or completely detect rare but serious side effects. Patients who receive a new treatment over the first few months to the first few years after initial marketing approval need to be regarded as part of the experiment. **Table 13-2** summarizes the roles that preclinical testing and phases 1, 2, 3, and 4 have traditionally played in the drug effectiveness and safety assessment process.

What Else Can Be Done?

Until recently, the FDA did not have authority to require follow-up studies of drugs once they were approved for clinical practice. In addition, as opposed to the preapproval process, the burden of proof was on the FDA to establish a safety hazard before an approved drug could be removed from the market. In addition, the FDA had limited authority over drug advertisements as long as they did not contradict FDA language. Other than including warning labels, or what have been called black box warnings, in the drug use instructions, the FDA had limited authority over the process of prescribing or monitoring drug use.

The Food and Drug Administration Amendment Act of 2007 provided a wide variety of new authorities for the FDA. These new authorities were designed as a response to a range of safety issues that have developed over several decades.[16] Congress provided the FDA with authority and a great deal of discretion over what should be done, how it should be done, and when it should be done. Many of the provisions of this law will take years or even a decade or more to be fully implemented.

The 2007 amendments to the FDA law provided the FDA with a wide range of new authority that it can use to monitor safety and act to reduce or eliminate side effects of drugs.[16] The use of this authority to protect against side effects while gaining the benefits of the drug use continues to be a difficult and controversial issue. Among the new authority granted to the FDA in the 2007 legislation are the following:

- The FDA was provided authority to require that more representative patients be included in randomized controlled trials with the aim to have randomized controlled trials more closely reflect the populations on whom the drug will be used.
- The FDA was given authority to require follow-up studies of drugs to monitor their performance in clinical practice.
- The FDA was given authority to develop large database systems to link pharmacy records with electronic medical records to assess side effects on an ongoing basis.
- The FDA was given authority to place increased restrictions on who can prescribe a particular drug and what conditions need to be fulfilled before it can be prescribed, including required testing prior to filling a prescription.
- The FDA was given increased authority to approve and monitor drug advertising to clinicians and directly to patients to ensure that they conform with FDA-approved language and accurately communicate risks.
- The FDA was given greater authority to withdraw drugs from the market when serious issues of safety are raised.

TABLE 13-2 FDA Process of Assessing Safety and Effectiveness of Drugs

	Definition	Objectives	Limitations
Preclinical testing	Safety assessment on at least two species at high dosages prior to initial use on humans.	Assess carcinogenic, teratogenicity, and fertility effects.	High-dose effects may not correlate with effects on humans. Species differences may result in missing effects that later appear in human testing or after widespread clinical use.
Phase 1	Initial testing of drug on humans may include healthy volunteers or terminally ill patients, but not necessarily those on whom drug will be used.	Designed to assess pharmacology, including metabolism and excretion, in an effort to establish dosage, timing, and route of administration. Safety assessed especially on vulnerable organs, including liver, kidney, testicles, and bone marrow.	Small numbers and short-term studies mean many effects may be missed. May not help predict side effects when patients are not representative of those the drug will be used on in practice.
Phase 2	Initial small-scale, controlled or uncontrolled, trial of efficacy with secondary assessment of safety.	Establishes that there is enough evidence of efficacy to warrant phase 3 randomized controlled trials.	Primary intent is assessment of efficacy.
Phase 3	Two independently performed randomized controlled trials unless not practical or ethical.	Establish efficacy for one indication among a homogeneous group of patients compared to conventional treatment. Investigate short-term safety relative to conventional treatment.	Randomized controlled trials may be too small, their duration too short, and their participants' conditions too simple or uncomplicated in terms of their disease(s) or their treatment(s) to observe side effects that will be seen in clinical practice.
Phase 4 Post-market surveillance	Assessment of safety based on the use of the drug in clinical practice. Spontaneous reporting system traditionally the basis for phase 4. Databases from clinical practice and formal studies of safety increasingly used to assess safety in clinical practice.	Designed to detect rare but serious side effects as well as increased frequency of known side effects. Once a drug is approved by the FDA for one particular indication, it may be used at different dosages, for different types of patients, and for other indications at the discretion of the prescribing clinician.	Spontaneous reporting system results may not detect side effects, especially if they simulate commonly occurring effects such as liver or kidney impairment. Interactions between drugs or between drugs and diseases are common, making it difficult to assess and attribute causation.

Today, a coordinated process of postmarket investigation of adverse effects of drugs has begun. The process relies not only on the spontaneous reporting system but also on follow-up of patients previously enrolled in randomized controlled trials. It also includes selective use of case-control studies and cohort studies, which take advantage of the greatly increased ability to link clinical and pharmacy records to investigate the relationship between drugs and adverse events.

Do All FDA-Regulated Products Receive the Same Effectiveness and Safety Assessment as Prescription and Nonprescription Drugs?

Vaccines undergo many of the same phases of testing and monitoring that are required for drug approval. Because vaccines are often given to millions of healthy people, additional monitoring for safety is often expected prior to and after approval. A "no fault" system of financial compensation exists for adverse side effects related to vaccines. This has resulted in more complete and more comprehensive reporting of side effects of vaccines.

Many substances taken regularly by millions of people are not subject to the types of evaluation that we have discussed for drugs and vaccines. The FDA regulates what are called **dietary supplements** under a different set of regulations than those covering "conventional" drug products (prescription and nonprescription).[17] Dietary substances include vitamins, minerals, and herbal treatments. The legal implication of dietary supplements that distinguishes them from drugs is that dietary supplements cannot be promoted as treatment for, or prevention of, a disease. Thus, when you hear about a dietary supplement, you will often see the disclaimer: "This product is not intended to diagnose, treat, cure, or prevent any disease."

As opposed to the makers of drugs and vaccines, the dietary supplement manufacturer is solely responsible for ensuring that a dietary supplement is safe before it is marketed. The FDA indicates that it is responsible for taking action against any unsafe dietary supplement product after it reaches the market. However, the burden of proof is on the FDA, making it very difficult to remove dietary supplements from the market.

Generally, manufacturers of dietary supplements need to register their products with the FDA. However, the FDA does not provide approval before the manufacturer may produce or sell dietary supplements. Manufacturers are responsible for making sure that product label information, including ingredients, is truthful and not misleading.

The FDA describes its postmarketing responsibilities for dietary supplements as monitoring safety through voluntary adverse event reporting similar to the spontaneous reporting system for drugs. As opposed to its authority over advertising for drugs and vaccines, the FDA does not have any authority over dietary supplement advertising. The Federal Trade Commission regulates dietary supplement advertising.

Thus today, drugs and vaccines are subject to careful premarket review and to increasingly active postmarket surveillance. Dietary supplements, on the other hand, undergo very limited premarket or postmarket evaluation.

What Other Products Does the FDA Regulate?

In addition to products classified as foods and drugs, the FDA has authority over a wide range of products. About 25% of every dollar spent by Americans is spent on products regulated by the FDA. The FDA regulates cosmetics, medical devices, biological products including the blood supply, and most recently tobacco products.

The FDA regulates the safety, labeling and manufacture of cosmetics. Medical devices are a broad category with their own set of regulations, which are currently under active review.

The FDA promulgates and enforces standards for blood collection and for the production of blood products. The FDA also inspects blood banks and monitors reports of errors, accidents, and adverse clinical events. Authority over tobacco products is relatively new, and the FDA is beginning to utilize its authority in this area, including the regulation of nicotine.

Food and drugs, as well as other health and cosmetic products, play an important role in modern society. The United States has developed a complex public health system designed to maximize the benefits of these products while identifying potential harms and minimizing their impact. The system is by no means perfect, but it continues to evolve and face new challenges. Do not expect these issues to go away. They have been a part of public health from the beginning and will continue to be key public health issues well into the future.

KEY WORDS

- **Micronutrients**
- **Cluster**
- **Outbreak**
- **Case definition**
- **Source traceback**
- **Food security**
- **Phase 1, 2, 3, and 4**
- **Surrogate endpoint**
- **Off-label prescribing**
- **Spontaneous reporting system**
- **Dietary supplements**

Discussion Questions

Take a look at the questions posed in the following scenarios, which were presented at the beginning of this chapter. See now whether you can answer them.

1. "We are what we eat," you hear said again and again. "Sure," you say, "too little is bad, too much is bad, but what other ways can food affect our health?"

2. An outbreak of hepatitis A occurs among employees eating in your cafeteria. To your surprise, the local health department and the CDC quickly investigate the outbreak and trace its source to seafood grown and harvested in an Asian country and to the factory that handled the food in the United States far from your home. *How is food being traced*, you wonder, *to allow outbreaks to be so rapidly and efficiently investigated*?

3. Jessica wondered why she needed a pregnancy test each month to refill her prescription for acne medication. She was not even currently sexually active. The pharmacist told her that she needed to come in with proof of a recent pregnancy test because serious birth defects are so common with this medication. *What a pain and what an embarrassment* she thought to herself. *Why is all this bureaucracy needed anyway*?

4. John's cancer was in remission but he was still taking chemotherapy and he often felt very sleepy. His doctor asked whether he wanted to try a new drug that was just approved by the FDA and showed evidence of reducing fatigue. John knew he was taking a chance but he readily agreed. The side effects were worse than expected and John's doctor told him some of them had never been reported before. "I guess I am part of the experiment," he told his doctor. "Yes, with new drugs, we are always on the lookout for surprises," his doctor said. John asked himself if it was worth it to be one of the first to try out a new drug.

5. Veronica saw it on TV and on the Web. It was a new dietary supplement that showed promise for reducing blood pressure, and that was just what Veronica needed. The fine print on the bottle said that it was not for the treatment or prevention of any disease. A low dose seemed to have some effect and a higher dose was even better. When Veronica started feeling a little dizzy, she went to the emergency room, where they found that she was losing blood in her stools. The dietary supplement was thought to be the cause of her bleeding and her reduced blood pressure. Veronica asked, "Do I need to treat dietary supplements as if they are drugs?"

6. Carlos's doctor told him he wanted to try him on a new treatment for his headaches because the standard treatment was not working. He told Carlos that the drug had been on the market for several years but was not officially recommended for headaches by the FDA. "I have been hearing that it works for headaches and I would like to try it out, if you agree," the doctor said. Carlos wondered, *Is that the way medicine is practiced*?

REFERENCES

1. U.S. Food and Drug Administration. Significant dates in U.S. food and drug law history. http://www.fda.gov/AboutFDA/WhatWeDo/History/Milestones/ucm128305.htm. Accessed June 28, 2013.

2. U.S. Food and Drug Administration. Food. http://www.fda.gov/Food/GuidanceRegulation/FSMA/ucm247559.htm. Accessed June 28, 2013.

3. About.com. The history of vitamins. http://inventors.about.com/library/inventors/bl_vitamins.htm. Accessed June 28, 2013.

4. Elmore JG, Feinstein AR. Joseph Goldberger: an unsung hero of American clinical epidemiology. *Annals of Internal Medicine.* 1994; 121:372–375.

5. MedlinePlus. Aflatoxin. http://www.nlm.nih.gov/medlineplus/ency/article/002429.htm. Accessed June 28, 2013.

6. Centers for Disease Control and Prevention. Estimates of foodborne illness in the United States. http://www.cdc.gov/foodborneburden. Accessed June 28, 2013.

7. Centers for Disease Control and Prevention. Foodborne outbreak investigations. http://www.cdc.gov/outbreaknet/investigations/investigating.html. Accessed June 28, 2013.

8. Centers for Disease Control and Prevention. Foodborne Diseases Active Surveillance Network (FoodNet). http://www.cdc.gov/foodnet. Accessed June 28, 2013.

9. U.S. Food and Drug Administration. FDA Food Safety Modernization Act (FSMA). http://www.fda.gov/food/guidanceregulation/fsma/default.htm. Accessed June 28, 2013.

10. World Health Organization. Food security. http://www.who.int/trade/glossary/story028/en. Accessed June 28, 2013.

11. United States Department of Agriculture. USDA programs and services. http://www.usda.gov/wps/portal/usda/usdahome?navid=PROGRAM_AND_SERVICE. Accessed June 28, 2013.

12. Institute of Medicine. *Preventing Medication Errors: Quality Chasm Series.* Washington, DC: National Academics Press; 2006.

13. United States Food and Drug Administration. Drugs. http://www.fda.gov/Drugs/ResourcesForYou/Industry/default.htm. Accessed July 28, 2013.

14. United States Food and Drug Administration. Drug applications for over-the-counter (OTC) drugs. http://www.fda.gov/drugs/developmentapprovalprocess/howdrugsaredevelopedandapproved/approvalapplications/over-the-counterdrugs/default.htm. Accessed June 28, 2013.

15. United States Food and Drug Administration. Postmarket drug safety information for patients and providers. http://www.fda.gov/Drugs/DrugSafety/PostmarketDrugSafetyInformationforPatientsandProviders/default.htm. Accessed June 2, 2013.

16. United States Food and Drug Administration. Food and Drug Administration Amendments Act (FDAAA) of 2007. http://www.fda.gov/regulatoryinformation/legislation/federalfooddrugandcosmeticactfdcact/significantamendmentstothefdcact/foodanddrugadministrationamendmentsactof2007/default.htm. Accessed June 28, 2013.

17. United States Food and Drug Administration. Dietary supplements. http://www.fda.gov/food/DietarySupplements/default.htm. Accessed June 28, 2013.

CHAPTER 14

From Single Solutions to Systems Thinking—The Future of Population Health

LEARNING OBJECTIVES

By the end of this chapter, the student will be able to:

- explain how systems thinking differs from reductionist thinking.
- identify characteristics of a system.
- identify the steps in systems analysis using systems diagrams.
- explain the meaning of interactions between factors.
- explain the meaning of bottlenecks and leverage points.
- identify and explain seven uses of systems thinking in public health.
- explain the requirements for successful systems analysis and the limitations of the approach.

You are pregnant and have a 10-year history of cigarette smoking. You are surprised that at your first prenatal visit, there is a big sticker on your chart saying "Smoker." Everyone in the doctor's office asks you what they can do to help, and they quickly enroll you in special services for smoking cessation for which you were not eligible before you got pregnant. When you ask why so much time, attention, and money is now coming your way, they tell you pregnancy is a leverage point for stopping smoking. *What do they mean by "leverage point"?* you ask yourself.

A patient with active TB is reported by the local hospital laboratory to the health department. The health department quickly connects with the patient to determine his close personal contacts.

They also ask him if they can test him for HIV. He turns out to be HIV positive, and permission is then requested to get in touch with his sexual contacts. You consider how you would describe the relationship between TB and HIV, and wonder how knowledge of this relationship can be used to reduce the risks of both TB and HIV.

A new type of large research study looks at four FDA-approved treatments for myocardial infarction. The study includes over 50,000 patients and is designed to determine not whether one treatment is better than another but instead whether there is any clinically important difference between the outcomes of the treatments. *What type of research is this,* you wonder, and why is it being done?

An expert panel reviews recent data in an effort to predict the incidence of HIV in 2020. They take into account the current data on incidence and prevalence as well as the effectiveness of known interventions. Unfortunately, within two years after the effort is completed, it is apparent that their estimates are quite inaccurate. *Why is prediction so difficult?* you wonder.

You hear that motor vehicle injuries, especially those due to automobile collisions, have been dramatically reduced in recent years. *Was there a magic bullet that accomplished this, you wonder, or was this reduction accomplished through a more complicated process?*

You love rare hamburgers. "Just wave them over the flame," you like to say. Recently, you have heard that ground beef is a high-risk food—even a health hazard. *What does that mean, and what is being done about it?* **you ask yourself.**

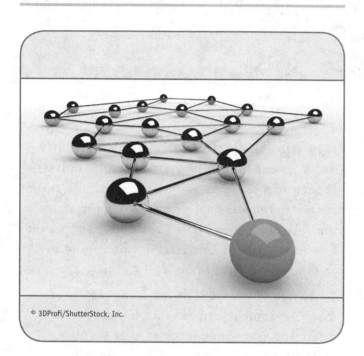

© 3DProfi/ShutterStock, Inc.

"Over the last 100 years, public health has evolved from having primarily a science focus to incorporating a problem focus and, most recently, a systems focus."

—Commission on Education of Health
Professionals for the 21st Century[1]

Let us take a look at how population health thinking is changing in the 2000s and gradually incorporating what we will call **systems thinking**. The focus on systems is so important that along with the population perspective, it is coming to define 21st century population health. The importance of systems thinking in public health education has been recognized by inclusion of systems thinking as a "cross-cutting" competency that is being included in the public health certifying examination.[2]

We begin by taking a look at what makes systems thinking different.

WHAT MAKES SYSTEMS THINKING DIFFERENT?

Traditional thinking in public health, like most science-based disciplines, has used what is called **reductionist thinking**. Reductionist thinking looks at one factor or variable at a time.[3] That is, it reduces the problem to one potential "cause" and one potential "effect."[a]

Reductionist thinking has often been used in public health and medicine to search for the one-and-only answer to the why, or etiology, and the one-and-only answer to what should be done to improve outcome. This approach may be called the magic bullet or miracle cure approach.

Reductionist thinking has been very useful for establishing specific factors as contributory causes of disease, such as cigarettes and lung cancer, high blood pressure and vascular disease, as well as aspirin and Reye's syndrome. However, it is increasingly important that we look at the impacts of multiple factors and see how they work together as parts of systems. Systems thinking, or a systems approach, often utilizes data derived from reductionist thinking but goes beyond reductionist thinking to look at multiple factors that cause disease and disease outcomes. Thus, it is the focus on multiple factors and how they fit together that distinguishes reductionist thinking from systems thinking.[4,b]

---

[a] When using reductionist thinking, other factors are traditionally included in public health studies in order to take them into account or control for them. These factors are called confounding variables when they are related to both the cause and the effect. Confounding variables may confound or confuse the investigation of the relationship between a single cause and a single effect. Confounding variables may be differences between groups in age, severity, or disease, or other risk factors that affect the chances of developing disease or experiencing a poor outcome. It is important to remember that confounding variables are not being included in the research in order to investigate their relationship to the disease or other outcome being investigated.

[b] The terminology can be confusing. We will use the term "systems thinking" to describe the thinking process of the systems approach. We will use the term "systems analysis" as a broad term describing a range of methods for operationalizing systems thinking. Systems diagrams illustrated in this chapter are one such method for operationalizing systems thinking. The simpler translational research model described in this chapter can be seen as another type of systems analysis. At times, the term "integrative" is used to describe systems thinking. "Integrative" describes the intention of systems thinking or the systems approach to bring together disparate influences into a coherent whole. Integrative thinking is at times used to distinguish systems thinking from reductionist thinking. Here we will use the term "systems thinking" as the broadest term, and "systems analysis" will be used as a term to describe a variety of methods to operationalize systems thinking. The definition chosen for the term "system," as indicated in the text, is an interacting group of items forming a unified whole. This definition was drawn and modified from a long list of potential definitions because it emphasizes the need to identify items or factors, their interactions, and how they fit together as a whole. We believe that these are the core elements of systems thinking.[5]

WHAT IS A SYSTEM?

There are a large number of definitions of a system. We will define a **system** as an interacting group of items forming a unified whole. According to O'Connor and McDermott, the key to identifying a system is that a system maintains its existence and functions as a whole through the interaction of its parts. They write:

> Your body is the perfect example. Your body consists of many different parts and organs, each acting separately, yet all working together and each affecting the others. Your thoughts affect your digestion and heart beat, the state of your digestion affects your thoughts—especially after a large lunch. The eye cannot see, nor the legs move without a blood supply, and the blood supply has to be oxygenated through the lungs. The movement of the legs helps pump the blood back to the heart. The body is a complex system.[6]

It is important to appreciate the features of a system and the implications of a system. O'Connor and McDermott distinguish a system from what they call a heap or collection of pieces as follows:

- A system is a series of interconnected parts which function as a whole. A heap is merely a collection of parts.
- A system changes if you take away or add pieces; if you cut a system in half, you do not get two smaller systems: you get a system that will not function. A heap can be divided into pieces, each of which can function on their own.
- In a system, the arrangement of the pieces is crucial, while in a heap, the arrangement is irrelevant.
- In a system, the parts are connected to each other and work together, while in a heap, the arrangement of the pieces is irrelevant.
- The behavior of a system depends on its overall structure, while in a heap, size rather than structure determines behavior.

As we have seen, the term "system" may be used to describe complex biological relationships. "System" may also be used to describe organizations' relationships or processes, such as a healthcare system, a public health system, or a research system. Alternatively, "system" may be used to describe the working of factors or influences that bring about disease and the outcome of disease. Each of these uses of the term "system" shares the intention of understanding how the pieces or items fit together in a coherent whole. In recent years, population health has increasingly turned to systems thinking to better understand the operation of organizations and processes, as well as the development and outcome of disease.[c]

Implementing or operationalizing systems thinking requires tools for analyzing the pieces and understanding how they fit together. This process is called **systems analysis**. There are a wide range of these tools. Often, systems analysis relies on diagrams or graphics that visually display the relationships between the parts and allow us to better understand how the parts fit together and work together.

Let us look at some important methods of systems analysis that are being used in population health.

HOW CAN SYSTEMS ANALYSIS BE USED TO UNDERSTAND THE HEALTH RESEARCH PROCESS?

In the research arena, population health research is now being viewed as part of an integrated continuum of research designed to focus on outcomes at the population as well as the individual level. This came about in large part because the National Institutes of Health has developed and used a systems analysis approach to develop what is being called **translational research**.

Translational research began as an effort to connect basic science with clinical care of individuals and was described as "from the bench to the bedside." More recently, this movement has been extended to the community and the population and may be described as "from the lab to the living room."[7]

We can view translational research as an attempt to bridge the gaps between basic research, clinical applications, and population health implications by seeing health research as a system. **Figure 14-1** outlines the key components of translational research, which are increasingly guiding the distribution of research funding through the National Institutes of Health and other health research funders.

Translational research is often thought of as having three components called T-1, T-2, and T-3. T-1 refers to the now traditional efforts to establish efficacy by using randomized controlled trials. T-2 distinguishes between efficacy under experimental conditions and effectiveness in public health or clinical practice. This concept of effectiveness includes not only how well an intervention works but also its potential harms and, at times, its costs. That is, it includes all of its outcomes.

---

[c] It may be argued that the U.S. healthcare and public health systems include many of the features of a heap rather than a system. While this is probably an overstatement, it points out the importance of thinking in systems and the potential contributions that thinking in systems can have on the development of healthcare and public health organizations.

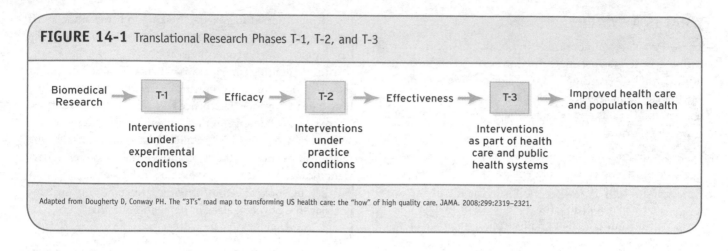

FIGURE 14-1 Translational Research Phases T-1, T-2, and T-3

Adapted from Dougherty D, Conway PH. The "3T's" road map to transforming US health care: the "how" of high quality care. JAMA. 2008;299:2319–2321.

T-2 research also now includes efforts to compare two or more interventions for the same conditions, or what is being called **comparative effectiveness research**. For instance, comparative effectiveness research may examine a series of FDA-approved treatments for diabetes or a series of drugs that are FDA-approved for anticoagulation but have different side effects and different costs.

A new type of very large randomized controlled trial called an **equivalence trial** or a **noninferiority trial** is increasingly being used to study the relative effectiveness of currently approved and utilized interventions. These studies are designed not to determine whether one treatment is better or superior to other treatments but instead to determine if their effectiveness differs in clinically important ways. If no important differences in effectiveness can be demonstrated, decisions can be made on other grounds, such as safety, convenience, and/or cost.[8]

T-3 research looks at the delivery of clinical and public health services. It asks what factors influence the success of interventions that appear to work in T-1 and T-2 studies. T-3 research is increasingly being guided by the RE-AIM framework, which seeks to evaluate the impact of research in practice. RE-AIM is a mnemonic that stands for reach, effectiveness, adoption, implementation, and maintenance. You can think of the "RE" factors as evaluating the potential of the intervention for those it is designed to include or reach. The "AIM" factors examine the realities for application of the intervention in clinical or public health practice. The RE-AIM framework may help us better understand how to translate new interventions into improved outcomes as part of a system. In describing the RE-AIM framework, Laurence Green, one of its developers, has written, "If we want more evidence-based practice, we need more practice-based evidence."[9]

The translational research framework can be viewed as a basic systems analysis diagram. It identifies the pieces, looks at how they should connect, and attempts to put the pieces together as a coherent whole. Despite the simplicity of the diagram, thinking in systems and backing the process up with financial support is having a major impact on how the research process is viewed and how population health in particular is integrated into the research system.

In addition to being useful for better understanding processes such as research, systems analysis is increasingly being used to understand the factors or influences that bring about disease as well as the outcomes of disease.

WHAT ARE THE INITIAL STEPS IN SYSTEMS ANALYSYS?

When using systems analysis to understand disease and its outcomes, we need to start by identifying the most important **influences** on the outcome(s) of interest. Influences are factors or determinants that interact with each other to bring about outcomes, such as disease or the results of disease.[d]

Let us see how we might identify influences on smoking cessation. Using one-at-a-time reductionist studies, the following interventions have been shown to be effective: smoking cessation programs, prohibitions on smoking in public places, social marketing, and cigarette taxes. In addition, measures of the strength of a relationship such as relative risk obtained from reductionist studies often help us measure the magnitude of the influence that a factor has on an outcome. Thus, the first two steps in systems thinking are often built on data derived using reductionist thinking.

---

[d] The term "influences," like the term "risk factors," does not imply that all the criteria for a contributory cause have been established. We need to be careful with the use of the term "determinant" because it is often used as a synonym for "influences," even though it sounds like its presence carries an inevitability of developing a condition or disease.

Rather than looking at one intervention at a time, however, systems thinking asks about the best combination of interventions and how they can be used together. Let us assume that smoking cessation programs, prohibition on smoking in public, social marketing, and higher taxes have been identified as the four most important interventions or influences on the rate of cigarette smoking. The question then becomes how they can be effectively and efficiently combined.

Reductionist thinking usually assumes a straight-line or linear relationship between influences, implying that increased levels of an intervention, such as increasing taxes on tobacco, will produce a straight-line decrease in the levels of tobacco use. However, it is possible that small increases in taxes have little effect, while somewhat larger increases have dramatic effects. In addition, reductionist thinking does not look at how the impact of one intervention may be affected by connecting it with other interventions, whereas systems thinking looks at these interactions. Thus, systems thinking would ask questions about how to most effectively utilize cigarette taxes by combining them with other approaches, such as using the taxes to support tobacco education programs, or reduce exposure to other causes of lung cancer, such as radon and asbestos.

The following summarizes the initial steps in a systems analysis:

- Step 1: Identify the key influences or interventions on an outcome such as disease or the outcome of disease.
- Step 2: Indicate the relative strength of the impact of each of the influences or interventions.
- Step 3: Identify how these influences or interventions interact—that is, how they work together or, alternatively, interfere with each other.

These three steps in systems analysis are basic to understanding the structure of a system.

WHAT ADDITIONAL STEPS ARE NEEDED TO COMPLETE A SYSTEMS ANALYSIS?

Increasingly, we are taking the process one step further. We are using systems analysis to better understand how systems function. Systems thinking requires not only an examination of multiple influences and their interaction at one point in time using a static approach but also encourages us to look at how these factors change over time. That is, systems thinking can lead to a dynamic approach. Let us see how this may be accomplished.

Systems analysis attempts to take into account changes in the overall system that occur over time due to changes in one or more of the factors or influences. These changes in a factor or influence are said to provide feedback into the process

producing what are called **feedback loops**. Feedback loops can have either positive or negative impacts on the outcome. For instance, in developing a systems analysis, we might ask: Does the reduction in the percentage of people who smoke due to higher taxes lead to changes over time in social attitudes, which themselves may set the stage for greater enforcement of public smoking regulations? This would be a positive feedback loop. Alternatively, raising cigarette taxes might reduce the money available to individuals to pay for smoking cessation programs if these services are not paid for by health insurance. This would be a negative feedback loop. Systems thinking does not view the impact of interventions as static. Rather, it tries to develop dynamic models, incorporating the feedback processes that reinforce or accelerate the impacts or alternatively dampen or reduce the impact.

Systems analyses encourage us to identify feedback loops, including positive feedback loops that reinforce or accentuate the process and negative feedback loops that dampen or slow down the process. Feedback loops are key to understanding how a system operates or functions. Complex systems, such as the human body, rely heavily on feedback loops in order to maintain stability. When one component gets out of control, such as body temperature or hydration, other components of the system respond to maintain the body within a tolerable range. This requires positive and negative feedback loops. Similarly, communicable disease in a population is controlled to a certain extent by responses or feedback, including voluntary isolation of sick individuals, development of immunity, and, unfortunately, death of affected individuals. Understanding these feedback loops can help us improve on the natural systems that exist while utilizing the positive aspects of existing systems.

Looking at the dynamic nature of systems and the changes that occur over time allows us to identify **bottlenecks** that limit the effectiveness of systems and **leverage points** that provide opportunities to greatly improve outcomes. For instance, systems analysis might identify a bottleneck such as the need to train large numbers of clinicians in smoking cessation methods so that they can address the demand for smoking cessation services created by social marketing, increased cigarette taxes, and better drug treatments. A leverage point that might be identified is pregnant women who smoke but are highly motivated to quit due to the severe impact on their offspring.

Thus, the additional steps in systems analysis can be described as follows:

- Step 4: Identify the dynamic changes that may occur in a system by identifying the feedback loops that occur in the system.

- Step 5: Identify bottlenecks that limit the effectiveness of the system.
- Step 6: Identify leverage points that provide opportunities to greatly improve outcomes.

HOW CAN WE USE A SYSTEMS ANALYSIS TO BETTER UNDERSTAND A PROBLEM SUCH AS CORONARY ARTERY DISEASE?

Let us use each of the six steps we have identified in a systems analysis to better understand the problem of coronary artery disease.

Step 1: Identify influences—We know from reductionist research that there are multiple factors that increase the risk of coronary artery disease, including high blood pressure, high LDL cholesterol, low HDL cholesterol, abdominal obesity, diabetes, cigarette smoking, physical inactivity, family history, etc. Recognizing each of these factors has been an important part of addressing the problem of coronary artery disease. Further progress, however, requires us to think about how these interventions connect to each other.

Step 2: Estimate the relative strength of the influences—We need to estimate the relative strength or magnitude of the impact of each of the influences. We might estimate the relative risk for each of these factors, or we might classify their impacts as weak, moderate, or strong. In the case of coronary artery disease, each of these factors is considered of moderate importance with relative risks in the range of 2 to 4.

Step 3: Examine the interactions between factors—Examining the interaction between factors helps us understand what happens when two or more of the factors are present. Risk factors for disease may add together to increase the risk of disease, such as high blood pressure plus high LDL cholesterol and low HDL cholesterol. Alternatively, one factor, such as physical activity, may have a protective effect against coronary artery disease in and of itself. Interactions between factors may multiply the risk rather than resulting in an additive impact. Risk factors for coronary artery disease are usually assumed to add together rather than to multiply the impact. However, a combination of risk factors known as the metabolic syndrome has been shown to interact and greatly increase the risk. Metabolic syndrome includes increased waist circumference, low HDL cholesterol, elevated triglycerides, hypertension, and elevated fasting blood sugar. When all or a number of these risk factors occur together, they greatly magnify the probability of coronary artery disease as well as other large blood vessel diseases such as strokes.

Step 4: Identify feedback loops that lead to dynamic changes in the functioning of the system—Understanding how systems operate over time requires us to identify feedback mechanisms, or feedback loops, that alter the likelihood of disease or impact its outcome. For instance, increased weight, especially increased abdominal girth, may lead to increased LDL cholesterol, diabetes, reduced exercise, reduced HDL cholesterol, and increased blood pressure. Alternatively, multiple interventions focused on weight, exercise, blood sugar control, and treatment of hypertension may work together to have a surprisingly positive impact on the probability of coronary artery disease.[e]

Step 5: Identify bottlenecks—Bottlenecks imply that there are points in the system that need to be addressed in order for the other factors or influences to have their potential impacts. For instance, in coronary artery disease, if severe narrowing of the coronary arteries already exists, it is unlikely that interventions such as reducing blood sugar, reducing LDL cholesterol, increasing exercise, or stopping cigarette smoking are going to have a dramatic impact. If the bottleneck, the narrowed artery, can be addressed using angioplasty or surgery, attention to the other risk factors may have a much greater impact.

Step 6: Identify leverage points—The systems analysis that we have done so far suggests some leverage points where interventions may have greater than expected impacts. For instance, increasing exercise post angioplasty or surgery may be safer than when severe disease is present. Patients may also be highly motivated to exercise after having angioplasty or surgery. Exercise then might be effective in helping patients stop smoking cigarettes and reduce abdominal girth, as well as having an impact on HDL cholesterol and blood sugar.

Table 14-1 summarizes the steps in the process, the meaning of each step, and the examples from cigarette smoking and coronary artery disease.

At times, we may be able to use the results of a systems analysis to display the structure and function of a system using what is called a **systems diagram**. A systems diagram is a graphic means of displaying the way we understand systems to be structured and/or to function. Let us see how we can use a systems diagram to display the functioning of a system.

---

[e] These dynamic effects may produce what are called stocks and flows. Stocks and flows can be thought of much like that of a dammed river system. The stocks are the reservoirs, or reserves, that we see. The flows represent the water coming into and out of the reservoir. Stocks and flows are especially important in systems analyses that address issues of the speed of events that occur when systems thinking is applied to organizational issues.

TABLE 14-1   Steps and Their Meaning in Systems Analysis

Step #	Meaning	Examples
1. Identify influences	Identify factors or determinants that are thought to affect or influence the probability of occurrence of a disease or the outcome of a disease.	Coronary artery disease—High LDL cholesterol, cigarette smoking, increased abdominal obesity, etc., increase occurrence. Cigarettes—Taxation of cigarettes, smoking cessation programs, prohibitions on public smoking, etc., improve outcome.
2. Estimate the relative strength of the influences	Estimate the relative risks of each of the influences or at least the relative strength, such as weak, moderate, or strong.	Coronary artery disease—Most important factors are of moderate strength with relative risks between 2 and 4. Cigarettes—Degree of addiction is a strong factor in determining outcome. Radon and asbestos each have relative risk of approximately 5.
3. Examine the interactions between factors	How is the occurrence of disease or the outcome of disease affected when two or more influences are present? Do the impacts of the influences add together, does one influence protect against another influence, does the presence of two influences multiply the impact?	Coronary artery disease—The metabolic syndrome is an example of interactions between factors in which the presence of multiple factors has more than an additive impact. The impacts of radon and asbestos on lung cancer are multiplied in the presence of cigarette smoking.
4. Identify feedback loops	Identify ways that an influence increases or decreases the impact of other factor(s) over time.	Coronary artery disease—Exercise can reduce weight, blood sugar, and blood pressure as well as having a protective impact in and of itself. Cigarettes—Reduction in the percentage of the population who smoke may encourage greater use of other interventions to further reduce the percentage who smoke.
5. Identify bottlenecks	Identify points in the system or constraints that need to be addressed in order for the other factors or influences to have their potential impacts.	Coronary artery disease—Severe constriction of major artery often needs to be addressed by angioplasty or surgery to enable other interventions to work effectively. Cigarettes—Addiction often needs to be addressed directly in order for other influences to be effective.
6. Identify leverage points	Identify points in the system that present opportunities for interventions to have greater than otherwise expected impacts.	Coronary artery disease—Exercise may have greater than expected impacts if used post angiography or surgery when exercise is safer and patients are motivated. Cigarettes—Interventions aimed at pregnant women may have greater than expected impacts short term and longer term because women are highly motivated to stop cigarette smoking during pregnancy.

HOW CAN WE USE SYSTEMS DIAGRAMS TO DISPLAY THE WORKINGS OF A SYSTEM?[10, 11]

Let us use an example to illustrate the development and use of systems diagrams. We will take a look at the etiology and outcomes of motor vehicle injuries, especially automobile injuries. **Box 14-1** presents the "facts" that we will use in developing our systems diagrams.

The development of systems diagrams begins with identifying the key factors that will be included in the systems. For each factor, we need to:

- Indicate the direction in which it operates, in other words, which way the arrow points
- Indicate whether the factor operates to reinforce or increase another factor or outcome, which is indicated

BOX 14-1   Background on Motor Vehicle Injuries as a Systems Issue

Overview

Motor vehicle injuries in the United States, and automobile injuries in particular, have been the leading cause of death for children and young adults for at least the last half century. Today, they remain a critical problem; however, the death rates from motor vehicle collisions, especially when measured as death per miles driven, have fallen so dramatically that the CDC classified highway safety as one of the 10 great public health achievements of the 20th century. This progress has not been due to any one intervention or magic bullet—it is the combination of systems thinking and coordinated interventions that have made the difference.

We might regard the dramatic fall in automobile-related deaths as a systems thinking success story. However, change brings new issues and new challenges. The widespread practice of texting while driving poses new safety hazards that need to be addressed.

We will use motor vehicle injuries as an example that allows us to illustrate principles of systems thinking. We will aim to analyze the issue of motor vehicle injuries from both an etiology and an outcome perspective. That is, we will look at both the reason for motor vehicle injuries and consequences of motor vehicle injuries. We will see how we can impact one, the other, or both of these. In using a systems thinking approach, we need to incorporate the following information. For purposes of this example, you need to act as if the following represents important factual information.

Etiology

In terms of etiology, motor vehicle collisions are greatly influenced by alcohol use, which has direct impacts on the risk of motor vehicle collisions but also leads to speeding, which itself strongly influences the chances of motor vehicle collision. Speeding greatly increases the likelihood of a collision

as well as reducing available response times. Efforts aimed at both speeding and alcohol use have been especially effective in reducing motor vehicle injuries.

Motor vehicle collisions are also increased by texting, which greatly increases the response time when potential hazards occur. In addition, it may directly produce motor vehicle collisions by the movements or mechanical issues produced by texting, which disrupt safe driving.

Motor vehicle collisions can be reduced by road safety technology such as wider shoulders, barriers, and straighter roads. Vehicle collision prevention technology such as more visible brake lights, occupied blind spot notification systems, and out of lane notification systems may reduce the probability of collisions. Vehicle collision safety technology such as crumple zones, which absorb impacts, roll-over protections, and safety glass can reduce injuries when collisions do occur. Passenger restraint systems including safety belts and airbags can reduce the chance of injury from motor vehicle collisions.

Outcome

In terms of outcome, an emergency response system can take advantage of the "golden hour," a period of time when emergency intervention can save many lives, which can reduce death and disability after injuries do occur. The emergency response system can be thought of as including first responders, emergency department preparedness, as well as a trauma triage system helping ensure that those injured get appropriate care as fast as possible. By eliminating the long delays in reaching care, the emergency response systems have been especially effective in reducing the rate of death and disability due to motor vehicle injuries.

A systems analysis of both etiology and outcome underlies the approaches that have been used to address motor vehicle injuries. The collaborative efforts of public health and clinical medicine have been an essential ingredient in this success.

by a (+), or operates to dampen or decrease another factor or outcome, which is indicated by a (−).

Figure 14-2 looks at the direction of two factors, emergency response system and injury, as well as their type of

impacts on death and disability. Note that both emergency response system and injury point toward death and disability because they presumably impact the frequency of occurrence of death and disability. However, emergency response has a negative sign because it hopefully reduces the frequency of death

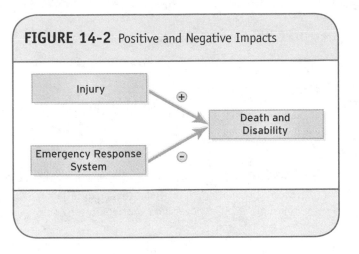

FIGURE 14-2 Positive and Negative Impacts

FIGURE 14-3 Strength of Response

and disability. Injury itself increases the frequency of death and disability.[f]

In addition to indicating the direction of influence and whether the influence is positive or negative, systems diagrams often indicate the strength or magnitude of the impact. The strength or magnitude of the impact is indicated by the width of the arrow used. The thicker the arrow, the greater the impact. **Figure 14-3** illustrates the strength or magnitude of two relationships. The thicker arrow between texting and slow response indicates a stronger impact while the thinner arrow between texting and motor vehicle collision indicates a weaker direct impact.

Texting has a strong impact on response time because those who are texting often fail to see and respond to hazards in a timely way. In addition, texting may in and of itself lead to collisions due to the movements or mechanical issues produced by texting, which disrupt safe driving, such as having one or both hands off the steering wheel while writing a text, or inadvertently swerving when reaching for the phone.

Figure 14-4 demonstrates what is called a positive feedback loop. In a positive feedback loop, one factor reinforces another to magnify the impact. Alcohol use reduces inhibitions and often leads to driving well beyond the speed limit. It also decreases response time, and together with the increased speed, greatly magnifies the effect of alcohol alone. A positive feedback loop can help us identify leverage points where extra efforts can have great benefits. Efforts to address

both alcohol use and speeding, often together, have been especially effective in having a major impact on the reduction of motor vehicle collisions.

Figure 14-5 demonstrates what is called a negative feedback loop. As shown in the figure, the occurrence of injuries leads to increased use of the emergency response system, which itself is intended to reduce the probability of death and disability. The increased use of the system may provide increased experience and increased competence for these health professions, so the increased use may actually improve outcome. A negative feedback loop can help us identify bottlenecks, which prevent later otherwise effective interventions from working. Efforts to eliminate long delays in reaching trauma care and taking advantage of the golden hour have largely removed this bottleneck. These interventions have been especially effective in reducing the deaths and disabilities due to motor vehicle injuries.[g]

Figure 14-6 represents a basic systems diagram putting together the impact of the positive and the negative feedback loops and indicating the direction of influence and the strength or magnitude of the impacts. This is the simplest type of full systems diagram.

---

[f] At times, arrows may point in both directions. Stoplights, for instance, may reduce the occurrence of injuries. The increased occurrence of injuries might also increase the frequency of placement of stoplights. When this occurs, expect there to be arrows in both directions. Each of these arrows may have a positive or a negative sign, and the magnitude or strength of the impacts may be different in the two directions.

---

[g] In systems analysis, positive and negative feedback loops are distinguished by the product of the signs. Two negative signs or two positive signs therefore produce a positive feedback loop. Three negative signs or two positive signs and one negative sign produce a negative feedback loop. In general, when the product of the signs is positive, the loop is considered a positive feedback loop, and when the product of the signs is negative, the loop is considered a negative feedback loop.

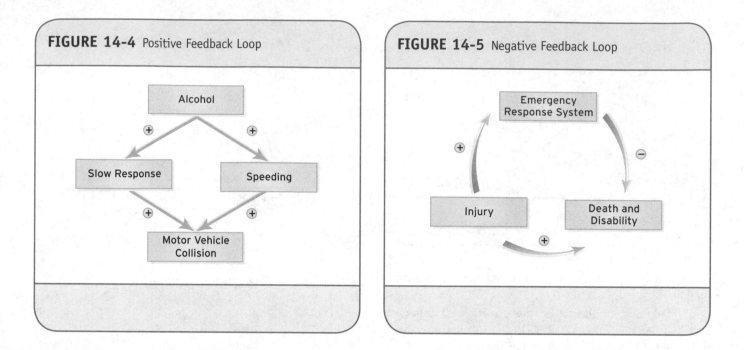

FIGURE 14-4 Positive Feedback Loop

FIGURE 14-5 Negative Feedback Loop

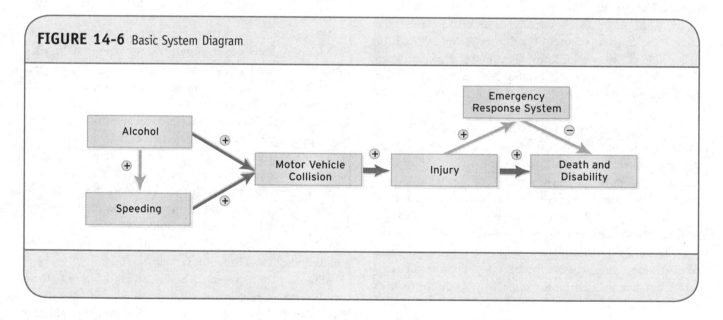

FIGURE 14-6 Basic System Diagram

Often additional factors can be included in the systems diagram. **Figure 14-7** diagrams the dampening or negative impact of a series of factors on the probability of motor vehicle collisions and also on the occurrence of injury once motor vehicle collisions occur. These factors are road safety technology, vehicle collision prevention technology, vehicle collision safety technology, and passenger restraint technology.

Figure 14-8 illustrates additional positive or accelerating/magnifying impacts of the combination of speeding and texting on motor vehicle collisions. It indicates how both speeding and texting have direct and indirect impacts that increase the probability of motor vehicle injury. Here it is assumed that texting has its major impact by slowing response time, while speeding has its greatest impact by directly increasing the chances of a collision.

Finally, **Figure 14-9** attempts to put all of these components together to develop a systems diagram incorporating all the factors or influences that we indicated have an impact

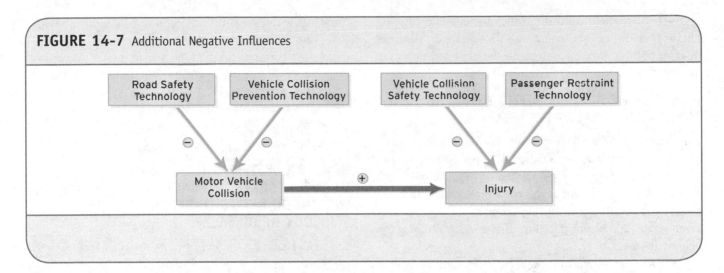

FIGURE 14-7 Additional Negative Influences

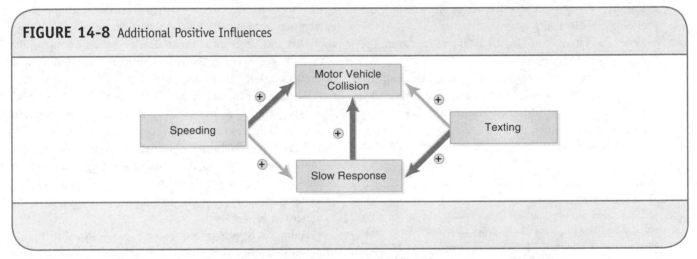

FIGURE 14-8 Additional Positive Influences

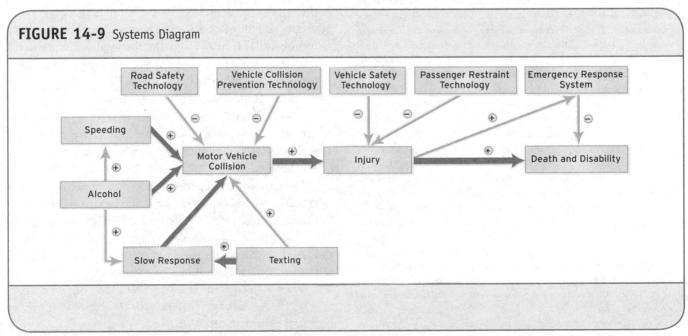

FIGURE 14-9 Systems Diagram

on the occurrence of collision or the outcome of collisions.[h] Figure 14-9 may be used as the basis for developing potential interventions or future research on the expected impact of interventions.[i]

HOW CAN WE APPLY SYSTEMS THINKING TO POPULATION HEALTH ISSUES?

Even when we do not have enough data to do a full systems analysis or develop a systems diagram, specific components of systems thinking can be applied to population health issues. Let us take a look at the roles that systems thinking can play in population health. In doing this, we will look at seven population health questions that systems thinking can help us answer.

- How can systems thinking help us incorporate interactions between factors to better understand the etiology of disease?
- How can systems thinking help take into account the interactions between diseases?
- How can systems thinking help us understand the impact of a disease over the life span?
- How can systems thinking help identify bottlenecks and leverage points that can be used to improve population health?

---

[h] Systems diagrams are designed to communicate the author's understanding or belief about the relationships that produce disease or impact the outcomes. Thus, there can be variations, with no single one serving as the correct version. Systems diagrams often do not include all the potential interactions that occur. Which interactions to include is often a judgment call. One consideration in drawing systems diagrams is to avoid having arrows cross each other, which makes the completed diagram more complicated and difficult to read and interpret. Because one of the aims of systems diagrams is to communicate efficiently, systems diagrams should not be any more complex than necessary to convey an appreciation of what the author believes are the key relationships.

[i] Systems diagrams at times can be converted into what is called a systems model if measureable variables are used to describe each factor. For instance, instead of using alcohol as a factor, a measure of alcohol consumption needs to be used, such as blood level of alcohol. Systems models aim to simulate the actual operation of a system. By developing a systems model, we may be able to use computerized methods to perform simulations of the operation of the model and quantitatively test the model to estimate how the outcome(s) may be altered by altering one or more of the factors. Simulations imply calculating quantitatively the outcome(s) of the model after making one or more changes in the model. The simulation may be "run" a large number of times based on chance selection of particular values from a possible distribution of values for each factor. The results of the simulation can then be presented as a range of values using the mean and standard deviations of each outcome. The process of running the model a large number of times allows us to determine whether the outcome is sensitive to the level or value of a particular factor. This process can help us judge the potential impact of a number of possible interventions, or, at times, changes that occur over time.

- How can systems thinking help us develop strategies for multiple simultaneous interventions?
- How can systems thinking help us look at processes as a whole to plan short-term and long-term intervention strategies?
- How can systems thinking help us predict the future frequency of diseases?

HOW CAN SYSTEMS THINKING HELP US INCORPORATE INTERACTIONS BETWEEN FACTORS TO BETTER UNDERSTAND THE ETIOLOGY OF DISEASE?

Understanding the interactions between factors, influences, or determinants has become central to population health, as illustrated by new approaches such as the social determinants of health. Let us examine a specific interaction that has received a great deal of attention in public health in recent years: the interaction between radon and cigarette smoking in causing lung cancer.[12] Radon is a naturally occurring radioactive gas. It is colorless and odorless. Radon is produced by the decay of uranium in soil, rock, and groundwater. It emits ionizing radiation during its radioactive decay. Radon is found all over the country, though there are areas of the country with substantially higher levels than other areas. Radon gets into the indoor air primarily by entering via the soil under homes and other buildings at the basement or lowest level.

Today, it is recognized based on high-quality epidemiological studies that radon causes lung cancer. Radon is the second most important cause of lung cancer after cigarettes and the most common cause of lung cancer among nonsmokers. The EPA estimates that radon accounts for over 20,000 cases of lung cancer, as compared with the over 100,000 cases attributed to cigarettes. The average indoor level in the United States is about 1.3pCi/L. The EPA has set a level of 2pCi/L as an attainable level and a level of 4pCi/L as the maximum recommended level. Approximately 15% of homes in the United States have basement radon levels above 4pCi/L.

Cigarette smoking and radon exposure are multiplicative; that is, when both are present, the hazard is multiplied. For instance, using the EPA's figures, the relative risk of lung cancer for the average smoker is approximately nine times the risk compared to a nonsmoker. The relative risk from radon when the level is 10pCi/L compared to 2pCi/L is over 4.5. When both cigarette smoking and a level of radon exposure of 10pCi/L are present, the relative risk of lung cancer increases almost 40 times.

The recognition that radon multiplies the impacts of cigarette smoking has had a key impact on the approaches used to address these potential hazards. For smokers with exposure to these hazards, the risk can be greatly reduced by reductions in radon as well as by stopping smoking. Because radon is a measurable and controllable environmental exposure, there has been a great deal of attention and effort given to control of this hazard. Thus, the recognition of interactions that multiply or greatly increase the risk have become an important tool for setting priorities and developing approaches to risk reduction.

HOW CAN SYSTEMS THINKING HELP TAKE INTO ACCOUNT THE INTERACTIONS BETWEEN DISEASES?

The classic connection between diseases was Edward Jenner's observation that children who develop cow pox were very unlikely to get smallpox even when exposed. This fundamental observation led to the concept and term "vaccination," from the Latin word "vacca," or cow. It also established that there is a relationship between diseases.

In recent years, it has been increasingly recognized that some diseases predispose to other diseases. In addition, there are patterns of risk factors or symptoms that tend to occur together. These are often called **syndromes**. As we have seen, the components of the metabolic syndrome frequently occur together and greatly increase the probability of coronary artery and other large blood vessel diseases. The recognition of the frequent occurrence of the metabolic syndrome has led to concerted efforts to identify individuals with the syndrome and make a multi-intervention approach to reducing the risk.

HIV provides a good example of the complex interactions that occur between diseases. A number of sexually transmitted diseases, especially those that interrupt the mucosal membranes lining the genital organs, such as syphilis and herpes genitalis, increase the risk of being infected with HIV if exposed. In addition, diseases such as gonorrhea greatly increase the level of the HIV virus that appears in semen, thus increasing the communicability of HIV.

HIV itself predisposes to a large number of infections, the most important of which from the public health perspective is tuberculosis. Finally, HIV is found in association with other conditions, including drug abuse and intimate partner violence, which greatly increases the burden of disease. These types of interactions of HIV with other diseases and conditions have been described as a **syndemic**. A syndemic is the occurrence together of two or more diseases that interact to magnify the occurrence and/or burden of disease.[13]

Disease interactions are not always detrimental. At times, one disease may provide protection against other diseases. Early infection with bacteria and other pathogens in environments such as that which occurs on farms has been shown to be associated with reduced incidence of food and skin allergies.

Systems thinking can not only help us understand the relationship between diseases, but it can also help us understand the impact that a disease has over the life span.

HOW CAN SYSTEMS THINKING HELP US UNDERSTAND THE IMPACT OF A DISEASE OVER THE LIFE SPAN?

Varicella, or chicken pox, provides a good example of the importance of understanding the impact of a disease over the life span. Chicken pox is a highly contagious viral disease that until the 2000s affected approximately 90% of children in the United States. It was considered a mild disease among young children. Healthy individuals who develop chicken pox as adolescents or adults often have far more severe disease, often resulting in pneumonia and other life-threatening conditions. Because the disease is so contagious and generally mild among young children, parents in the United States often held "chicken pox parties." Children were intentionally exposed to other children with chicken pox to try to ensure early infection.

Chicken pox can result in a range of complications, including life-threatening skin infections, pneumonia, and encephalitis, or infection of the brain, especially among immunosuppressed individuals and pregnant women. In addition, women who develop chicken pox in early pregnancy can pass it on to their fetus, producing a 1 to 2% probability of congenital deformities including physical deformities and learning disabilities.

Naturally acquired chicken pox provides long-lasting immunity, which prevents recurrent chicken pox, but the virus remains within the sensory nerve roots that supply areas of the skin surface called dermatomes. As immunity wanes with age, the virus can emerge as a disease called shingles in the area supplied by these nerves. An estimated 50% of individuals who live to be 85 years old, the most rapidly growing age group in the United States, will experience shingles. Shingles produces chicken pox–like sores and severe pain that can become chronic severe pain.

Thus, chicken pox is truly a disease that affects people and populations from the fetus to the elderly. When considering interventions to prevent or treat chicken pox, it is important to recognize that this is a disease that spans the life span.[14]

As we have discussed, identifying bottlenecks and leverage points is a fundamental goal of systems analysis. Let us take a look at how these points can be identified and used to improve population health.

HOW CAN SYSTEMS THINKING HELP IDENTIFY BOTTLENECKS AND LEVERAGE POINTS THAT CAN BE USED TO IMPROVE POPULATION HEALTH?

Looking at the dynamics of systems helps us identify two types of points that benefit from special attention. The first of these is called a bottleneck or a constraint. A bottleneck is a point at which events are slowed down, presenting obstacles to success of an intervention. We have already identified some important bottlenecks. In the 1960s, it was recognized that after trauma, such as injuries from war or motor vehicle collisions, many victims are able to physiologically respond and temporarily tolerate blood loss and other injuries before rapidly deteriorating. This early period became known as the golden hour.

Few victims of motor vehicle injuries before the 1970s were reaching emergency care during the golden hour. To address this bottleneck, a sophisticated system of emergency response was put into place in the United States, which, as we have discussed, greatly reduced the response time and resulted in a large reduction in deaths and disabilities from motor vehicle collisions.

We identified another example of a bottleneck in the course of cigarette smoking. The vast majority of cigarette smokers start before age 18 and often many years earlier. These smokers often have a great deal of difficulty stopping smoking, even when they are intellectually committed to stopping in later years. Addiction to nicotine in cigarettes has been recognized as a key bottleneck to successful control of cigarette smoking. Recent interventions are addressing this bottleneck, including new authority for the FDA to regulate the quantity of nicotine in cigarettes. On the other hand, leverage points are points in systems in which successful interventions produce better than expected outcomes. We can see them as opportunities to make major improvements in outcomes. At leverage points, there is no bottleneck, but the conditions are right to take advantage of the interactions that exist between factors. For instance, with cigarette smoking, pregnant women who smoke are at greatly increased risk of delivering premature infants. In addition, they are highly motivated to stop smoking and often have encouragement to do so by family and friends. New efforts to put extra resources and extra efforts into smoking cessation for pregnant women are having a large payoff for their newborns and themselves. In addition to helping us identify bottlenecks and leverage points, systems thinking can help us develop a coordinated approach or strategy for combining multiple simultaneous interventions.

HOW CAN SYSTEMS THINKING HELP US DEVELOP STRATEGIES FOR MULTIPLE SIMULTANEOUS INTERVENTIONS?

As we have seen, the approach to coronary artery disease has successfully utilized multiple simultaneous interventions for several decades. Today, we are moving to a coordinated strategy of utilizing primary, secondary, and tertiary interventions. Primary interventions include control of high blood pressure, cholesterol, cigarette smoking, obesity, diabetes, and a growing list of other contributory causes of coronary artery disease. Secondary interventions designed to prevent heart damage and death, including interventions in the early hours of a myocardial infarction, have become an increasingly successful part of an overall strategy. Drug treatment and post myocardial exercise rehabilitation are now a standard part of medical care. Finally, tertiary interventions to prevent sudden death in public places have now become a population health intervention, with placement of automated defibrillators in places where people congregate, such as airports and sporting events.

New approaches to disease often combine primary, secondary, and tertiary interventions. For instance, efforts to address HIV increasingly include primary prevention through barrier protection, circumcision, precoital and intracoital treatment, and eventually vaccination. Postexposure treatments are being extensively investigated as well. Detection during the first few weeks, when transmissibility is greatest, is being investigated as an important new intervention. In addition, early and continuous drug treatment of HIV has been found not only to help the individual but also to reduce his or her infectivity. The success of these efforts among sexually active individuals remains to be seen, but for maternal to child transmission, there is already strong evidence of success. **Box 14-2** discusses the success of the multiple intervention approach to prevention of maternal–child transmission of HIV.

The strategy of coordinated use of multiple simultaneous complementary interventions has become a highly successful population health strategy. For many years, interventions were studied and applied one intervention at a time, with little thought to how they interact or how they could be used in combination to produce the best results. In recent years, systems thinking and systems analysis approaches have contributed to the development of increasingly effective strategies that combine multiple interventions.

Fully developed systems thinking approaches, when feasible, can also be used to help us see entire processes to help us plan short-term as well as long-term intervention strategies.

BOX 14-2 Success of the Multiple Intervention Approach to Maternal–Child Transmission of HIV

Prevention of maternal–child transmission of HIV in the United States has been highly successful. Today, infection with HIV by the maternal–child route should be considered a failure of public health and medicine. HIV can be transmitted via the placenta during pregnancy. The higher the level of virus in the mother's blood, the greater the probability of transmission. Thus, early testing and active treatment of pregnant women is fundamental to prevention of maternal–child transmission. In addition, there is an increased risk during vaginal delivery. Selective use of Cesarean delivery can reduce this risk. Early treatment of infants has been shown to reduce the risk still further. Finally, breastfeeding carries a small but important risk of transmission. Avoidance of breastfeeding or active maternal drug treatment during breastfeeding among women with HIV can greatly reduce this risk as well.

HOW CAN SYSTEMS THINKING HELP US LOOK AT PROCESSES AS A WHOLE TO PLAN SHORT-TERM AND LONG-TERM INTERVENTION STRATEGIES?

Efforts to see the entire processes rather than pieces of the pie have become key to planning interventions and have been incorporated into the "health in all policies" approach. The drug regulatory process has moved beyond a focus on premarket studies designed to establish efficacy and acceptable levels of safety in low-risk patients. Today, we are increasingly looking at postmarket studies examining safety in practice as well as longer term effectiveness and safety. In addition, comparative effectiveness studies of FDA-approved treatments conducted as part of comparative effectiveness research are asking questions about the effectiveness, safety, acceptance, and cost of the existing treatments.

Systems thinking approaches to food safety have developed in recent years.[15] Initially, systems thinking has focused on identifying interventions for high-risk food one type of food at a time. This process has been called the Hazard Analysis and Critical Control Points (HACCP) system. **Box 14-3** takes a look at the HACCP approach and the efforts to control the hazard of ground beef.

New approaches to food safety build on the HACCP system and its big picture look at the process as a whole. In

BOX 14-3 The HACCP System and Ground Beef

Hazard Analysis and Critical Control Points (HACCP) is a systems approach that looks for key leverage or **control points** to manage food safety issues. It is built upon a series of prerequisite conditions designed to first ensure basic environmental and operating conditions. These prerequisite conditions might be viewed as efforts to remove the bottlenecks to an effectively functioning system. These include facilities that maintain sanitary conditions; proper equipment construction, installation, and maintenance; personal hygiene by employees; etc.

Once these basic conditions of food safety are accomplished, HACCP looks for options for interventions at multiple leverage or control points and institutes a series of safeguards at these specific points.

Meat safety issues reflect this approach. Ground beef, which often combines meat from leftover portions of multiple animals, has been identified as a high-risk product or hazard. Toxin-producing strains of *E. coli* are widespread in ground beef products and have been responsible for a number of

fatal outbreaks of foodborne illness in the past. The threats to health have led to a more coordinated systems thinking approach using the HACCP system. Let us take a look at the HACCP process and the ground beef example.

The systems thinking approach known as HACCP attempts to understand, monitor, and quickly respond to breakdowns in the food safety system. This methodology, originally developed for the U.S. space program, is based on the principle that risks to food safety exist from the field to the fork. HACCP is increasingly being adopted for such products as seafood, meat, poultry, and fruit juices. HACCP includes the following seven steps:

- *Analyze hazards*. Potential hazards associated with a food and potential interventions to control those hazards are identified. The hazard could be biological, such as a microbe; chemical, such as a toxin; or physical, such as ground glass or metal fragments.

(continues)

BOX 14-3 The HACCP System and Ground Beef (*continued*)

- *Identify critical control points*. These are points in a food's production—from its raw state through processing and shipping to consumption by the consumer—at which the potential hazard can be controlled or eliminated. Examples are cooking, cooling, packaging, and metal detection.
- *Establish preventive measures with critical limits for each control point*. For a cooked food, for example, this may include setting the minimum cooking temperature and time required to ensure the elimination of any harmful microbes.
- *Establish procedures to monitor the critical control points*. Such procedures may include determining how and by whom cooking time and temperature should be monitored.
- *Establish corrective actions to be taken when monitoring shows that a critical limit has not been met*. An example is reprocessing or disposing of food if the minimum cooking temperature is not met.
- *Establish procedures to verify that the system is working properly*. An example is testing time- and temperature-recording devices to verify that a cooking unit is working properly.
- *Establish effective recordkeeping to document the HACCP system*. This would include records of hazards and their control methods, the monitoring of safety requirements, and actions taken to correct potential problems. Each of these principles must be backed by sound scientific knowledge—for example, published microbiological studies on time and temperature factors for controlling foodborne pathogens.

Key control points at which ground beef may be contaminated in the meatpacking process have been identified. Monitoring by testing now includes a random testing process on all batches of ground beef. The process uses rapid testing of a sample of the finished ground beef and holding up distribution until the results are available. Education of consumers about the danger of eating rare or raw ground beef is also a key component of this strategy. In addition, separating beef products from other food preparation, especially from food products eaten raw, is an important educational effort.

The HACCP process has already had a major impact on the incidence of disease associated with ground beef. It is not a cure-all but looking at the process as a whole has helped us come up with effective interventions.

an emerging systems thinking approach, most food's detailed location and time of production down to the level of the farm or factory are being identified on the label. This allows public health officials to trace the food back to where and when the problem occurred. Adding this approach to the HACCP provides a mechanism for quickly responding to early indications of foodborne outbreaks, regardless of the type of food involved. The combination of the HACCP system and food tracing provides the potential for a fully developed systems thinking approach to food safety.

Finally, let us take a look at the use of systems thinking to predict the future.

HOW CAN SYSTEMS THINKING HELP US PREDICT THE FUTURE FREQUENCY OF DISEASES?

We would like to be able to predict the future frequency and course of a disease. This could help us focus on the big problems of the future to find better approaches or at least get ready for what is coming. Systems thinking approaches are being used to try to make these estimates. For instance, considerable effort has gone into estimating the future prevalence of Alzheimer's disease, including stages of severity. Researchers have then made estimates of the impact of better interventions and better ways to take care of Alzheimer's patients. Similar efforts are underway to understand the AIDS epidemic.

Estimates of the future are always difficult and need to rest on the big assumption that only the factors we are focusing on will change in the future. Of all the goals we have in public health, and other applied sciences such as economics, politics, meteorology, as well as biological systems, the most difficult task is prediction, especially long-term prediction. Understanding the factors that influence current conditions and the feedback processes that affect the dynamics of a system, we can hope to predict short-term outcomes in the range of months or a few years. Long-term outcomes are particularly difficult to predict, as new factors come into play and old relationships and feedback loops change over time. Small current changes can make large future differences like a slight misalignment of an auto tire can have major implications after many miles of travel.

In addition, current models of systems are built on past data. Data by definition reflects the past state of affairs. Unless new data is constantly collected and incorporated into our analysis, the evidence we incorporate into our systems analysis will literally be obsolete the day we include it. For example, we often use life expectancy to reflect the health status of populations. Yet life expectancy reflects the population health status at one point or year in time in the past. When used to predict the future, it makes the big and unrealistic assumption that nothing will change either for the better or for the worse. Life expectancy may help us predict the short-term future, but the longer we look into the future, the less it helps us predict.

Thus, a systems thinking approach can help us think through and develop plans for a wide range of population health problems, but we should not count on it alone to solve our most difficult challenge, that of predicting the future.

Having reviewed the list of applications of systems thinking to public health, let us step back and try to put these approaches into three basic categories that allow us to see the contribution that systems thinking can make to public health as well as the limitations of systems thinking.

WHAT CAN SYSTEMS THINKING CONTRIBUTE TO PUBLIC HEALTH, AND WHAT ARE ITS LIMITATIONS?

The contributions of systems thinking to population health can be classified as assisting in explanation, operation, and prediction. While systems thinking helps us think through each of these issues, it also has substantial limitations, often related to inadequate data and incomplete understandings of how systems actually work.

Explanation asks: What are the factors that influence the development and outcome of a disease or other problem as part of a system? Multiple factors may influence the development and course of disease. The influences on disease and disease outcomes are complicated, and we need to consider the interactions between factors. Systems thinking brings to bear evidence from multiple sources and allows us to examine multiple causal relationships at the same time. In addressing issues of explanation, systems thinking is limited by our limited knowledge of the factors that actually cause disease as well as the interactions between factors.

Operation asks: How can an intervention be combined with other interventions to maximize the overall impact? Systems operate in dynamic and changing ways to produce disease and the outcomes of disease or other conditions. Looking at systems may allow recognition of bottlenecks that interfere with maximum outcome and leverage points that should be utilized as ways to facilitate optimal outcomes. Recognizing bottlenecks and leverage points requires an understanding of the dynamic ways that systems operate, including feedback loops producing changes over time. Once again, systems thinking is of limited use if we do not understand the way feedback loops act to influence the operation of the system. Taking advantage of these understandings still requires the adequate resources and well-developed collaborations.

Prediction asks: What changes in systems can be expected and how can they be channeled to improve future outcomes? Prediction of the future is the ultimate challenge of systems thinking and the most difficult to achieve. Linear or straight-line prediction based on current trends is commonly used but is very dangerous because it fails to take into account the multiple changes that are likely to occur over time. Prediction by necessity is based on past data, and by definition, past data is not the same as future reality. Our less than complete knowledge and understanding makes prediction very difficult. Short-term prediction measured in months or a few years is often more reliable than predictions that extend over multiple years or decades.

Population health is increasingly making systems thinking a core component rivaling in importance the population perspective itself. Therefore, to understand the future of population health, we need to understand principles of systems thinking and their application to population health problems.

KEY WORDS

- **Systems thinking**
- **Reductionist thinking**
- **System**
- **Systems analysis**
- **Translational research**
- **Comparative effectiveness research**
- **Equivalence trial or noninferiority trial**
- **Influences**
- **Feedback loops**
- **Bottlenecks**
- **Leverage points or control points**
- **Systems diagram**
- **Syndromes**
- **Syndemic**

Discussion Questions

Take a look at the following discussion questions and see how well you can apply principles of systems thinking.

1. You are pregnant and have a 10-year history of cigarette smoking. You are surprised that at your first prenatal visit, there is a big sticker on your chart saying "Smoker." Everyone in the doctor's office asks you what they can do to help, and they quickly enroll you in special services for smoking cessation for which you were not eligible before you got pregnant. When you ask why so much time, attention, and money is now coming your way, they tell you pregnancy is a leverage point for stopping smoking. *What do they mean by "leverage point"*? you ask yourself.

2. A patient with active TB is reported by the local hospital laboratory to the Health Department. The department quickly connects with the patient to determine his close personal contacts. They also ask him if they can test him for HIV. He turns out to be HIV positive, and permission is then requested to get in touch with his sexual contacts. You consider how you would describe the relationship between TB and HIV, and wonder how knowledge of this relationship can be used to reduce the risks of both TB and HIV.

3. A new type of large research study looks at four FDA-approved treatments for myocardial infarction. The study includes over 50,000 patients and is designed to determine not whether one treatment is better than another but instead whether there is any clinically important difference between the outcomes of the treatments. *What type of research is this*, you wonder, *and why is it being done*?

4. An expert panel reviews recent data in an effort to predict the incidence of HIV in 2020. They take into account the current data on incidence and prevalence as well as the effectiveness of known interventions. Unfortunately, within two years after the effort is completed, it is apparent that their estimates are quite inaccurate. *Why is prediction so difficult*? you wonder.

5. You hear that motor vehicle injuries, especially those due to automobile collisions, have been dramatically reduced in recent years. *Was there a magic bullet that accomplished this*, you wonder, *or was this reduction accomplished through a more complicated systems thinking process*?

6. You love rare hamburgers. "Just wave them over the flame," you like to say. Recently, you have heard that ground beef is a high-risk food—even a health hazard. *What does that mean, and what is being done about it*? you ask yourself.

REFERENCES

1. Frenk J, Chen L, et al. Health professionals for a new century: transforming education to strengthen health systems in an interdependent world. *Lancet*. 2010;376:1923–1958.

2. Association of Schools and Programs of Public Health. MPH core competency development project. http://www.asph.org/document.cfm?page=851. Accessed November 29, 2013.

3. Meadows H. *Thinking in Systems: A Primer*. White River Junction, Vermont: Chelsea Green Publishing; 2008.

4. National Cancer Institute–United States Department of Health and Human Services. Greater Than the Sum: Systems Thinking in Tobacco Control—Executive Summary. Washington, DC: U.S. Department of Health and Human Services–National Institutes of Health; 2007.

5. Merriam-Webster. System. http://www.merriam-webster.com/dictionary/system. Accessed July 26, 2013.

6. O'Connor J, McDermott I. *The Art of Systems Thinking: Essential Skills for Creativity and Problem Solving*. Phoenix, AZ: Premium Source Publishing; 2006.

7. Dougherty D, Conway PH. The "3T's" road map to transforming US health care: the "how" of high quality care. *JAMA*. 2008;299:2319–2321.

8. Piaggio G, Elbourne DR, et al. CONSORT group. Reporting of non-inferiority and equivalence randomized trials: an extension of the CONSORT statement. *JAMA*. 2006;295(10):1152–1160.

9. Green L. Guidelines and categories for classifying participatory research projects in health. http://www.lgreen.net/guidelines.html. Accessed July 26, 2013.

10. Kirkwood CW. System dynamic methods: a quick introduction. http://www.public.asu.edu/~kirkwood/sysdyn/SDIntro/SDIntro.htm. Accessed July 26, 2013.

11. The Open University. Systems thinking and practice: diagramming. http://systems.open.ac.uk/materials/T552. Accessed July 23, 2013.

12. U.S. Environmental Protection Agency. Radon. http://www.epa.gov/radon. Accessed July 26, 2013.

13. Centers for Disease Control and Prevention. CDC grand rounds: the TB/HIV syndemic. http://www.cdc.gov/mmwr/preview/mmwrhtml/mm6126a3.htm. Accessed July 26, 2013.

14. Centers for Disease Control and Prevention. Chickenpox (Varicella). http://www.cdc.gov/chickenpox/about. Accessed July 26, 2013.

15. United States Food and Drug Administration. Hazard analysis & critical control points (HACCP). http://www.fda.gov/Food/Guidance Regulation/HACCP. Accessed July 26, 2013.

SECTION V

Cases and Discussion Questions

PUBLIC HEALTH DEPARTMENTS—GETTING THE LEAD OUT

A series of articles appears in your local newspaper investigating reports of elevated lead levels and reduced academic performance among students in a local grade school. The series ends with an editorial asking: "Where was the health department and what are they going to do now?"

The health department was aware of these reports and had sent a letter to each parent alerting them to the dangers of increased lead levels and letting them know of doctors and local clinics that could follow up and provide treatment through a health department-funded program. The mayor is not satisfied. He asks: "But isn't public health about prevention? How can we prevent this from happening again?" He asks the health department for a full report within a month.

The health department sets out to evaluate the range of potential sources of lead exposure in the community. They find the following possible factors: a local factory releases fumes that contain lead, local playgrounds are still contaminated by lead from gasoline despite the fact that lead was completely removed from gasoline well over a decade ago, lead paint in older homes, possible exposure from lead used in water pipes, and lead from painted toys and glazes on homemade pottery. The health department's report to the mayor concludes that prevention of lead exposure requires not just the health department's role, but also the cooperation of schools, parks, the environmental protection agency, the water system, the housing agency, as well as local industry and merchants. "We cannot do it alone," the report concludes.

"Okay," says the mayor, "it sounds like this is a job for the whole city. I am issuing an order requiring all city agencies to cooperate with the health department to find the sources of lead and develop a plan to reduce them." Then he turns to you, a new health department employee. "Work on this and write me a report by next month, but I want a press release out this afternoon."

Discussion Questions

1. How would you recommend reducing or eliminating the hazard from each of the sources of lead identified by the health department? Explain.

2. How does this case reflect the role that the media and effective communications play in public health? Explain.

3. How does this case reflect the multiple collaborations that are needed to practice public health effectively? Explain.

4. How does this case reflect the relationship between public health agencies and clinicians? Explain.

5. How does this case illustrate the inherently political nature of public health? Explain.

COMMUNITY-ORIENTED PRIMARY CARE (COPC)

A community-oriented primary care team was developed in a large Hispanic/Latino community defined by census tracks. The vast majority of the community is employed, and over half of the working population receive minimum wage and have no health insurance. There are a large number of immigrants from Central America. Over 25% of the community is estimated to be undocumented aliens, most of whom live in crowded conditions. A high percentage of those over 18 are married with an average family size of 5—considerably larger than other communities in the same city. The population of the community is generally younger than the surrounding more affluent communities. The vast majority of the community receives its health care at one community clinic.

The community's priority issues according to community residents include tuberculosis (TB), HIV/AIDS, a lack of recreational facilities for children, a lack of dental services, and a lack of Spanish-speaking healthcare professionals. The COPC team, consisting of health professionals, public health experts, a clinical administrator, and members of the community, identified tuberculosis for further study. They found CDC evidence-based guidelines that recommend the following:

- Early and accurate detection, diagnosis, and reporting of TB cases leading to initiation and completion of treatment
- Identification of contacts of patients with infectious TB and treatment of those at risk with an effective drug regimen
- Identification of other persons with latent TB infection at risk for progression to TB disease and treatment of these persons with an effective drug regimen
- Identification of settings in which a high risk exists for transmission of Mycobacterium tuberculosis and application of effective infection-control measures

To implement these recommendations, risk factors for tuberculosis were identified in the community, including crowded conditions, HIV infections, high numbers of recent immigrants from endemic areas, and poor follow-up of treatment.

The COPC team found data on the estimated prevalence of a positive skin test for TB, the prevalence of active TB, the percentage of HIV-positive patients among those with active

TB, and the percentage of active TB patients who completed a full course of treatment. The team recommended interventions for those factors that are most amenable to change, including intensive testing and follow-up of HIV-positive patients and special home health assistance to ensure completion of TB treatment.

The team recommended monitoring the percentage of HIV patients who were given tuberculosis skin tests and the percentage of TB patients who completed a full course of treatment. They also recommended measuring the prevalence of active TB before and after the interventions. Finally, they advised working closely with the local health department so that recommended TB follow-up practices are successfully performed. This included making sure that whenever active TB is diagnosed, all those in contact with the individual are offered TB skin testing and preventive treatments if they convert to positive.

Discussion Questions

1. Identify how the COPC team accomplished each of the six steps in the COPC process.

2. What factors would you consider in selecting a particular condition, such as tuberculosis, for special intervention efforts?

3. Identify one of the community's other priority issues and suggest interventions that you would use for addressing it and assessing, monitoring, and evaluating the impact of your intervention.

4. What are the strengths and limitations of the COPC approach?

HURRICANE KARL AND THE PUBLIC HEALTH SUCCESS IN OLD ORLEANS

Hurricane Karl, a category 4 hurricane, made landfall last August 29th on the gold coast of the state of Good Fortune. The state is home to the town of Old Orleans, a historical community built below sea level and home to a large community from a range of socioeconomic backgrounds. Old Orleans has a model health department that seeks to provide the 10 essential public health services.

Before Hurricane Karl made its impact on the community, preparation for hurricanes had been an ongoing activity of the health department, which worked closely with first responders to ensure safe evacuation and protection from fire and looting. The department also worked with the local TV and radio stations to advise citizens on the purchasing

and storing of essential food, water, and first aid supplies. It organized a community-wide emergency care network to ensure that 911 calls were responded to as quickly as possible in the event of a hurricane and worked with local hospitals to ensure that a triage system was in place to allocate patients to available emergency facilities, while not overwhelming any one healthcare institution.

When Hurricane Karl did strike, the damage was more extensive than expected. Leaks in the public sewer system led to water contamination. A local chemical plant experienced a major chemical discharge. Almost 200 residents were stranded in their homes without adequate food. Nearly half of the homes experienced water damage and rapid growth of mold. Many older residents did not have access to their daily medications.

The local health department had prepared for disasters like Hurricane Karl. After testing the water for contamination, supplies of stockpiled bottled water were distributed to homes in the contaminated areas by the National Guard. The police department had purchased specially equipped vehicles on the recommendation of the health department and was able, with the help of community organizations, to evacuate the stranded residents. The health department also sent out trained teams to diagnose the type and extent of hazards related to chemical contamination. With the help of the emergency radio system and cell phones, all individuals in the contaminated areas were notified and educated about methods for protecting themselves and their children.

Based on the emergency plan, the health department set up temporary healthcare sites and pharmacies staffed by nurses, physicians, and pharmacists who had been certified as emergency responders. The department also worked with representatives of the building industry to test water-exposed homes for mold and provided assistance to minimize the damage.

After the emergency, the health department joined with the local schools of public health and medicine to evaluate the response to Hurricane Karl and make recommendations for future emergencies. The data on infections, injuries, and deaths, as well as the use of services during the emergency, was collected and published. A national network was set up as a result to coordinate efforts for future disasters and learn from the experience in dealing with Hurricane Karl.

Discussion Questions

1. Which of the 10 essential services did the health department of Old Orleans fulfill? Explain.

2. What efforts beyond those of the health department were needed to accomplish the 10 essential public health services? Explain.

3. In addition to providing the 10 essential public health services, to what extent are efforts required to deal with a disaster such as Hurricane Karl? Explain.

4. How does this case illustrate the complementary relationship between public health and medicine? What are the benefits of working together?

LUNG CANCER: OLD DISEASE, NEW APPROACHES

Lung cancer in the United States today is the most commonly diagnosed life-threatening cancer among both men and women, with over 150,000 deaths per year. Cases of lung cancer increase with advancing age, with the disease rarely occurring before age 50. Lung cancer is usually diagnosed at a late stage. The duration of the disease after diagnosis is often measured in months, and the chance of death once the diagnosis is made is well above 90%.

Cigarette smoking has been recognized as the most important contributory cause of lung cancer since 1964, when the data was sufficient for the U.S. surgeon general to publish the first of a series of reports on smoking and health concluding that cigarette smoking is a cause of lung cancer and that interventions are needed to reduce the rate of cigarette smoking.

A large number of specific interventions have been studied and implemented, many with some success. Nearly 50% of men and 25% of women smoked cigarettes in the United States in the early 1960s. Initial efforts to reduce smoking included public service announcements and warning labels on cigarettes. The rate of smoking in the 1960s was modestly reduced among men, but little or no change occurred among women. In fact, over the subsequent decades, the rates of cigarettes smoking increased among young women. During these years tobacco companies advertised Virginia Slims and other products which associated smoking with weight loss and may have led to increased smoking among young women.

During the 1980s and early 1990s, efforts included increased taxes on cigarettes and restrictions of cigarette smoking in public places, including airplanes and increasingly in the workplace justified by evidence of the hazards of second-hand smoking. Evaluation efforts indicated a gradual reduction in smoking, with rates falling to less than 25% among both adult men and women.

The evaluation data indicated that the rates among adolescents were increasing to above 35% by the mid-1990s. In addition, it was recognized that nearly 90% of adult smokers began smoking before age 18 and most at a much earlier age. This led to a better understanding of the addictive nature of smoking and the need for interventions aimed at preventing addiction and addressing it through behavioral modification and drug treatments.

By the late 1990s, efforts were directed at reducing the rate of smoking among adolescents. A range of interventions was introduced. Peer education, even higher taxes on cigarettes, and laws preventing advertising of cigarettes and selling cigarettes to minors, such as the Joe Camel campaign, were among the interventions used. The subsequent rates of cigarette smoking among adolescents gradually fell to approximately the same rates as those of adults.

Data suggests that most of the approximately 20% of the population who continue to smoke are strongly addicted to nicotine and that education and even motivation are not likely to be effective. Recent efforts have turned to the regulation of nicotine in cigarettes, and the Food and Drug Administration now has authority to regulate but not eliminate nicotine in cigarettes. Pregnant women have been recognized as a group who are highly motivated to stop smoking to prevent the adverse effects on their offspring. Efforts to stop smoking during pregnancy have the potential to carry over beyond delivery.. Early detection, extra attention, and insurance coverage for cessation efforts have become widespread strategies for addressing smoking during pregnancy.

The declining rate of cigarette smoking in the United States has been coupled with a better recognition of other factors that today play roles in the development of lung cancer. A large number of Americans have been exposed to asbestos, a substance used as insulation in building, in brake linings, and in many other applications. It was widely used in the shipbuilding industry during World War II, where several million workers were heavily exposed. Restrictions on the use of asbestos and regulations of renovation and demolition of asbestos-containing buildings have greatly reduced exposures to asbestos.

Uranium miners in several countries have been found to have an increased risk of developing lung cancer even in the absence of cigarette smoking. Radon, a naturally occurring invisible, odorless gas that is produced by the breakdown of uranium, was found to be widely present in homes in many geographic areas not just those with uranium mines. Public health investigators began to examine whether there was a connection between radon gas exposure and lung cancer. Approximately 20,000 cases of lung cancer per year are now attributed to radon exposure by the Environmental Protection Agency. About 1 in 15 homes currently have radon exposures above the levels at which the Environmental Protection Agency recommends action. The EPA recommends voluntary routine home testing. However, the major effort to successfully control radon exposure has been laws requiring testing prior to sale of a property and compulsory reductions in levels when high levels are detected.

The importance of asbestos and radon exposures have been apparent based on data indicating that these risk factors for lung cancer have multiplicative effects on the risk when combined with cigarette smoking. For instance, when the relative risk of asbestos is 5 and the relative risk of cigarette smoking is 10, the risk when there is exposure to both is nearly 50. Thus reductions in either of these risk factors can have dramatic impacts on the overall risk of lung cancer among those who also smoke cigarettes.

Early detection and treatment of lung cancer by chest X rays have been shown to have little if any impact. Studies of routine chest X rays for long-term smokers have been shown to produce a slightly earlier diagnosis, but to merely extend the time between diagnosis and death. Once evident on chest X ray, the lung cancer is nearly always beyond the point of cure. Recent studies have confirmed that a newer type of X ray test called a spiral computerized tomogram, or spiral CT, is capable of diagnosing lung cancer at an earlier stage. The test is expensive and has false positives as well as false negatives. However, it has been shown to reduce the deaths due to lung cancer by about 20%. Controversy continues over if and when to use spiral CT for screening for lung cancer.

An appreciation of the causes of lung cancer has led to multiple efforts to reduce exposure and to detect and treat it early. The rates of lung cancer in recent years have begun to fall, but the disease remains the most common cause of cancer deaths in both men and women. Increasingly, a systems thinking approach is being used to develop a coherent approach to reducing the incidence rate and the mortality rate due to lung cancer.

Discussion Questions

1. Identify the interventions discussed for cigarette smoking in this case as primary, secondary, and tertiary, and discuss the advantages and disadvantages of using each of these types of interventions.

2. Identify the interventions discussed in this case for cigarette smoking as using education, motivation, or obligation, and discuss the advantages and disadvantages of using each of these types of interventions.

3. Discuss how the systems analysis approach of identifying multiple factors and investigating their interactions is illustrated in this case.

4. Discuss how systems analysis goals of identifying bottlenecks and leverage points are illustrated in this case.

RESTORITAL—HOW DO WE ESTABLISH SAFETY?

The family wanted to know what went wrong. The FDA had approved the drug; her doctor had prescribed it; and her local pharmacy had filled the drug. Why had they been told in the ER that it looked like their mother, Noreen, had a bad drug reaction and may not survive?

The Food and Drug Administration had approved a new drug called Restorital to prevent fractures due to osteoporosis that did not respond to other available treatments. Restorital worked by blocking action of a newly recognized enzyme that was central to bone destruction. Animal studies showed no evidence of teratogenic, carcinogenic, or fertility problems except at doses well beyond the range that would be used for treating patients. Phase 1 studies on 30 healthy patients established dosage levels and did not detect side effects in vulnerable organs, including the liver, kidneys, and bone marrow. Phase 2 studies supported the efficacy of Restorital and suggested that randomized controlled trials with approximately 1,000 patients, 500 each in the study and in the control groups, would be adequate for establishing the efficacy of Restorital.

The results of two randomized controlled trials conducted on approximately 1,000 patients each demonstrated that the drug was able to modestly increase bone density for postmenopausal women with osteoporosis who had failed on other existing treatments. The drug was tested over a one-year period on patients with severe osteoporosis who were taking no other prescription drugs. The only side effects observed more frequently in the study group were occasional nausea and diarrhea.

The drug was approved by the FDA and widely advertised for prevention of fractures due to osteoporosis. The advertisement noted in small print that Restorital had been approved for treatment of osteoporosis when all other available treatments had failed.

Physicians were impressed with Restorital's rapid improvement in bone density, its once-a-day dosage, its apparent lack of side effects, and its acceptance by patients. Patients found that most of the nausea and diarrhea could be avoided if they took their medicine with food. The success of the treatment encouraged many physicians to use Restorital as initial treatment for osteoporosis.

Noreen had begun Restorital four years ago, along with five other medications. She was pleased that Restorital did not seem to have any side effects and was successful in slowing down her bone loss, according to the follow-up tests ordered by her doctor.

Over the next few months, there seemed to be a subtle change in Noreen. She did not have her usual energy or enthusiasm and just wanted to stay home. When her family checked her medication, they found that she had been taking double the prescribed dose of Restorital. When they finally got her to her doctor, he ordered a series of blood tests. The next day, he called, saying, "Meet me in the ER. We need to look into this right away. Noreen's liver is not doing well."

Her doctor was worried about whether Restorital could have been the problem. He went so far as to file a report with the FDA's spontaneous reporting system, the first time he had ever done this in 20 years of practice. The FDA told him that they now had a series of 10 such reports suggesting that Restorital can cause life-threatening liver failure when used for 3 or more years at higher than recommended dosages, usually along with other drugs that can injure the liver. The FDA, he was told, was reviewing whether to put a black box warning label on Restorital, recommending liver function tests on patients taking it for more than a year.

It was too late to help Noreen, her doctor thought, but he was not going to prescribe Restorital again. "I guess even wonder drugs are not always so wonderful for every patient," he said to himself.

Discussion Questions

1. What does this case study illustrate about the limitations of safety testing of drugs in animal studies?

2. What does this case study illustrate about the limitations of phase one and phase two drug testing?

3. What does this case study illustrate about the limitations of safety testing of drugs using randomized controlled trials?

4. What does this case study illustrate about the potential dangers of using approved drugs?

5. How could the FDA use its new authority provided in the 2007 amendments to prevent this type of problem from occurring?

THE FUTURE OF HIV/AIDS

It is 2020 and maternal-to-child transmission of HIV has become a very rare event, its occurrence is now defined as a hallmark of poor medicine and poor public health. HIV transmitted by blood transfusion likewise has all but disappeared.

Transmission by contaminated needles and homosexual transmission have been greatly reduced. However, heterosexual HIV transmission remains a major source of disease transmission.

Overall, HIV remains an important cause of mortality and morbidity in the United States. The overwhelming percentage of new cases occur as a result of heterosexual intercourse. A large number of interventions has been studied one at a time to determine if they can prevent heterosexual transmission of HIV. These interventions have been shown to have efficacy under research conditions as well as effectiveness under practice conditions. Imagine that a summary of these findings indicated:

- The recently FDA-approved HIV vaccine has been found to have 40% efficacy in clinical practice in preventing HIV transmission but no impact once transmission has occurred. The vaccine reliably produces HIV antibodies and results in a positive HIV antibody test. It is an inactivated vaccine, so it can safely be administered to pregnant women.
- Early detection of HIV within 2 weeks of exposure using expensive HIV antigen testing linked with rapid follow-up of sexual contacts has been shown to reduce by 50% the high incidence of HIV infection among those recently sexually exposed.
- Pre-exposure drug treatment for HIV-negative individuals exposed to HIV-positive partners reduces by 30% the rate of HIV transmission. Widespread use of this intervention is expected to produce HIV drug resistance.
- Use of male or female latex condoms has been shown to reduce by 80% the rate of transmission of HIV.
- Intra-coital protections, including antiviral vaginal drug gels, reduces transmission by 40% when used alone and by 95% when used with male or female condoms. HIV drug resistance is expected to be low with this intervention.
- Post-coital treatment within 24 hours has been found to reduce by 75% the occurrence of heterosexual HIV transmission. Its potential for drug resistance if widely used is unknown.
- Active HIV drug treatment for those with chronic HIV has been shown to reduce by approximately 50% the rate of transmission.
- Male circumcision has been found to reduce by approximately 50% the rate of transmission to males through heterosexual intercourse.

Controlling the spread of heterosexual transmission has become a national priority. Short-term cost considerations are considered secondary to the development of a success-ful national strategy to reduce the incidence of heterosexual transmission of HIV.

Discussion Questions

1. What other data would you like to have in order to make recommendations about the use of these interventions?

2. Which of these interventions are likely to have positive interactions with each other? Is it likely that any of the interventions have negative interactions with other interventions?

3. Based only on the information included in this exercise, decide whether you would recommend or not recommend each of the interventions listed. Explain.

4. For those interventions that you would recommend, for what population of individuals should the intervention be recommended? Explain.

5. How could these interventions be combined into an effective national strategy for controlling HIV/AIDS? What other interventions would you add to the ones previously outlined as part of an effective national strategy? Explain.

Glossary

Absolute risk—The actual chances or probability of developing the disease expressed as a probability, such as 0.01, or a percentage, such as 1%.

Academic health center—An organization that includes a medical school, one or more other health profession schools, and an affiliated hospital.

Accreditation—A process applied to educational institutions, healthcare institutions, and governmental health departments, to define and enforce required structures, processes, and outcomes.

Actual causes—Modifiable factors that lead to major causes of mortality.

Administrative regulations—In the United States, the type of law produced by executive agencies of federal, state, and local governments.

Affordable Care Act—U.S. legislation passed in 2010 that makes major changes to the U.S. health insurance system.

Age adjustment—Taking into account age distribution of a population when comparing populations or when comparing the same population at two different points in time.

Age distribution—The number of people in each age group in a population.

All-hazards approach—An approach to public health preparedness that uses the same approach to preparing for many types of disasters, including use of surveillance systems, communications systems, evacuations, and an organized healthcare response.

Altered environment—The impact of chemicals, radiation, and biological products that humans introduce into the environment.

Ancillary criteria—Criteria that may be used to argue for a cause-and-effect relationship when the definitive requirements have not been fulfilled (Synonym: supportive criteria).

Antibody—A protein produced by the body in response to a foreign antigen that can bind to the antigen and facilitate its elimination.

Artifactual association—An association observed in the data that is actually the result of the method of data collection.

Artifactual difference or changes—Differences between populations or changes in a population over time due to changes in interest in identifying the disease, change in ability to recognize the disease, or changes in the definition of the disease.

Assessment—A core public health function that includes obtaining data that defines the health of the overall population and specific groups within the population, including defining the nature of new and persisting health problems.

Association—The occurrence together of two factors, such as a risk factor and a disease, more often than expected by chance alone.

Assurance—A core public health function that includes governmental public health's oversight responsibility for ensuring that key components of an effective health system, including health care and public health, are in place even though the implementation will often be performed by others.

Asymptomatic—Without symptoms. When referring to screening for disease, it implies the absence of symptoms of the disease being sought.

Asymptomatic transmission—The ability to transmit the disease while humans or animals are free of symptoms of the disease.

At-risk population—The group of people who have a chance or probability of developing a disease.

Attenuated vaccines—Use of a living organism in a vaccine. Living organisms included in vaccines are expected to be attenuated or altered to greatly reduce the chances that they will themselves produce disease (Synonym: live vaccines).

Attributable risk percentage—The percentage of the disease or disability that can potentially be eliminated, among those with the factor being investigated, assuming a contributory cause and assuming the impact of the "cause" can be immediately and completely eliminated (Synonym: percent efficacy).

Authoritative decision—A decision made by an individual or a group that has the power to implement the decision.

Bayes' theorem—A mathematical formula that can be used to calculate posttest probability of disease based on the pretest probability of the disease plus the test's sensitivity and specificity.

Belmont Report—The commonly used name for a report of the National Commission for the Protection of Human Subjects of Biomedical and Behavioral Research that established key principles upon which the current approach to protection of human subjects is based.

Beneficence—An ethics principle that states that persons are treated in an ethical manner not only by respecting their decisions and protecting them from harm, but also by making efforts to secure their well-being.

BIG GEMS—A mnemonic that summarizes the determinants of disease, including behavior, infection, genetics, geography, environment, medical care, and socioeconomic-cultural status.

Bioethics—Lies at the intersection of health law and policy and attempts to apply individual and group values and morals to controversial issues.

Biological plausibility—An ancillary or supportive criteria for contributory cause in which the disease can be explained by what is currently known about the biology of the risk factor and the disease.

Bottlenecks—Factors that limit the effectiveness of systems.

Branding—A marketing concept for creating identification with a product or service that is also used in social marketing.

Built environment—The physical environment constructed by human beings.

Burden of disease—Generically, an analysis of the morbidity and mortality produced by disease. Often used to refer to the use of DALYs to estimate the burden of morbidity and mortality.

Cap—A limit on the total amount that the insurance will pay for a service per year, per benefit period, or per lifetime.

Capitation—A system of reimbursement for health care based upon a flat payment per time period for each person for whom a provider of care assumes responsibility for providing healthcare services, regardless of the services actually provided.

Case-control studies—A study that begins by identifying individuals with a disease and individuals without a disease. Those with and without the disease are identified without knowledge of an individual's exposure or nonexposure to the factors being investigated (Synonym: retrospective study).

Case definition—A set of criteria used to define which persons will be considered to have a disease as part of an outbreak.

Case-fatality—The chances of dying from a condition once it is diagnosed.

Case finding—As used in public health, an effort to identify and locate contacts of individuals diagnosed with a disease and evaluate them for possible treatment.

Case law—Law made by courts when applying statutory or administrative law to specific cases (Synonyms: judicial law, common law).

Cell-mediated immunity—Immunological protection that is produced by t-lymphocytes and other white blood cells that combats intracellular pathogens and tumor cells.

Certainty effect—A risk-taking attitude in which the decision maker favors the status quo rather than a probability of obtaining a better or a worse outcome.

Certification—A nongovernmental process designed to ensure competence by individual health professionals based upon completion of educational requirements and performance on an examination or other evaluation procedure.

Chance node—A circle in a decision tree that indicates that once a decision is made, outcomes occur with known probabilities indicated in the decision tree.

Choice node—A square in a decision tree that indicates that a selection needs to be made.

Chronic carriers—Those individuals without symptoms of the disease but with the ability to chronically transmit the disease.

Cluster—Occurrence of an increased number of cases of a disease over a defined time period.

Cohort study—An investigation that begins by identifying a group that has a factor under investigation and a similar group that does not have the factor. The outcome in each group is then assessed (Synonym: prospective study).

Coinsurance—The percentage of the charges that the insured is responsible for paying.

Common law—Law made by courts when applying statutory or administrative law to specific cases (Synonyms: judicial law, case law).

Communicable disease—A disease due to an organism such as bacteria or a virus that is transmitted person-to-person or from animals or the physical environment to humans by a variety of routes, including from air and water, contaminated articles or fomites, and insect bites and animal bites. Here considered a subset of infectious disease.

Community-based participatory research (CBPR)—Research in which community members are involved in all phases of the research process, contributing their expertise while sharing ownership and responsibility over the research.

Community-oriented primary care (COPC)—A structured six-step process designed to move the delivery of health services from a focus on the individual to an additional focus on the needs of communities.

Community-oriented public health (COPH)—An effort on the part of governmental health agencies to reach out to the community and to the healthcare delivery system to address specific health issues.

Community rating—Insurance rates set the same for all eligible individuals and families based on the previous expenses in a defined community.

Comparative effectiveness research—Research that compares two or more approved and utilized interventions for the same conditions.

Concierge practice—A form of private practice of medicine that aims to provide personalized health care to those who can afford to pay for additional access and services out of pocket.

Confounding variable—A difference in the groups being compared that makes a difference in the outcome being measured.

Consecutive testing—A screening strategy that uses one test followed by one or more additional tests if the first test is positive (Synonym: sequential testing).

Consistency—A supportive or ancillary criteria implying that the relationship has been observed in a wide range of populations and settings.

Constitutional law—In the United States, a form of law based upon the U.S. Constitution or the constitution of a state.

Contributory cause—A definition of causation that is established when all three of the following have been established: (1) the existence of an association between the "cause" and the "effect" at the individual level, (2) the "cause" precedes the "effect" in time, and (3) altering the "cause" alters the probability of the "effect."

Control points—Points or locations in a system in which interventions can have substantial impacts (Synonym: leverage points).

Copayment—An amount that the insured is responsible for paying even when the service is covered by the insurance.

Core public health functions—Describes governmental public health functions that cannot be delegated and remain the responsibility of governmental public health. The Institute of Medicine has defined these functions as assessment, assurance, and policy development.

Cost-effective—A measure of the cost of an intervention relative to its benefit. In interventions, implies that any additional benefit is considered worth the cost. The term can also imply that a large cost savings is worth a small reduction in net effectiveness.

Cost sharing—An effort to reduce healthcare costs in the United States by shifting the costs of health care to individuals on the assumption that individuals will spend less when the costs are coming out of their pockets.

Course of disease—A description of a disease or other condition often using incidence, prevalence, and case-fatality.

Covered service—A service for which health insurance will provide payment if the individual is otherwise eligible.

Credentialing—A general term indicating a process of verifying that an individual has the desirable or required qualifications to practice a profession.

Customary, prevailing, and reasonable—These standards are used by many insurance plans to determine the amount that will be paid to the provider of services.

Data—Facts or the representation of facts as opposed to information.

Database—A collection of data organized in such a way that a computer program can select and compile the desired pieces of data.

Dead vaccine—Injection of a nonliving organism or antigens from an organism designed to develop antibodies to protect an individual from the disease (Synonym: inactivated vaccine).

Decision analysis—A process that compares the outcomes of two or more interventions based on principles of expected utility.

Decision maker—A generic term that can be applied to a range of individuals and organizations that make health decisions, including individuals, health professionals, and organizations ranging from nonprofits to corporations to government agencies.

Decision tree—A graphic method for displaying the benefits and harms of two or more options for intervention.

Deductible—The amount that an individual or family is responsible for paying before being eligible for insurance coverage.

Demographic transition—Describes the impact of falling childhood death rates and extended life spans on the size of populations and the age distribution of populations.

Determinants—Underlying factors that ultimately bring about disease.

Dietary supplements—A category within FDA law that includes vitamins, minerals, and many herbal remedies.

Diffusion of innovation theory—A theory that identifies stages of dissemination and types of adopters of new technology and other changes, including behavioral change.

Disability-adjusted life years (DALYs)—A population health status measure that incorporates measures of death and disability and allows for measurement of the impact of categories of diseases and risk factors.

Discounting—A process in which we place greater importance on events that are expected to occur in the immediate future than on events that are expected to occur in the distant future.

Distribution of disease—How a disease is spread out in a population, often using factors such as person, place, and time.

Dose–response relationship—A relationship that is present if changes in levels of an exposure are associated with changes in frequency of the outcome in a consistent direction.

Downstream factors—Factors affecting behavior that directly involve an individual and can potentially be altered by individual interventions, such as an addiction to nicotine.

Dread effect—Perception of an increase in the probability of occurrence of an event due to its ease of being able to be visualized and its feared consequences.

Ecological approach—As used here, an evidence-based approach to problem solving that considers a range of possible interventions, including health care, traditional public health, and social interventions (Synonyms: population health approach, socioecological approach).

Ecological assessment—An assessment of the impact of an alteration of the physical environment on plants and animals.

Ecological association—Two factors, such as a characteristic and a disease, occur together more often than expected by chance alone in the same group or population. Does not require that the investigator have data on the characteristics of the individuals that make up the group or population (Synonym: group association).

Ecological studies—A type of investigation in which groups are compared without having information on the individuals within the group (Synonym: population comparisons).

Effectiveness—An intervention has been shown to increase the positive outcomes or benefits in the population or setting in which it will be used.

Efficacy—An intervention increased positive outcomes or benefits in the population on which it is investigated.

Eligible—An individual may need to meet certain criteria to be eligible for enrollment in a health insurance plan.

Endemic—A term that implies that a disease is present in a community at all times but at a relatively low rate.

Epidemic—A term used when a disease has increased in frequency in a defined geographic area far above its usual rate.

Epidemiological transition—A concept indicating the change that has been historically observed as part of social and economic development, from mortality and morbidity dominated by infections, to morbidity and mortality dominated by what has been called noncommunicable disease or degenerative and man-made diseases (Synonym: public health transition).

Epidemiological treatment—Treatment of contacts of an individual with a disease even in the absence of evidence of transmission of the disease.

Epidemiologist—An investigator who studies the occurrence and control of disease or other health conditions or events in defined populations.

Equivalence trial—Research being used to study the relative effectiveness of currently approved and utilized interventions, hypothesizing that there are no clinically important differences in outcome (Synonym: noninferiority trial).

Essential public health services—The 10 services that have come to define the responsibilities of the combined local, state, and federal governmental public health system.

Estimation—A statistical term implying a measurement of the strength of an association or the size of a difference.

Etiology—The cause of a disease or health condition.

Evidence—Reliable quantitative or qualitative information or data upon which a decision can be based.

Expected utility—In decision analysis, the probability multiplied by the utility to produce a probability that takes into account the utility of the outcome.

Experience rating—Health insurance rates set on the basis of a group's past history of healthcare expenses (Synonym: medical underwriting).

Experimental study—An investigation in which individuals are assigned to study or control groups using a process of randomization (Synonym: randomized controlled trial).

Exposure assessment—A step of risk assessment which assesses who has been exposed to a pollutant and the extent to which exposure took place.

False negative—Individuals who have a negative result on a screening test but turn out to have the disease.

False positive—Individuals who have a positive result on a screening test but turn out not to have the disease.

Fee-for-service—A system of reimbursement for health services provided based on charges for health services actually provided to patients.

Feedback loops—In systems analysis, the impact of changes in one influence or factor on other influences or factors in a positive or negative direction.

Food desert—A geographic area that lacks grocery stores and other establishments in which low-income individuals are able to purchase nutritious food due to high prices or inaccessibility.

Food security—As defined by the World Health Organization, requires that all people at all times have access to sufficient, safe, nutritious food to maintain a healthy and active life.

Gini index—A measure of income distribution. The index, ranging from 0 to 1, measures the extent of deviation between an economy's distribution of income among individuals or households and that of perfectly equal distribution or an index of 0.

Group association—Two factors, such as a characteristic and a disease, occur together more often than expected by chance alone in the same group or population. Does not require that the investigator have data on the characteristics of the individuals that make up the group or population (Synonym: ecological association).

Hazard—A measure of the inherent capability of a substance to produce harm.

Hazard identification—A step in risk assessment that looks at the health effects caused by a pollutant.

Health-adjusted life expectancy (HALE)—A population health status measure that combines life expectancy with a measure of the population's overall quality of health.

Health belief model—A model of behavioral change that posits that personal beliefs influence health behavior and people will be more likely to take action if they believe they are susceptible to the condition; the condition has serious consequences; taking action would benefit them, with the benefits outweighing the harms; people are exposed to factors that prompt action; and people believe in their ability to successfully perform the action.

Health communications—The full range of uses of information in health, from data collection to decision making.

Health disparity—A type of difference in health that is closely linked with social or economic disadvantage. Health disparities negatively affect groups of people who have systematically experienced greater social or economic obstacles to health. These obstacles stem from characteristics historically linked to discrimination or exclusion, such as race or ethnicity, religion, socioeconomic status, gender, mental health, sexual orientation, or geographic location. Other characteristics include cognitive, sensory, or physical disability.

Health equity—When all people have the opportunity to attain their full health potential and no one is disadvantaged from achieving this potential because of his or her social position or other socially determined circumstance.

Health in all policies—A comprehensive approach where private and public entities, across sectors, work toward common goals to achieve improved health for all and reduce health inequities.

Health inequalities—Differences, variations, and disparities in the health achievements of individuals and groups of people.

Health inequity—A difference or disparity in health outcomes that is systematic, avoidable, and unjust.

Health insurance exchanges—Web-based competitive marketplaces established by the Affordable Care Act at which eligible individuals can obtain information, obtain subsidies if qualified, and purchase insurance policies.

Health literacy—The degree to which individuals have the capacity to obtain, process, and understand basic health information and services needed to make appropriate health decisions.

Health-related quality of life (HRQOL)—A health status measure that reflects the number of unhealthy days due to physical plus mental impairment. HRQOL provides an overall quality of health measure, but it does not incorporate the impact of death.

Health system—The healthcare system plus the public health system.

Healthcare delivery system—A linkage of institutions and healthcare professionals that together take on the responsibility of delivering coordinated care.

Healthcare disparity—Racial or ethnic differences in the quality of health care that are not due to access-related factors or clinical needs, preferences, and appropriateness of intervention.

Healthcare safety net—The provision of services for those who cannot afford to purchase the healthcare services.

Healthcare system—A healthcare delivery system plus the financial system that pays for the delivery of health care.

Herd immunity—Protection of an entire population from a communicable disease by obtaining individual immunity through vaccination or natural infections by a large percentage of the population (Synonym: population immunity).

Heuristics—Rules of thumb for decision making that often allow more rapid decision making based on a limited amount of information.

High-risk approach—Focuses on those with the highest probability of developing disease and aims to bring their risk close to the levels experienced by the rest of the population.

Home rule—Authority granted to local jurisdictions, such as cities or counties, by state constitutions or state legislative actions.

Immunization—The strengthening of the immune system to prevent or control disease through exposure to antigens or administration of antibodies.

Imposed risk—A potential threat to the health of individuals and populations that is out of their direct control, such as exposure to environmental toxins from a local factory.

Improving-the-average approach—Assumes that everyone is at some degree of risk and the risk increases with the extent of exposure.

Inactivated vaccine—Injection of a nonliving organism or antigens from an organism designed to develop antibodies to protect an individual from the disease (Synonym: dead vaccine).

Incidence—Rates that measure the chances of occurrence of a disease or other condition over a period of time, usually one year.

Incremental cost-effectiveness—A measurement of the additional cost relative to the additional net-effectiveness (See: net-effectiveness).

Infant mortality rate—A population health status measure that estimates the rate of death in the first year of life.

Infections—Invasion of host's bodily tissues by an organism such as bacteria or a virus.

Infectious disease—A disease caused by an organism such as bacteria or a virus. Here used to include communicable diseases as well as other infections that are not communicable.

Infectivity—The ability of a pathogen to enter and multiply in a susceptible host.

Inference—A statistical term used to imply the drawing of conclusions about a population based upon data from a sample using statistical significance testing.

Influences—As used in systems thinking, factors or determinants that interact with each other to bring about outcomes, such as disease or the results of disease.

Inform of decision—A decision-making approach in which a clinician is merely expected to inform the patient of what is planned.

Informed consent—A decision-making approach in which a clinician is expected to provide information and obtain agreement to proceed from the patient.

Inpatient facility—A healthcare facility in the United States in which an individual may remain for more than 24 hours. Examples include hospitals and nursing homes.

Institutional review board (IRB)—An institution-based group that is mandated by federal regulations to review human research conducted at the institution and determine whether it meets federally defined research standards.

Intentional injuries—Injuries that are brought about on purpose, whether the injury is self-inflicted or meant for others.

Interaction analysis—An approach to environmental health assessment that looks at the consequences of two or more exposures.

Interventions—The full range of strategies designed to protect health and prevent disease, disability, and death.

Judicial law—Law made by courts when applying statutory or administrative law to specific cases (Synonyms: case law, common law).

Justice—An ethical principle based on a sense of fairness in distribution of what is deserved.

Koch's postulates—Four postulates that together definitely establish a cause and effect for a communicable disease: the organism must be shown to be present in every case of the disease; the organism must not be found in cases of other diseases; once isolated, the organism must be capable of replicating the disease in an experimental animal; and the organism must be recoverable from the animal (See: Modern Koch's postulates).

Lead-time bias—The situation in screening for disease in which early detection does not alter outcome but only increases the interval between detection of the disease and occurrence of the outcome, such as death.

Legislative statutes—In the United States, the type of law that includes statutes passed by legislative bodies at the federal, state, and local levels.

Leverage points—Points or locations in a system in which interventions can have substantial impacts (Synonym: control points).

Licensure—Granted by a governmental authority that provides permission to engage in an activity, such as the practice of a health profession.

Life expectancy—A population health status measure that summarizes the impact of death in an entire population utilizing the probability of death at each age of life in a particular year in a particular population.

Live vaccines—Use of a living organism in a vaccine. Living organisms included in vaccines are expected to be attenuated or altered to greatly reduce the chances that they will themselves produce disease (Synonym: attenuated vaccines).

Long-shot effect—A decision-making attitude in which a decision maker perceives the status quo as intolerable and is willing to take an action with only a small chance of success and a large chance of making the situation worse.

Mainstream factors—Factors affecting behavior that result from the relationship of an individual with a larger group or population, such as peer pressure to smoke or the level of taxation on cigarettes.

Market justice—The philosophy that market forces should be relied upon to organize the delivery of healthcare services.

Medicaid—A federal–state program that covers groups defined as categorically needy as well as groups that may be covered at the discretion of the state, including those defined as medically needy, such as those in need of nursing home care.

Medical home—A concept of primary care that includes a team approach as part of a larger healthcare system.

Medical loss ratio—The ratio of benefit payments paid to premiums collected, indicating the proportion of the premiums spent on medical services.

Medical malpractice—A body of state civil law designed to hold practitioners accountable to patients for the quality of health care.

Medical underwriting—Health insurance rates set on the basis of a group's past history of healthcare expenses (Synonym: experience rating).

Medicare—A federal health insurance system that covers most individuals 65 and older as well as the disabled and those with end-stage renal disease.

Medigap—A supplemental health insurance linked to Medicare and designed to cover all or most of the charges that are not covered by Medicare, including the 20% copayment required for many outpatient services.

Mental health—A state of successful performance of mental function, resulting in productive activities, fulfilling relationships with other people, and the ability to adapt to change and to cope with challenges.

Micronutrients—Vitamins and minerals that in small quantities are considered essential to good health.

Model—A combination of ideas and concepts taken from multiple theories and applied to specific problems in particular settings.

Modern Koch's postulates—A set of criteria for establishing that an organism is a contributory cause of a disease, requiring evidence of an epidemiological association, isolation, and transmissions (See: Koch's postulates).

Morbidity—A public health term to describe the frequency of impairments or disability produced by a disease or other condition.

Mortality—A public health term to describe the frequency of deaths produced by a disease or other condition.

Multiple risk factor reduction—Simultaneous efforts to reduce more than one risk factor.

Multiplicative interaction—A type of interaction between two or more exposures such that the overall risk when two or more exposures are present is best estimated by multiplying the relative risk of each of the exposures.

Natural experiment—A change that occurs in one particular population but not another similar population without the intervention of an investigator.

Necessary cause—If the "cause" is not present, the disease or "effect" will not develop.

Negative constitution—The principle that the U.S. Constitution allows but does not require government to act to protect public health or to provide healthcare services.

Negligence law—A body of law designed to protect individuals from harm.

Net benefit—A measure of the benefits minus the harms of an intervention (Synonym: net-effectiveness).

Net-effectiveness—A measure of the benefits minus the harms of an intervention (Synonym: net benefit).

No-duty principle—The principle of U.S. law that healthcare providers, either individuals or institutions, do not have an obligation to provide health services.

Nongovernmental organization (NGO)—An entity that is funded, at least partially, by the government but acts independently from the government.

Noninferiority trial—Research being used to study the relative effectiveness of currently approved and utilized interventions, hypothesizing that there are no clinically important differences in outcome (Synonym: equivalence trial).

Nutritional transition—Countries frequently move from poorly balanced diets often deficient in nutrients and calories to a diet of highly processed food including fats, sugars, and salt.

Odds ratio—A measure of the strength of the relationship that is often a good approximation of the relative risk. This ratio is calculated as the odds of having the risk factor if the disease is present divided by the odds of having the risk factor if the disease is absent.

Off-label prescribing—Prescribing of FDA-approved products for indications, dosages, or durations other than those specifically approved by the FDA.

Outbreak—An increased number of cases of a disease over a defined time period in which affected individuals share a characteristic in common.

Outcome measures—Measures of quality that imply a focus on the result of health care, ranging from rates of infection to readmissions with complications.

Out-of-pocket expenses—Payments for health services not covered by insurance that are the responsibility of the individual receiving the services.

Outpatient facility—A healthcare facility in the United States in which patients can remain for fewer than 24 hours. These facilities include the offices of clinicians, general and specialty clinics, emergency departments, and a range of new types of community-based diagnostic and treatment facilities.

Pandemic—An epidemic occurring worldwide, or over a very wide area, crossing international boundaries and affecting a large number of people.

Parallel testing—A screening strategy that uses two tests initially, with follow-up testing if either test is positive (Synonym: simultaneous testing).

Passive immunity—Short-term protection against a disease provided by administration of antibodies.

Percent efficacy—The percentage of the disease or disability that can potentially be eliminated, among those with the factor being investigated, assuming a contributory cause and assuming the impact of the "cause" can be immediately and completely eliminated (Synonym: attributable risk percentage).

P.E.R.I.E. process— A mnemonic that comes from the first letters in the steps of the evidence-based public health approach.

Phase 1, 2, 3, and 4—The FDA phases of drug approval. Phases 1, 2, and 3 occur prior to approval, while phase 4, often referred to as postmarket surveillance, occurs after the drug is approved by the FDA.

Phenotypic expression—The clinical presentation of a disease, which may be quite variable despite the same genetic composition, or genotype.

Place—A component of social marketing which identifies the target audiences and how to reach them.

Point of service plans (POS)—A type of health plan that is a modification of staff model HMOs. POS plans allow enrollees to obtain care outside the HMO but require that the patient pay for a portion of the cost of the care received.

Police powers—Authority of governmental public health based on the power of state government to pass legislation and implement actions to protect the common good.

Policy development—A core public health function that includes developing evidence-based recommendations and other analyses of options, such as health policy analysis, to guide implementation, including efforts to educate and mobilize community partnerships to implement these policies.

Population comparisons—A type of investigation in which groups are compared without having information on the individuals within the group (Synonym: ecological study).

Population health approach—As used here, an evidence-based approach to problem solving that considers a range of possible interventions, including health care, traditional public health, and social interventions (Synonyms: ecological approach, socioecological approach).

Population health status measures—Quantitative summary measures of the health of a large population, such as life-expectancy, HALEs, and DALYs.

Population immunity—Protection of an entire population from a communicable disease by obtaining individual immunity through vaccination or natural infections by a large percentage of the population (Synonym: herd immunity).

Portability—The ability to continue employment-based health insurance after leaving employment, usually by paying the full cost of the insurance. A federal law known as COBRA generally ensures employees 18 months of portability.

Posttest probability of disease—The probability of the disease after the results of the test are known.

PRECEDE-PROCEED—A planning framework that provides a structure to design and evaluate health education and health promotion programs through a diagnostic planning process followed by an implementation and evaluation process.

Prediction rule—A quantitative formula designed to increase the ability to predict the outcome of a condition and thereby guide the use of interventions.

Predictive value of a negative—The posttest probability that the disease is absent when the test results are negative.

Predictive value of a positive—The posttest probability of the disease when the test results are positive.

Preferred provider organization (PPO)—An insurance system that works with a limited number of clinicians. These providers agree to a set of conditions that usually includes reduced payments and other conditions. Patients may choose to use other clinicians, but they often need to pay more out of pocket.

Premium—The price paid by the purchaser for the insurance policy on a monthly or yearly basis.

Preponderance of the evidence—A legal term implying that a trial is decided based upon the conclusion that the evidence is more supportive of the plaintiff than the defendant or vice versa.

Pretest probability of disease—The probability of the disease before the test results are known. An estimate based on prevalence of the disease, the presence of risk factors for the disease, and, if present, signs or symptoms suggestive of the disease.

Prevalence rate—A measurement of the number of individuals who have a disease at a particular point in time divided by the number of individuals who could potentially have the disease.

Price—A component of social marketing that refers to identifying the benefits, the barriers and financial costs of a behavior or innovation.

Primary care—Traditionally refers to the first contact providers of care who are prepared to handle the great majority of common problems for which patients seek care.

Primary intervention—An intervention that occurs before the onset of the disease.

Procedural due process—A form of due process that prohibits governments from denying individuals a right in an arbitrary or unfair way.

Process measures—Measurements of quality that focus on the procedures and formal processes that go into delivering care, from procedures to ensure credentialing of health professionals to procedures to ensure timely response to complaints.

Product—A component of social marketing that refers to the behavior or innovation being marketed.

Proportion—A fraction in which the numerator is made up of observations that are also included in the denominator.

Promotion—A component of social marketing that includes organizing a campaign or program to reach the target audience(s).

Prospective study—An investigation that begins by identifying a group that has a factor under investigation and a similar group that does not have the factor. The outcome in each group is then assessed (Synonym: cohort study).

Protective factor—A factor that is associated with a reduced probability of disease.

Provider—A term used to include a wide range of health professionals who provide health services.

Proximal cause—A legal concept of causation that asks whether the injury or other event would have occurred if the negligent act had not occurred.

Public health assessment—A formal assessment that incorporates risk assessment but also includes data on the actual exposure of a population to a hazard.

Public health surveillance—Collection of health data as the basis for monitoring and understanding health problems, generating hypotheses about etiology, and evaluating the success of interventions (Synonym: surveillance).

Public health transition—A concept indicating the change that has been historically observed as part of social and economic development, from mortality and morbidity dominated by infections, to morbidity and mortality dominated by what has been called noncommunicable disease or degenerative and man-made diseases (Synonym: epidemiological transition).

Quality adjusted life-year (QALY)—A measurement that asks about the number of life-years saved by an intervention rather than the number of lives.

Quarantine—The compulsory physical separation of those with a disease or at high risk of developing a disease from the rest of the population.

Random assignment—As part of a randomized clinical trial, assignment of participants to study and control groups using a chance process in which the participants are assigned to a particular group with a known probability (Synonym: randomization).

Randomization—As part of a randomized clinical trial, assignment of participants to study and control groups using a chance process in which the participants are assigned to a particular group with a known probability (Synonym: random assignment).

Randomized controlled trial—An investigation in which individuals are assigned to study or control groups using a process of randomization (Synonym: experimental study).

Rates—Used here as a generic term to describe measurements that have a numerator and a denominator.

RE-AIM—A mnemonic that comes from the first letters of the steps in a fully developed evaluation process.

Reciprocal determinism—A component of social cognitive theory describing the dynamic interplay among personal factors, the environment, and behavior.

Recommendations—Statements based upon evidence indicating that actions, such as cigarette cessation, will improve outcomes, such as reducing lung cancer.

Reductionist thinking—An approach to problem solving that looks at each of the components of a problem one at a time.

Relative risk—A ratio of the probability of the outcome if a factor known as a risk factor is present compared to the probability of the outcome if the factor is not present.

Reproduction ratio (R_0)—The number of new cases one individual with the disease generates on average over the course of the disease's communicable period.

Respect for persons—An ethical principle that incorporates two ethical convictions: first, that individuals should be treated as autonomous agents, and second, that persons with diminished autonomy are entitled to protection.

Retrospective study—A study that begins by identifying individuals with a disease and individuals without a disease. Those with and without the disease are identified without knowledge of an individual's exposure or nonexposure to the factors being investigated (Synonym: case-control studies).

Reverse causality—The situation in which the apparent "cause" is actually the "effect."

Rights—Protections afforded to individuals on the basis of the U.S. Constitution, a state constitution, or legislative actions.

Ring vaccination—As used in the smallpox eradication program, immediate vaccination of populations in surrounding geographic areas after identification of a case of disease.

Risk assessment—A process used in environmental health to formally assess the potential for harm due to a hazard, taking into account factors such as the likelihood, timing, and duration of exposure.

Risk avoider—A decision maker who consistently favors avoiding an action even when a decision analysis utilizing probabilities, utilities, and timing argues for the action.

Risk characterization—A step in risk assessment that looks at the extra risk of health problems in an exposed population.

Risk factor—A characteristic of individuals or an exposure that increases the probability of developing a disease. It does not imply that a contributory cause has been established.

Risk indicator—A characteristic, such as gender or age, that is associated with an outcome but is not considered a contributory cause (Synonym: risk marker).

Risk marker—A characteristic, such as gender or age, that is associated with an outcome but is not considered a contributory cause (Synonym: risk indicator).

Risk taker—A decision maker who consistently favors taking an action even when a decision analysis utilizing probabilities, utilities, and timing argues against the decision.

Risk-taking attitudes—A decision-making attitude in which an individual or group consistently favors taking actions or avoiding actions that differ from the recommendations of a decision analysis utilizing probabilities, utilities, and the timing of events.

Route of transmission—The anatomical and physiological methods for transmission from person to person or from animal species to humans.

Score—In the context of evidence-based recommendations, a measurement of the quality of the evidence and a measurement of the magnitude of the impact.

Screening—As used here, testing individuals who are asymptomatic for a particular disease as part of a strategy to diagnose a disease or identify a risk factor.

Secondary care—Refers to specialty care provided by clinicians who focus on one or a small number of organ systems or on a specific type of service, such as obstetrics or anesthesiology.

Secondary intervention—Early detection of disease or risk factors and intervention during an asymptomatic phase.

Self-imposed risk—A potential threat an individual knowingly and willingly takes on through his or her own actions, such as choosing not to wear a motorcycle helmet while riding a motorcycle.

Sensitive—In decision analysis, indicates that changes in a particular factor within a realistic high and realistic low range result in changes in the recommendation of the decision analysis.

Sensitivity—The probability of a positive test when the disease is present.

Sequential testing—A screening strategy that uses one test followed by one or more additional tests if the first test is positive (Synonym: consecutive testing).

Shared decision making—A decision-making approach in which a clinician is expected to directly or indirectly provide information and options for intervention to a patient and then rely on the patient to synthesize the information and make his or her own decision.

Simultaneous testing—A screening strategy that uses two tests initially, with follow-up testing if either test is positive (Synonym: parallel testing).

Single payer—A healthcare system with one source of payment, usually a governmental source.

Skimming—Enrolling predominating healthy individuals into a health plan to reduce the costs to the plan.

Social cognitive theory—An interpersonal theory of behavior change that focuses on the interaction between individuals and their social systems.

Social determinants of health—The complex, integrated, and overlapping social structures and economic systems including the social environment, physical environment, health services, and structural and societal factors.

Social justice—A philosophy that aims to provide fair treatment and a fair share of the reward of society to individuals and groups.

Social marketing—The use of marketing theory, skills, and practice to achieve social change, e.g., in health promotion.

Socioecological approach—As used here, an evidence-based approach to problem solving that considers a range of possible interventions, including health care, traditional public health, and social interventions (Synonyms: population health approach, ecological approach).

Socioeconomic gradient—A phenomenon describing the hierarchical differences in health outcomes among a population based on the value that society places on certain characteristics, whether it be income, job, educational attainment, etc. This can be viewed as a ladder in that moving down the social ladder, more ill health and shorter life expectancy are experienced at each rung.

Socioeconomic status—In the United States, a measurement using scales reflecting education, income, and professional status.

Source traceback—A process used in foodborne outbreak investigations to trace the origin of food suspected of causing an outbreak.

Specificity—The probability of a negative test when the disease is absent.

Spontaneous reporting system—An FDA system for reporting adverse events that occur while taking medications.

Stages of change model—A model of behavioral change that hypothesizes five steps in the process of behavioral change, including precontemplation, contemplation, preparation, action, and maintenance (Synonym: transtheoretical model).

Standard population—The age distribution of a population that is often used as the basis for comparison with other populations. The age distribution of the U.S. population in the year 2000 is generally used.

State Child Health Insurance Program (SCHIP)—A federally funded health insurance program that provides funds to the states to use to expand or facilitate the operation of Medicaid or for other uses to serve the health needs of lower income children.

Strength of the relationship—Supportive or ancillary criteria implying that a measurement of the strength of an association, such as a relative risk or odds ratio, is large or substantial.

Structure measures—Measure of quality of health care focused on the physical and organizational infrastructure in which care is delivered.

Substantive due process—A type of due process in which state and federal governments must justify the grounds for depriving an individual of life, liberty, and property.

Sufficient cause—If the "cause" is present, the disease or "effect" will occur.

Supportive criteria—Criteria that may be used to argue for a cause-and-effect relationship when the definitive requirements have not been fulfilled (Synonym: ancillary criteria).

Surrogate endpoint—Use of substitute measures of outcomes that do not necessarily reflect the clinically important outcomes that a drug or other therapy intends to improve.

Surrogate outcome—A measurement of outcome that looks at short-term results, such as changes in laboratory tests, that may not reflect longer term or clinically important outcomes.

Surveillance—Collection of health data as the basis for monitoring and understanding health problems, generating hypotheses about etiology, and evaluating the success of interventions (Synonym: public health surveillance).

Syndemic—A systems thinking approach that focuses attention on how health problems interact as part of larger systems.

Syndrome—A pattern of risk factors or symptoms that tend to occur together.

System—An interacting group of items forming a unified whole.

System error—Problems resulting from deficiencies in the system for delivering health care or other services.

Systems analysis—A variety of methods that operationalize the investigation of systems.

Systems diagram—A graphic means of displaying the way we understand systems to be structured and/or to function.

Systems thinking—An approach that examines multiple influences on the development of an outcome or outcomes and attempts to bring them together in a coherent whole.

Tertiary care—A type of health care often defined in terms of the type of institution in which it is delivered, often an academic or specialized health center. This type of care may also be defined in terms of the type of problem that is addressed, such as trauma centers, burn centers, or neonatal intensive care.

Tertiary intervention—An intervention that occurs after the initial occurrence of symptoms but before irreversible disability occurs.

Theory—A set of interrelated concepts that presents a systematic view of relationships among variables in order to explain and predict events and situations.

Theory of planned behavior—A theory of behavior change that posits that behavioral intention is influenced by individuals' attitudes toward performing a behavior, their beliefs about whether people important to them approve or disapprove of the behavior, and their beliefs about their control over performing the behavior.

Translational research—An attempt to bridge the gaps between basic research, clinical applications, and population health implications by seeing health research as a system.

Transtheoretical model—A model of behavioral change that hypothesizes five steps in the process of behavioral change, including precontemplation, contemplation, preparation, action, and maintenance (Synonym: stages of change model).

True positive—Individuals who have a positive result on a screening test and turn out to have the disease.

True rate—A measurement that has a numerator that is a subset of the denominator and a unit of time, such as a day or a year, over which the number of events in the numerator is measured.

Unaltered environment—The natural environment.

Uncontrollability effect—Perception of increased probability of occurrence of an event due to the perceived inability of an individual to control or prevent the event from occurring.

Under-5 mortality—A population health status measure that estimates the probability of dying during the first 5 years of life.

Undergraduate medical education—Refers to the four years of medical school leading to a MD or DO degree, despite the fact that an undergraduate, or bachelor's, degree is generally required for admission.

Unfamiliarity effect—Perception of increased probability of an event due to an individual's absence of prior experience with the event.

Unintentional injuries—Injuries that occur not on purpose, such as most motor vehicle collisions, drowning, falls, fires, and poisonings.

Upstream factors—Factors affecting behavior that are grounded in social structures and policies, such as government-sponsored programs that encourage tobacco production.

Utility scale—A scale that goes from zero to one, with zero reflecting immediate death and one reflecting full health. This scale is used to measure the value or importance that an individual or a group places on a particular outcome.

Victim blaming—Placing the responsibility or blame for a bad outcome on the individual who experiences the bad outcome due to his or her behavior.

Note: Page numbers followed by *b*, *f*, *t*, and *n* indicate material in boxes, figures, tables, and footnotes respectively.

reciprocal determinism, 88, 88*f*
recommendations, 32
  classification of (score), 33–34, 34*f*
  develops, 35*b*
  evidence-based versus eminence-based, 33
  in P.E.R.I.E process, 22
Red Cross, 244
reductionist thinking, 268, 271
reference interval, 122
registered nurses (RNs), 184
regulation, role in reducing healthcare costs, 222
relative risk, 29*n*
  interventions reducing, 33*n*
  for measuring strength of relationship, 29*n*
religion, may affect health, 79, 80*t*
reproduction ratio (R_0), 138, 139
research ethics, 106
residency programs, in medical education, 183*b*
residual pesticides, 255
respect for persons, in ethical research, 106
retrolental fibrosis (RLF), 48
retrospective studies, 28
reverse causality, 28*n*
rewards, for health professionals, 186, 187*t*–188*t*
Reye's syndrome, 268
ribonucleic acid (RNA) virus, 147
rights
  balancing individual and societal needs, 104
  to health care, 103
  Supreme Court role in, 103
  U.S. Constitution and, 99
ring vaccination, 142
risk assessment, 155
  addressing environmental diseases, 156–158
  benzene, 157, 157*b*
  steps in, 157, 158, 158*b*, 158*t*
risk avoiders, 68, 68*b*
risk factors, 24*n*, 28
  distribution of disease and, 24
  multiple risk factor reduction, 124–127, 126*b*–127*b*
  versus protective factors, 30*n*
  public health and, 11
  risk indicators compared with, 24
risk indicators, 24, 24*n*
risk markers, 24, 24*n*
risk takers, 68, 68*b*
risk-taking attitudes, 67
RLF. *See* retrolental fibrosis
RNs. *See* registered nurses
Robert Wood Johnson Foundation, 244

Rockefeller Foundation, 244
route of exposure, environmental risks and, 156*b*
route of transmission, 138
  for HIV/AIDS, 145*t*
rule of three, 260*n*

S

SADS. *See* sudden adult disability syndrome
safety, 162–165
"safety net" services, 196
SAMHSA. *See* Substance Abuse and Mental Health Services Administration
sanitarium movement, for TB, 137*b*
SCHIP. *See* State Child Health Insurance Program
scientific inquiry and reasoning skills (SIRS), 183*b*
scope, of environmental diseases, 152, 152*f*
score, 33
scoring healthcare systems, 219
screening, 120, 169–170
  genotypic-based, 129–130
  for heart disease and cancer, 125*t*
  multiple risk factors reduction and, 127
  reducing burden of communicable diseases, 140
  reducing burden of noncommunicable diseases, 124–127
scurvy, 6
secondary care, 186
secondary interventions, 35, 280
self-imposed risk, 104
Semmelweis, Ignaz, 6
sensitive, 66*b*
  to environmental risks, 156*b*
  false positives and, 123*b*
sentinel monitoring, as source of public health data, 56*t*
sequential testing, in screening, 122
Severe Acute Respiratory Syndrome (SARS) epidemic, 243*b*
sexual practices, approaches to public health and, 6
sexually transmitted diseases, barriers to, 140
shared decision making, clinical decision making approaches, 67, 69*t*
side effects, of vaccines, 147
SIDS. *See* sudden infant death syndrome
Silent Spring (Carson), 158, 160
simultaneous testing (parallel testing), 122*n*
single payer, 221
SIRS. *See* scientific inquiry and reasoning skills
skimming, 213*n*
smallpox, 141–142
smoking
  cessation programs, 34, 39*b*, 46, 101, 270–271
  continuing problem, 45–46

traditional public health, 11
traditional thinking in public health, 268
training. *See* education, and training
translational research, 269–270, 270*t*
transportation, social determinants of health, 81
Transtheoretical Model, 84
trauma triage system, 274*b*
treatment
   epidemiological treatment, 141
   multiple risk factors and, 124–127
Treatment for Emergency Medical Conditions and Women
      in Labor Act, 1986, 103
TriCare system, 211*n*
true positives, 122
true rates, 23*b*
truth˙ campaign, The, 90
TSS. *See* toxic shock syndrome
tuberculosis (TB), 172
   burden of, 136
   treatment as means of reducing risk of transmission, 141
Tuskegee Syphilis Study, 106
Tylenol (acetaminophen), 83

U

UNAIDS. *See* United Nations Programme on AIDS/HIV
unaltered environment, impact on disease, 152
uncontrollability effect, perception of health
      information, 60
under-5 mortality, 58
undergraduate medical education, 183*b*
undernutrition, 253
unfamiliarity effect, perception of health information, 60
UNICEF. *See* United Nations Children's Fund
unintentional injuries, environmental health and safety, 162
United Kingdom's healthcare system, 217–218, 219*t*
United Nations Children's Fund (UNICEF), 242
United Nations Programme on AIDS/HIV (UNAIDS), 242
United States (U.S.)
   actual causes of death in the United States, 118*t*
   inpatient facilities in, 194–196
   mechanisms for monitoring/ensuring quality of care, 203
   outpatient facilities in, 196
United States Agency for International Development
      (USAID), 242
United States Department of Agriculture (USDA), 256,
      257–258

Universal Declaration of Human Rights and the
      Constitution of the World Health Organization, 103
upstream factors, in behavioral change, 83
U.S. Constitution, role in public health and health care, 99
U.S. healthcare system, 217–218, 217*t*
USAID. *See* United States Agency for International
      Development
utility scale, decision analysis, 61

V

VA. *See* Veterans Administration
vaccines, 264
   Bacillus Calmette-Guérin (BCG) vaccine, 137
   history of public health and, 6
   immunization and, 140
   National Vaccine Plan, 245*b*
   for rabies, 147
   side effects of, 147
   for smallpox, 142
vehicle collision safety technology, 274*b*
VERB˙ campaign, The, 90, 91*b*, 91*n*
Veterans Administration (VA)
   health care provided by, 211*n*
   as healthcare delivery system, 199, 200*b*
victim blaming, 36
vital statistics, as source of public health data, 56*t*
vitamins deficiency, 253, 254*b*, 255
vulnerable groups
   public health and, 4
   social justice and, 6
vulnerable populations
   changes in understanding of, 10
   as focus of public health, 10–11

W

WHO. *See* World Health Organization
work, social determinants of health, 81
World Bank, 242
World Health Organization (WHO), 121*b*, 257–258
   role of global health agencies, 242
   smallpox eradication campaign, 142

X

X rays, for TB, 84, 137*b*